Energy Balance and Cancer

Volume 15

Series Editor:
Nathan A. Berger
Case Western Reserve University, School of Medicine,
Cleveland, OH, USA

More information about this series at http://www.springer.com/series/8282

David Berrigan • Nathan A. Berger
Editors

Geospatial Approaches to Energy Balance and Breast Cancer

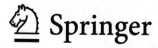 Springer

Editors
David Berrigan
Division of Cancer Control
and Population Sciences
National Cancer Institute
Bethesda, MD, USA

Nathan A. Berger
Center for Science, Health and Society
Case Comprehensive Cancer Center
Case Western Reserve University
Cleveland, OH, USA

ISSN 2199-2622   ISSN 2199-2630   (electronic)
Energy Balance and Cancer
ISBN 978-3-030-18410-0   ISBN 978-3-030-18408-7   (eBook)
https://doi.org/10.1007/978-3-030-18408-7

This Springer imprint is published by the registered company Springer Nature Switzerland AG
The registered company address is: Gewerbestrasse 11, 6330 Cham, Switzerland

Putting Cancer in Its Place: Geospatial Approaches to Energy Balance and Breast Cancer

Cancer occurs in specific places and spaces, each of which has identifiable geographical coordinates and all of which have specific natural, built, and social characteristics. Cancer research has a long history of attention to both space and place, and in recent years, there has been renewed focus on better using concepts and tools of spatial thinking to improve etiological and prevention research along the entire cancer control continuum. Such thinking has made substantial contributions to etiological, public health, and health-care delivery research, and with rapid advances in technology and data sciences coupled with a focus on applying spatial thinking to health research, there is an emerging view that this "spatial turn in health research" can advance efforts to address health and health disparities (Richardson et al. 2013).

This volume has its origins in the NCI's Transdisciplinary Research in Energetics and Cancer Initiative (https://cancercontrol.cancer.gov/brp/hbrb/trec/index.html) which inspired the initiation of the Springer series titled "Energy Balance and Cancer" (https://www.springer.com/series/8282). In the first volume of this series, *Cancer and Energy Balance, Epidemiology and Overview*, published in 2010, diverse authors reviewed the developing obesity pandemic and its association with cancer risk and progression, noting that the problems of energy balance and cancer were unlikely to be solved by individual scientists or even by interdisciplinary or multidisciplinary teams but that a transdisciplinary approach would almost certainly be necessary. About 10 years later, continued growth in geospatial approaches to energetics and cancer suggested a need for further review and synthesis. Accordingly, considerable geospatial research is now being focused on lung, colorectal, breast, and many other malignancies. Because of the explosion in this approach and because breast cancer appeared to be the site for which spatial thinking was most advanced, this volume will focus on breast cancer, while future volumes will consider other tumor systems. This new volume continues to epitomize the need for a transdisciplinary approach, by bringing together teams and concepts representing diverse disciplines, including epidemiology, geography, environmental sciences, medicine, and other disciplines.

A chapter in Volume 1 of that series provided an analysis of geographic and contextual effects on energy balance-related behaviors and cancers (Berrigan et al.

2010). That chapter identified the importance of expanding the traditional approach to environmental sciences to include factors such as built, social, and policy aspects of the environment and how they affect obesity and physical activity. At that time, the rapid development in Geospatial Information Systems (GIS) and the use of data from the Global Positioning System (GPS) were noted as sources of information for better understanding spatially related influences on cancer. However, it was also emphasized that the study of spatial variation in diet, weight, and physical activity as causes of cancer and targets for cancer prevention efforts was in the early stages of development. The chapter emphasized a critical research gap related to better understanding spatial variation in physical, toxicological, behavioral, and social environment and their associations with disease etiology and management.

Since 2010, there has been considerable research adopting a geospatial approach to diverse issues across much of the cancer control continuum, from etiological studies through primary prevention and diverse aspects of health-care delivery research. This expansion in the study of geospatial factors impacting health and disease, especially cancer, has included the development of multiple new techniques, analytic approaches, and focused investigators. Progress in this area and its importance in enhancing cancer control efforts at the community level resulted in a 2016 NCI-sponsored conference on Geospatial Approaches to Cancer Control and Population Sciences attended by almost 300 investigators ((https://epi.grants.cancer.gov/events/geospatial/). The conference also resulted in a focused issue of the journal *Cancer Epidemiology Biomarkers & Prevention* titled, "Geospatial Approaches to Cancer Control and Population Sciences" (http://cebp.aacrjournals.org/content/26/4#CEBPFocusGeospatialApproachestoCancerControlandPopulatio nSciences). Moreover, a recent review of publications arising from NCI-Designated Cancer Centers indicates rapid increase in the number of papers involving geospatial approaches especially since 2000 (Korycinski et al. 2018).

Contributions to this volume address energetics and breast cancer across the entire cancer control continuum. The first theme is a focus on key methodological issues concerning spatial analysis, including a review of geospatial approaches to breast cancer (Chap. 1 Wilson, Chap. 2 Jacquez, Chap. 3 Tatalovich and Stinchcomb, Chap. 4 Jankowska et al., Chap. 5 Lynch, Chap. 6 Reynolds et al., Chap. 7 Thompson et al.). These chapters address the major ingredients of geospatial health research and some of its key challenges (Thompson et al.) as well as a series of methods that are central to spatial analysis of breast cancer or among promising new directions. Chapters 2, 3, 4 discuss integrated analysis of space and time, advances and resources for mapping cancer incidence and mortality, and efforts to better understand built environment influences on energy balance-related health behaviors via simultaneous measurement of physical activity behavior (with accelerometry), location (with GPS), and environment (with GIS). These three chapters emphasize how technological and data science advances have led to new insights into causes of cancer and potential interventions related to the environment, broadly defined, to include toxic, natural, built, social, and policy features. Aspects of spatial thinking, such as ideas about proximity, access, and clustering, may apply to digital as well as spatial environments. This possibility has not yet been explored in much detail in literature addressing cancer, despite the potential role of the digital environment in mediating and moderating human relationships with environments and health-care systems (Stokols 2017). Chapter 5 describes the neighborhood-wide association approach to understand environmental influences on behavioral risk factors and cancer characteristics. This extension of GWAS to systematically explore high-dimensional data related to environments is a fascinating new approach but to date has only been attempted in a handful of studies. Chapter 6 gives an invaluable over-view of the challenge of reconstructing residential histories, ambient air pollutants, and their integration for exposure assessment. This chapter should be a real boon for leaders of other cohorts wishing to emulate the California Teachers Study pioneer-ing work in this area. The last of these methodological and overarching chapters (Chap. 7) presents a systematic review of recent papers using geospatial approaches to breast cancer. Together with Korycinski et al. (2018) and other recent papers reviewing geospatial research on cancer, we have a valuable overview of what is happening in the field and a convincing call for a continued emphasis on multidis-ciplinary collaboration.

Combining methodological and etiological topics, a second major theme addresses environmental, neighborhood, and contextual influences on breast cancer as well as physical activity and weight loss (Chap. 8 Conroy et al., Chap. 9 Dupre et al., Chap. 10 DeRouen et al., and Chap. 11 Zenk et al.). Chapters 8, 9, 10 explore environmental and contextual factors influencing breast cancer, with a substantial focus on social determinants of health and on novel environmental exposures, including the green environment, air pollution, and light at night. Despite major advances in analytical techniques and data resources, these three chapters illustrate substantial heterogeneity in the presence and strength of associations between envi-ronmental variables and behavior or cancer outcomes. Two recent and important articles further discuss the challenges in understanding neighborhood effects (Kwan 2018) and mobile sensing for neighborhood research (Chaix 2018) exemplified in the chapters in this book at several spatial and temporal scales. Notably, Conroy et al. emphasize disentangling the effects of neighborhood change for residents ver-sus neighborhood change from residential relocation. This topic emphasizes the need for residential history data as discussed in Chap. 6 and awareness that the neighborhood effects can take many years to manifest themselves (Powell-Wiley et al. 2014; Xiao et al. 2018). The final paper in this section takes a somewhat dif-ferent approach from the epidemiological analyses in the first three chapters. Zenk et al. review evidence that environmental factors moderate responses to behavioral interventions, a critical factor in the dissemination and implementation of such interventions for cancer control. They report scant evidence for such moderation, albeit their review covers a small number of studies. This somewhat counterintuitive result demands greater attention.

Three chapters (Chap. 12 Elkin et al., Chap. 13 Boscoe and Hutchinson, Chap. 14 Tsui et al.) explore screening, diagnosis, and beyond. Elkin emphasizes difficulties in synthesizing the literature because of heterogeneity in data sources, cohort defini-tions, measures of access and boundaries, and analytic methods. Here, and in many of the topics addressed in this book, one conclusion is that efforts are needed to adopt core sets of measures or common data elements to enhance comparability of studies. In a provocative analysis, Boscoe and Hutchinson examine trends in stage at diagnosis to argue for limited benefits of screening mammography and further use spatial scan statistics to characterize disparities in stage at diagnosis. Further comparisons from New York state suggest that differences between middle and upper income respondents rather than contrasts with the poorest populations. Both papers serve to highlight widespread disparities in the use of even well-supported aspects of cancer control. Tsui et al.'s discussion of medical neighborhoods in relation serves as an important reminder that each of us inhabits multiple "neighborhoods such as our school, work, and home neighborhoods." These neighborhoods may overlap or not, and each may have distinct associations with health and health outcomes (Matthews and Yang 2013).

The final section (Chap. 15 Beyer et al., Chap. 16 McLafferty, Chap. 17 Rosen et al., and Chap. 18 Onega) examine crosscutting and emerging topics. Beyer et al. highlight both the persistence of racial disparities in breast cancer and the geographic variation in their magnitude. Spatial approaches to breast cancer have done much to rigorously document disparities, and Beyer's chapter demonstrates that spatial thinking can connect disparities to underlying causes, such as racism, housing discrimination, segregation, and their health consequences (Kreiger 2017). This work vividly illustrates the need to address both the physical and social contexts of exposure and outcomes to understand more deeply the historical, social, and environmental correlates and causes of cancer disparities. McLafferty further addresses health disparities, applying a spatial lens to rural-urban differences in diverse aspects of breast cancer. These observations are especially timely, considering the increased interest in rural cancer control (Kennedy et al. 2018) and research challenges related to small populations (Srinivasan et al. 2015). As with several chapters in this volume, McLafferty's chapter highlights the need for further collaboration between cancer control researchers and geographers to integrate more advanced spatial thinking and analysis into cancer prevention and control.

Chapter 17 (Rosen et al.) addresses microenvironmental influences on team performance. The chapter focuses on sensor-based analysis of team performance and its social and behavioral underpinnings. This work is really exciting as improved team performance is vital to address health equity and health outcomes. Future work in this area could connect to larger spatial scales, including health-care practices or systems with multiple sites as well as entire "medical neighborhoods" discussed in Chap. 14. An additional connection between this chapter and the more traditional environmental approaches addressed in this book involves the use of sensors to describe location, exposure, affect, and physiology (e.g., Chap. 4). We hope the presence of Rosen et al.'s work in this book will spur further collaboration relating to environmental influences on team performance at different scales as well as the creative use of objective monitoring of behavior.

The final chapter in this section (Chap. 18 Onega) summarizes opportunities and challenges that this volume on geospatial approaches to energy balance and breast cancer will be important to all oncologists, endocrinologists, and behavioral scientists engaged in patient care to better understand their patients in the context of their environments. It should also provide an important consideration for physician, scientist, and public health officials planning clinical trials and community interventions as well as for community developers to plan environmental support to promote health, prevent disease, and eliminate cancer disparities. The volume will likewise be of value to all transdisciplinary researchers who need to better understand the potential role of geospatial studies and environmental factors and interventions in targeting and disrupting the linkage between obesity and cancer.

References

Berrigan D, McKinnon R, Dunton G, Huang L, Ballard-Barbash R. Geographic and contextual effects on energy balance-related behaviors and cancer. In: Berger N, editor. Cancer and energy balance, epidemiology and overview. New York: Springer; 2010. p. 267–97.

Chaix B. Mobile sensing in environmental health and neighborhood research. Ann. Rev. Public Health. 2018;39:367–84.

Kennedy AE, Vanderpool RC, Croyle RT, Srinivasan S. An overview of the national cancer institute's initiatives to accelerate rural cancer control research. Cancer Epidemiol Biomarkers Prev. 2018 Nov;27(11):1240–4.

Korycinski RW, Tennant BL, Cawley MA, Bloodgood B, Oh AY, Berrigan D. Geospatial approaches to cancer control and population sciences at the United States cancer centers. Cancer Causes Control. 2018 Mar;29(3):371–7.

Kreiger N. Follow the North Star: Why space, place, and power matter for geospatial approaches to cancer control and health equity. Cancer Epidemiol Biomarkers Prev. 2017 Apr;26(4):476–9.

Kwan MP. The limits of the neighborhood effect: Contextual uncertainties in geographic, environmental health, and social science research. Ann. Assoc. Am. Geogr. 2018;108(6):1482–90.

Matthews SA, Yang TC. Spatial polygamy and contextual exposures (SPACEs): Promoting activity space approaches in research on place and health. Am Behav Sci. 2013;57(8):1057–81.

Pickle LW. A history and critique of U.S. mortality atlases. Spat Spatiotemporal Epidemiol. 2009;1(1):3–17.

Pickle LW, Szczur M, Lewis DR, Stinchcomb DG. The crossroads of GIS and health information: a workshop on developing a research agenda to improve cancer control. Int J of Health Geographics. 2006;5:51.

Powell-Wiley TM, Ayers C, Agyemang P, Leonard T, Berrigan D, Ballard-Barbash R, Lian M, Das SR, Hoehner CM. Neighborhood-level socioeconomic deprivation predicts weight gain in a multi-ethnic population: longitudinal data from the Dallas Heart Study. Prev Med. 2014 Sep;66:22–7.

Richardson DB, Volkow ND, Kwan M-P, Kaplan RM, Goodchild MF, Croyle RT. Spatial turn in health research. Science. 2013;339:1390–2.

Srinivasan S, Moser RP, Willis G, Riley W, Alexander M, Berrigan D, Kobrin S. Small is essential: importance of subpopulation research in cancer control. Am J Public Health. 2015 Jul;105(Suppl 3):S371–3.

Stokols D. Social Ecology in the Digital Age. London UK: Elsevier Academic Press; 2017.

Xiao Q, Berrigan D, Powell-Wiley TM, Matthews CE. Ten-Year change in neighborhood socioeconomic deprivation and rates of total, cardiovascular disease, and cancer mortality in older US adults. Am J Epidemiol. 2018 Dec 1;187(12):2642–50.

Acknowledgments

We thank Calvin Tribby and Lilian Perez for assistance with reviewing several chapters of this book. We gratefully acknowledge the leaders of the NCI DCCPS Multilevel Geospatial and Contextual Interest group Gary Ellison, Stephen Taplin, Sallie Weaver, and April Oh for encouraging this research agenda, Linda Pickle for her mentorship in geospatial thinking, and Christina Keely for the overall organizational coordination. Finally, we thank the Springer team for all their patience in shepherding this book forward.

Bethesda, MD, USA   David Berrigan
Cleveland, OH, USA   Nathan A. Berger

Contents

Contributors

Julie Von Behren University of California San Francisco, San Francisco, CA, USA

Amin Bemanian Institute for Health & Equity, Medical College of Wisconsin, Milwaukee, WI, USA

Kirsten M. M. Beyer Institute for Health & Equity, Division of Epidemiology, Medical College of Wisconsin, Milwaukee, WI, USA

Francis P. Boscoe New York State Department of Health, New York State Cancer Registry, Albany, NY, USA

Iona Cheng Department of Epidemiology and Biostatistics, University of California, San Francisco, CA, USA

Helen Diller Family Comprehensive Cancer Center, University of California, San Francisco, CA, USA

Shannon M. Conroy Department of Epidemiology and Biostatistics, University of California, San Francisco, San Francisco, CA, USA

Helen Diller Family Comprehensive Cancer Center, University of California, San Francisco, CA, USA

U. S. C. Dana USC Dana and David Dornsife College of Letters, Arts and Sciences, University of Southern California, Los Angeles, CA, USA

Mindy C. DeRouen Department of Epidemiology & Biostatistics, University of California San Francisco, San Francisco, CA, USA

UCSF Helen Diller Family Comprehensive Cancer Center, San Francisco, CA, USA

Michelle Doose Department of Population Science, Rutgers Cancer Institute of New Jersey, New Brunswick, NJ, USA

Rutgers, School of Public Health, Rutgers, The State University of New Jersey, New Brunswick, NJ, USA

David Dornsife USC Dana and David Dornsife College of Letters, Arts and Sciences, University of Southern California, Los Angeles, CA, USA

Natalie DuPré Brigham and Women's Hospital, Channing Division of Network Medicine, Boston, MA, USA

Department of Epidemiology and Population Health, University of Louisville, School of Public Health and Information Sciences, Louisville, KY, USA

Elena B. Elkin Department of Epidemiology and Biostatistics, Memorial Sloan Kettering Cancer Center, New York, NY, USA

Joseph Gibbons Department of Sociology, San Diego State University, San Diego, CA, USA

Center for Human Dynamics in the Mobile Age, San Diego State University, San Diego, CA, USA

Scarlett Lin Gomez Department of Epidemiology & Biostatistics, University of California San Francisco, San Francisco, CA, USA

Helen Diller Family Comprehensive Cancer Center, University of California, San Francisco, CA, USA

Jaime E. Hart Channing Division of Network Medicine, Department of Medicine, Brigham and Women's Hospital and Harvard Medical School, Boston, MA, USA

Department of Environmental Health, Harvard T.H. Chan School of Public Health, Boston, MA, USA

Kevin A. Henry Department of Geography and Urban Studies, Temple University, Philadelphia, PA, USA

Fox Chase Cancer Center, Temple University, Philadelphia, PA, USA

Susan Hurley University of California San Francisco, San Francisco, CA, USA

Lindsey Hutchison New York State Department of Health, New York State Cancer Registry, Albany, NY, USA

Sindana Ilango School of Public Health, San Diego State University, San Diego, CA, USA

Department of Family Medicine and Public Health, University of California San Diego, San Diego, CA, USA

Geoffrey M. Jacquez BioMedware, Inc., and The University of Michigan, Ann Arbor, MI, USA

Jennifer Jain Department of Epidemiology and Biostatistics, University of California, San Francisco, San Francisco, CA, USA

Peter James Division of Chronic Disease Research Across the Lifecourse (CoRAL), Department of Population Medicine, Harvard Medical School and Harvard Pilgrim Health Care Institute, Boston, MA, USA

Marta M. Jankowska Calit2/Qualcomm Institute, University of California San Diego, La Jolla, CA, USA

Sadaf Kazi Armstrong Institute for Patient Safety and Quality, Johns Hopkins University School of Medicine, Baltimore, MD, USA

Jacqueline Kerr Department of Family Medicine and Public Health, University of California San Diego, La Jolla, CA, USA

Salar Khaleghzadegan Armstrong Institute for Patient Safety and Quality, Johns Hopkins University School of Medicine, Baltimore, MD, USA

Amber N. Kraft University of Illinois at Chicago, Chicago, IL, USA

Shannon M. Lynch Fox Chase Cancer Center, Philadelphia, PA, USA

Loïc Le Marchand Population Sciences in the Pacific Program, University of Hawaii Cancer Center, Honolulu, HI, USA

Sara McLafferty Department of Geography and GIScience, University of Illinois at Urbana-Champaign, Champaign, IL, USA

Atsushi Nara Center for Human Dynamics in the Mobile Age, San Diego State University, San Diego, CA, USA

Department of Geography, San Diego State University, San Diego, CA, USA

David O. Nelson Cancer Prevention Institute of California, Fremont, CA, USA

Tracy Onega Departments of Biomedical Data Science, of Epidemiology, The Dartmouth Institute for Health Policy & Clinical Practice at the Geisel School of Medicine at Dartmouth, Lebanon, NH, USA

Norris Cotton Cancer Center, Lebanon, NH, USA

Peggy Reynolds University of California San Francisco, San Francisco, CA, USA

Michael A. Rosen Armstrong Institute for Patient Safety and Quality, Johns Hopkins University School of Medicine, Baltimore, MD, USA

Salma Shariff-Marco Department of Epidemiology and Biostatistics, University of California, San Francisco, San Francisco, CA, USA

Helen Diller Family Comprehensive Cancer Center, University of California, San Francisco, CA, USA

Yurii B. Shvetsov Population Sciences in the Pacific Program, University of Hawaii Cancer Center, Honolulu, HI, USA

David G. Stinchcomb Westat, Inc., Rockville, MD, USA

Elizabeth Tarlov Edward Hines Jr. VA Hospital, Chicago, IL, USA

University of Illinois at Chicago, Chicago, IL, USA

Zaria Tatalovich Surveillance Research Program, Division of Cancer Control and Population Sciences, National Cancer Institute, Bethesda, MD, USA

Caroline A. Thompson School of Public Health, San Diego State University, San Diego, CA, USA

Department of Family Medicine and Public Health, University of California San Diego, San Diego, CA, USA

Ming-Hsiang Tsou Center for Human Dynamics in the Mobile Age, San Diego State University, San Diego, CA, USA

Department of Geography, San Diego State University, San Diego, CA, USA

Jennifer Tsui Department of Population Science, Rutgers Cancer Institute of New Jersey, New Brunswick, NJ, USA

Rutgers, School of Public Health, Rutgers, The State University of New Jersey, New Brunswick, NJ, USA

Margaret M. Weden RAND Corporation, Santa Monica, CA, USA

Lynne R. Wilkens Population Sciences in the Pacific Program, University of Hawaii Cancer Center, Honolulu, HI, USA

John P. Wilson Spatial Sciences Institute, Dana and David Dornsife College of Letters, Arts and Sciences, University of Southern California, Los Angeles, CA, USA

Juan Yang Department of Epidemiology & Biostatistics, University of California San Francisco, San Francisco, CA, USA

Jiue-An Yang Calit2/Qualcomm Institute, University of California San Diego, La Jolla, CA, USA

Staci Young Center for Healthy Communities and Research, Department of Family and Community Medicine, Medical College of Wisconsin, Milwaukee, WI, USA

Shannon N. Zenk University of Illinois at Chicago, Chicago, IL, USA

Part I
Overview and Spatial Methods

Chapter 1
Connecting Population, Health and Place with Geospatial Tools and Data

John P. Wilson

Abstract This chapter traces how the growth of geographic information science and the potential for using the accompanying geospatial tools and data to advance our understanding of disease prevalence, etiology, transmission, and treatment. Two major and interrelated topics are addressed. The first describes current geospatial tools and data along with a framework for their use in health applications, and the second documents several conceptual and methodological challenges that are likely to frustrate our efforts to use these geospatial tools and data to connect population, health and place in meaningful ways. The chapter closes by noting some new opportunities and predictions for the future.

Keywords Geographic information · Geospatial tools · Place-based genetic geographic information science · Conceptual and methodological challenges

1.1 Introduction

An argument can be made that the connections between population, health and place have come full circle since John Snow's use of a map to discover the source of the contaminated water that spawned the cholera outbreak in Soho, England in 1854 [75]. The origins of epidemiology and public health as academic pursuits are often traced to this and similar events around the same time. Thus epidemiology and public health research are grounded in map-based analysis and visualization and technological advances have resulted in a growing place for spatial and place-based analysis of health and health outcomes.

Public health has blossomed during the past 175 years and most of the world's leading research universities now support large public health units focusing on

J. P. Wilson (✉)
Spatial Sciences Institute, Dana and David Dornsife College of Letters, Arts and Sciences, University of Southern California, Los Angeles, CA, USA
e-mail: jpwilson@usc.edu

© Springer Nature Switzerland AG 2019
D. Berrigan, N. A. Berger (eds.), *Geospatial Approaches to Energy Balance and Breast Cancer*, Energy Balance and Cancer 15, https://doi.org/10.1007/978-3-030-18408-7_1

disease and well-being. Diverse public health subspecialties increasingly incorporate spatial perspectives across the entire human disease and health spectrum, from the basic science of disease causation to health disparities across space and among different racial and socio-economic groups, and the impact of health interventions at a global scale.

Some of these same observations can be made about demography, whose beginnings can be traced back to the work of John Graunt in 1662. Graunt analyzed the Bills of Mortality in London, England and found very high mortality since there were just 16 people still alive at age 36 for every 100 people born in some parts of London during the seventeenth Century [84]. The study of demography has long incorporated the study of health and place and more recently, demography or population studies, a more modern and inclusive term, has become a multi-disciplinary venture, including in its ranks economists, geographers, historians, sociologists, gerontologists, and researchers from several of the public health subspecialties.

The origins of many of the spatial methods available today can be traced to the work of geographers, who have also made seminal contributions to the study of health and place. This work includes Stamp's [78] seminal book on the geography of life and death, Melinda Meade's [47] book review essay in which she described a series of recent books and demonstrated that the geography of life and death is deeper, broader and much more complicated than Stamp portrayed, and a fascinating book by Mitchell et al. [53] which used map-based analysis and visualization to explore the inequalities in life and death and what Britain would look like if it were more equal.

The past 50 years has also witnessed the emergence of geographic information science as a separate field of study focused on all the ways in which location can be used to gather, organize, analyze, model, and visualize information [19, 24, 25]. The growth of geographic information science and the deployment of the accompanying geospatial tools and data to help advance our understanding of disease prevalence, etiology, transmission, and treatment has led recently to calls for the establishment of a distributed, interoperable spatial data infrastructure to integrate health research data across and within disparate health research programs to realize the full benefits of these new geospatial capabilities (e.g. [63]).

These threads provide the foundation for the discussion documenting the use of geospatial tools and data for connecting population, health, and place in the remainder of this chapter. This discussion is divided into four parts. The first offers a framework within which the use of geospatial tools and data for connecting population, health, and place might be best situated. The second describes the large number and variety of geospatial tools and data that are available for use today. The third discusses several conceptual and methodological challenges that are likely to frustrate our efforts to connect population, health and place using geospatial tools and data moving forward, and the fourth and final section describes some new opportunities and offers some predictions for the future.

1.2 Guiding Principles

To start, we need a framework to clarify how geospatial tools and data can be used to connect population, health and place and for this, we are fortunate that Jacquez et al. [33] recently proposed a place-based genetic geographic information science founded on the exposome, genome+, and behavome (Fig. 1.1). Dr. Jacquez' chapter later in this volume further expands on some of these themes. The exposome in this vision described the totality of environmental exposures over the life course [90, 91]. The genome+ described an individual's biology, which includes the genome (genetic composition), regulome (which controls gene expression), proteome (the entire complement of amino acids and proteins), and the metabolome (which supports metabolism and homeostasis). The behavome described the totality of an individual's health behaviors over the life course which mediate the exposome and interactions between the exposome and the genome+. These three concepts, in turn, describe the three primary determinants of health, both in terms of illness and well-being, and they act through place, which was defined as the geographic, environmental, social, and societal milieus experienced over a person's life course.

Jacquez et al. [33] also argued that the implementation and use of this framework would require a mathematical foundation for emergent theory, process-based models that bridge biological and geographic scales, and biologically plausible estimates of space-time disease lags. They noted and illustrated how compartmental models may represent a possible path forward and the work of Daniel et al. [13] and Gehlert et al. [22] is used next, to illustrate how this might work.

In the first example, Daniel et al. [13] proposed a conceptual model that integrated time and two plausible pathways by which geospatial clustering of disadvantage might be viewed as causally related to the development of cardiovascular and glycemic disease (Fig. 1.2). This framework distinguishes environmental risk conditions that influence the expression of individual behavioral and psychosocial characteristics on the one hand, and the socio-economic and material conditions that influence regulatory systems through conscious and non-conscious mechanisms on the other hand.

Fig. 1.1 Schematic representation of the genetic geographic information science vision offered by Jacquez et al. [33]

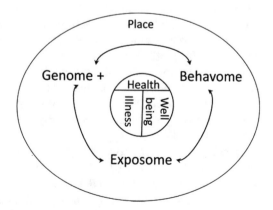

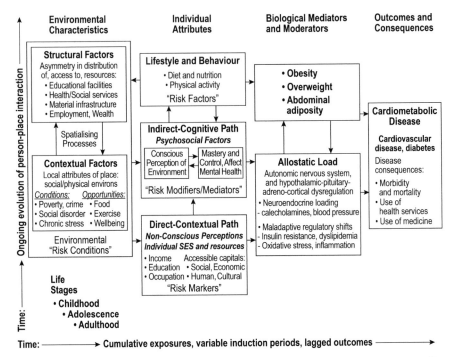

Fig. 1.2 Proposed causal indirect-cognitive and direct-contextual paths linking place to cardio-metabolic disease [13]

Gehlert et al. [22] also tried to link biology and place, using a mutually informative, multi-level and multi-modal model of African-American and white breast cancer health disparities. Their approach incorporated genes, hormones, psychological state and behavior patterns, social circumstances (social isolation, social support), housing and environmental exposures, and community and neighborhood (crime, collective efficacy, social ecology, etc.) across six distinct levels.

These two case studies are exemplary because they illustrate how: (1) the causal inference regarding the impact of place on health will be enhanced by paying attention to the biological plausibility of associations; and (2) the need for the chosen place-based exposures to precede the effects on health for the associations to be plausible in specific instances as well.

However, the discussion to this point has not adequately brought to light all of the subtleties of place and for this we turn to the work of Kemp [38]. She has advocated using a "relational" view of place because this conceptualizes place as a process – a fluid dynamic field of constantly interacting elements, within and beyond itself – rather than an entity.

Drawing on work by Popay et al. [61], Pred [62] and Cummins et al. [12], among others, Kemp [38] advocates the need to study the trajectories of both individuals and places over time. We need to understand the intimate place histories and memories of individuals and groups as well as the larger historical patterns that these individual patterns are nested within and linked to, which means we need to conceptualize place as inherently fluid, changing and on the "move" … in a state of "becoming" that is constantly being made and remade by individual, collective, and institutional practices, and by structural forces.

This conceptualization of place has some important consequences for how geospatial tools and data can be invoked and used to clarify the role of place in human disease and well-being because:

1. A relational approach to place necessarily involves the consideration of place trajectories, examined on multiple, interlocking dimensions from the structural to the personal (cf. [13, 22]).
2. An adequate understanding of place must grapple with not only the relationality of people and place but also the implications of these interactions over time, collectively and within individual lives (cf. [15, 58, 74]; and [14]).
3. The realization that place histories are not experienced uniformly and that multiple histories (and historical trajectories) are likely to coexist in each and every place (cf. [59, 60]; and [76]).

This said, we are fortunate that an increasing number of scholars have argued that the conceptualization of place along these lines is fundamental to improving our understanding of the connections between health and place. However, the vast majority of studies to date are cross-sectional and present focused. Therefore, the ways in which the more fluid conceptualization of place would shape the use of the geospatial tools and data described in the next section in health studies moving forward have not been clearly articulated in many instances.

We will describe the current status of geospatial tools and data next, and take up the methodological challenges brought by the conceptualization of place offered above in the following section.

1.3 Geospatial Tools and Data

There is a need here to provide a working definition of "place" as the location and immediate vicinity in which some human activity occurs – this could be the primary residence, the workplace, a seat on a local bus or train, a tennis court, or a beach for the moment – and let us assume that the immediate goal is to describe the physical, toxicological, behavioral, and social environments, and their association with disease etiology and management (i.e. primary prevention and the health care delivery system). This view mirrors current practice although it falls considerably short of the conceptualization of place offered by Kemp [38] and others.

The good news here is the availability of increasing numbers and kinds of methods to help with the aforementioned tasks and to move towards a more relational description of place. The University Consortium for Geographic Information Science has sponsored an ongoing project to describe the various components of this new and rapidly evolving field of study [92]. This dynamic web-based resource divides the field into 10 knowledge areas – foundational concepts, the knowledge economy, computing platforms, programming and development, data capture, data management, analytics and modeling, cartography and visualization, and domain applications – and then describes each knowledge area using a series of topics. One of the topics in the Domain Applications knowledge area addresses Geographic Information Science & technology and epidemiology [87]. This particular entry aside, the most relevant topics for the work at hand are those in the Data Management, Analytics and Modeling, and Cartography and Visualization knowledge areas.

The Data Management knowledge area includes 57 topics in six groups (Table 1.1). The topics in the six groups – spatial databases, representation of spatial objects, spatial access methods, spatial data quality, georeferencing systems, and spatial data infrastructures – cover a series of fundamental concepts and ideas that are crucial to managing and using spatial data wisely. The topics that focus on the

Table 1.1 The 57 topics currently included in the geographic information science & technology body of knowledge's data management knowledge area (see https://gistbok.ucgis.org/all-topics? term_node_tid_depth=95 for additional details)

Spatial databases	Spatial access methods	Georeferencing systems
Spatial database management systems	Data retrieval strategies	Approximating the Earth's shape with geoids
Use of a relational DBMS	Spatial indexing	Geographic coordinate system
Object-oriented DBMS	Space-driven structures: Grid, linear quadtree & z-ordering tree files	Planar coordinate systems
Extensions of the relational model	Data-driven structures: R-trees & cost models	Tessellated referencing systems
Topological relationships	Modeling unstructured spatial data	Linear referencing systems
Database administration	Modeling semi-structured spatial data	Vertical datums
Conceptual data models	Query Processing	Horizontal datums
Logical data models	Optimal I/O algorithms	Map projections
Physical data models	Spatial joins	Georegistration
NoSQL databases	Complex queries	
Problems with large spatial databases		**Spatial data infrastructures**
	Spatial data quality	Metadata
Representation of spatial objects	Modeling uncertainty	Content standards
	Vagueness	Data warehouses
Raster data model	Mathematical models of vagueness: Fuzzy sets & rough sets	Spatial data infrastructures
Hexagonal model	Error-based uncertainty	U.S. National Spatial Data Infrastructure
Triangulated irregular network model	Spatial data uncertainty	Common ontologies for spatial data & their applications
Hierarchical data models		
Spaghetti model		
Topological model		
Vector data models		
Network model		
Entity-based models		
Modeling 3-D entities		
Field-based models		
Fuzzy models		
Events and processes		
Genealogical relationships, lineage & inheritance		
Conflation & related spatial data integration techniques		
Standardization & exchange specifications		

representation of spatial objects and georeferencing, for example, are likely to be employed whenever spatial data are used in health studies.

The Analytics and Modeling knowledge area includes 96 topics in 11 groups (Table 1.2). The first four groups – conceptual frameworks, methodological context, data manipulation, and building blocks – cover the guiding principles and many simple but widely used concepts and functions, such as buffering and distance operations. The next five groups – data exploration and spatial statistics, surface and field analysis, network and location analysis, space-time analysis and modeling, and geocomputation methods and models – include many of the spatial analysis methods

Table 1.2 The 96 topics currently included in the geographic information science & technology body of knowledge's analytics and modeling knowledge area (see https://gistbok.ucgis.org/all-topics?term_node_tid_depth=96 for additional details)

Conceptual frameworks	Exploratory spatial data analysis	Space-time analysis & modeling
Basic primitives	Kernels & density estimation	
Spatial relationships	Spatial interaction	Time geography
Neighborhoods	Cartographic modeling	Capturing spatiotemporal dynamics in computational modeling
First & second laws of geography	Multi-criteria evaluation	GIS-based computational modeling
Spatial statistics	Spatial process models	Computational movement analysis
	Grid-based statistics & metrics	Accounting for errors in modeling
Methodological context	Landscape metrics	
Spatial analysis as a process	Digital elevation models & terrain metrics	**Geocomputation methods & models**
Geospatial analysis & model building	Point pattern analysis	
Changing context of GIS&T	Hot spot & cluster analysis	Cellular automata
	Global indicators of spatial autocorrelation	Agent-based modeling
Data manipulation	Local indicators of spatial autocorrelation	Simulation modeling
Point, line, & area generalization	Simple regression & trend surface analysis	Simulation & modeling systems for agent-based modeling
Coordinate transformations	Geographically weighted regression	Artificial neural networks
Data conversion	Spatially autoregressive models	Genetic algorithms & evolutionary computing
Impacts of transformation	Spatial filtering models	
Raster resampling		**Big data & geospatial analysis**
Vector-to-raster & raster-to-vector conversions	**Surface & Field analysis**	
Generalization & aggregation	Modeling surfaces	Problems of conducting geospatial analysis with large spatial databases
Transaction management	Surface geometry	Pattern recognition & matching
	Intervisibility	Artificial intelligence approaches
Building blocks	Watersheds and drainage	Data mining approaches
Spatial & spatiotemporal models	Gridding, interpolation, and contouring	Rule learning for spatial data mining
Length & area operations	Deterministic interpolation models	Machine learning approaches
Polyline & polygon operations	Inverse distance weighting	CyberGIS
Overlay & combination operations	Radial basis and spline functions	
Areal interpolation	Triangulation	**Analysis of errors & uncertainty**
Aggregation of spatial entities	Polynomial functions	
Classification & clustering	Core concepts in geostatistics	Problems of currency, source, & scale
Boundaries & zone membership	Kriging interpolation	Problems of scale & zoning
Tessellations & triangulations		Theory of error propagation
Spatial queries	**Network & location analysis**	Propagation of error in geospatial modeling
Distance operations	Introduction to network & location analysis	Fuzzy aggregation operators
Buffering	Network route & tour problems	Mathematical models of uncertainty
Directional operations	Location & service area problems	
Grid operations & map algebra	Modeling accessibility	
	Location-allocation modeling	
Data exploration & spatial statistics	The classic transportation problem	
Spatial sampling for spatial analysis		

that have found the most use in health studies to date. These topics include kernels and density estimation, spatial interaction, cartographic modeling, hot spot and cluster analysis, geographically weighted regression, kriging, accessibility, and location-allocation modeling for example. The tenth group of topics speaks to the role of big data and geospatial analysis in data science, and the eleventh and final group in the Analytics and Modeling knowledge area tackles the analysis of error and uncertainty. The topics in the second of these groups are important today (e.g. [26, 28]) and are likely to feature prominently in future health studies as the role of big data and data science in health science is further clarified [63, 94].

The Cartography & Visualization knowledge area includes 40 topics in six groups (Table 1.3). The first two and sixth and last of these groups – history and trends, data considerations, and map use – cover the foundational principles and the other three groups – map design fundamentals, map design techniques, and interactive design techniques – cover the concepts and methods one needs to make effective maps and other kinds of geovisual displays. The concepts and methods included in the scale and generalization, statistical mapping, map projection, bivariate and multivariate maps, flow maps, cartograms, geovisual analytics, and mobile maps and responsive design topics have found widespread use in health studies over the past three or four decades for example.

This said, there is a tremendous number and variety of software systems available today to support map-based analysis, modeling, and visualization. Some offer a full range of spatial tools and services whereas others focus on specific methods and/or applications. Some are proprietary and some offer free and/or open source solu-

Table 1.3 The 40 topics currently included in the geographic information science & technology body of knowledge's cartography and visualization knowledge area (see https://gistbok.ucgis.org/all-topics?term_node_tid_depth=97 for additional details)

History and trends	Map design techniques	Map use
Cartography & science	Common thematic map types	Map reading
Cartography & power	Bivariate & multivariate maps	Map interpretation
Cartography & art	Terrain representation	Map analysis
Cartography & education	Mapping time	Map critique
	Representing uncertainty	
Data considerations	Flow maps	
Vector formats & sources	Cartograms	
Raster formats & sources	Narrative & storytelling	
Metadata, quality, & uncertainty	Icon design	
Map design fundamentals	**Interactive design techniques**	
Scale & generalization	User interface & user experience	
Statistical mapping	(UI/UX) design	
Map projections	Web mapping	
Visual hierarchy & layout	Virtual & immersive environments	
Symbolization & the visual	Big data visualization	
variables	Geovisualization	
Color theory	Geovisual analytics	
Typography	Geocollaboration	
Aesthetics & design	Usability engineering & evaluation	
Map production & management	Basemaps	
	Mobile maps & responsive design	

tions. Some have a long history and software releases that span several decades whereas other systems were launched in the past few years. Some still look like the full geographic information systems of old and as such, offer systems of record, insight, and engagement which we will see later may help in building better health management systems. A full proprietary GIS, such as Esri's ArcGIS offers greater functionality, larger and more active user communities, and more substantial support in terms of supporting documentation, help, etc. but at the cost of higher license fees and a steeper learning curve (in terms of finding appropriate tools, crafting solutions, etc.) for those new to the field.

The computational power that is available across a variety of computing platforms (i.e. server, desktop, tablet, and mobile devices) has also grown enormously during the past 25 years as well. In those cases where software development and application have stalled, this has occurred more often than not, because there were not sufficient resources to reinvent the enabling software as the computer hardware and relevant computer operating system paradigms and languages evolved throughout this period.

Today's leading commercial GIS platform, ArcGIS, has evolved tremendously during the past 25 years. The capabilities and "look-and-feel" of the original command-line ArcInfo workstation flagship product was first combined with the Windows-based ArcView product and then merged and rebranded in the Windows-based ArcGIS platform launched in 1999. Various programming languages and related tools have been supported over the years, ranging from the application-specific Arc Macro Language (AML) and Avenue languages for ArcInfo and ArcView, respectively, in the early years to C++ and Visual Basic and most recently Python. Bridges have also been provided to support collaborative work using a variety of complementary products such as R and SAS. The ArcInfo coverage that served as the dominant file format 10–15 years ago was first replaced by the shapefile, which quickly became the de facto standard for storing and supporting geographic information, and then the geodatabase, which uses an object-relational database approach for managing and storing spatial data.

The ways in which the Esri software components are bundled and therefore, the ways in which the users interact with the software, has changed as well. The focus of Esri has now shifted to the development of ArcGIS Professional and ArcGIS Online, which provide a connected desktop in the first instance and a rich repository of both traditional and user-generated geospatial information in the second instance, and a rapidly expanding number of ArcGIS Apps that are aimed at specific communities of users and incorporate selected subsets of the core functionality. The latter include apps for the field (i.e. Collector for ArcGIS and Survey123 for ArcGIS), apps for the office (i.e. ArcGIS Business Analyst, ArcGIS Community Analyst, Insights for ArcGIS), apps for specific communities (i.e. ArcGIS Earth, ArcGIS Hub, ArcGIS Urban, Esri Story Maps), and app builders so users can quickly and easily build their own custom applications.

However, there are many other options that include several proprietary (e.g. Maptitude, MapInfo, Oracle Spatial) as well as numerous open source geographic information systems (GRASS, QGIS, SAGA) and online mapping platforms (Epi Info, OpenStreetMap), two proprietary remote sensing systems (ENVI, ERDAS

IMAGINE), three mapping systems that provide rich geospatial datasets and numerous analysis and mapping capabilities (e.g. Bing Maps, Google Maps, Google Earth), and numerous general purpose and specialty statistical software systems that include spatial analysis and mapping capabilities in the same systems (see MATLAB, R, SAS, and SPSS for examples of generic statistical software platforms and BoundarySeer, ClusterSeer, SpaceStat, and StatScan for examples of specialty software products) or through partnerships including two or more software providers (e.g. Alteryx and Tableau).

Many of the abovementioned software systems have followed similar trajectories to ArcGIS and perhaps the most important message thus far in terms of software tools, is that more changes can be expected across all of these platforms in the years ahead since the rate and magnitude of the changes in information technology show no signs of slowing down. The rapid advances in computational power and changing models of computing (i.e. cloud computing, cyberinfrastructure, interoperability, and software-as-a-service) offer new opportunities to develop new analytical tools and expand the geographic extent and heft of health applications moving forward.

Another major change in the last 50 years is that the world is suddenly awash with geospatial data. These data cover the natural and built environments along with the structural factors, socio-economic conditions, lifestyles and behaviors which frame the human experience, and the environmental risk factors that threaten human well-being.

There are now many geospatial data sources which can be used to describe the natural environment (i.e. climate, weather, geology, elevation, soil, land cover and land use) for virtually every part of the Earth. In addition, the rapid emergence and use of satellite imagery for Earth observation has spawned applications that monitor conditions continuously in real-time place. The National Water Model, for example, draws on meteorology, elevation, land use/land cover and hydrography to continuously predict stream flow in 2.3 million catchments spanning the conterminous U.S. at time intervals ranging from 3 h to 30 days (see http://water. noaa.gov/about/nwm for additional details). These kinds of data resources have not been fully integrated into exposure modeling for epidemiology thus far.

The same is true for the built environment. Building footprints and 3D models can be acquired from local government portals, private companies (i.e. Esri, Google and Microsoft) and not-for-profits (i.e. OpenStreetMap). Many of these datasets come with a rich collection of attribute data which include the building history, building layout, and the current uses (i.e. commercial, institutional, and residential). The transportation systems as well as other infrastructure (i.e. electrical transmission, municipal water and wastewater systems, oil and gas pipelines, telecommunications), parks and other kinds of green infrastructure, and large numbers and kinds of points-of-interest can be described in similar detail. The information for some of these phenomena and particularly points-of-interest are likely to have been gathered and shared purposively or passively by volunteers nowadays (see [83]) which may raise new concerns in terms of currency and/or quality. However, unlike the case with environmental information, there is a lack of national and integrated data sets about the built environment, and this poses a barrier for epidemiology and evaluation studies because each study has to laboriously compile appropriate data.

The structural factors include the asymmetry in the distribution of and access to the resources associated with educational facilities, health and social services, employment and wealth (see Fig. 1.2). These kinds of phenomena can be spatialized relatively easily nowadays and used to characterize the geographic variability. Shi et al. [73], for example, examined the spatial access and local demand for major cancer care facilities in the U.S. and generated a high resolution map which documented the spatial variation in the potentially unfilled demand for these facilities. Similarly, Bell et al. [4] used a modification of the two-step floating catchment method with natural neighborhood units in Mississauga, Canada to measure potential access to health care based on several spatial and aspatial (social) characteristics of the population and the physicians, including the numbers of physicians, the languages spoken by physicians and patients, and whether the physicians were accepting new patients or not. More broadly, Heinrich et al. [29], describe the Wellbeing Toronto tool and data which they used to explore the role of standardization and outlier removal in helping to make area-based composite indices that were comparable over time. This interactive online Wellbeing Toronto tool includes 11 categories of indicators – demographics, civics, economics, education, environment, health, housing, recreation, safety, transport, and culture – and was designed to serve government, decision makers, community organizations, and local businesses. The current version enables users to create their own area-based composite indices of neighborhood well-being across multiple time periods.

Socio-economic characteristics incorporated in such public health resources can be gathered from the census in many parts of the world and typically include data tabulated at two or more levels (census block groups, census tracts) and for a variety of other geographic reporting units (see Fig. 1.3 for examples from the State of Arizona). The U.S. used short- and long-forms to collect household information up

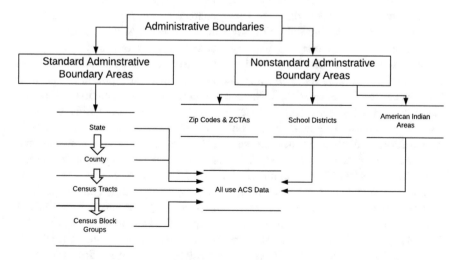

Fig. 1.3 Potential administrative boundary types that could be used to describe geospatial contents in the State of Arizona [42]

to and including the 2000 decennial census. After 2000, the 'long form' was replaced with the American Community Survey (ACS), which uses a small national sample and collects and reports data socio-economic data continuously. This approach provides more up-to-date information but the relatively sparse sample density means that some of the data for small geographic areas such as census tracts will suffer from large margins of error. There data can be acquired from the Census Bureau itself or from one of an increasing number of organizations that have compiled and shared these data using geospatial portals and services. This same approach has been used to share business data (cf. Esri's Business and Community Analyst products).

All of the aforementioned options provide aggregate data from which we typically want to infer individual level characteristics. In some instances, we may have individual data from which we want to infer population level characteristics. Large NIH-funded cohort studies like the Los Angeles Family and Neighborhood Survey (LA FANS; [69]), which collected detailed socio-economic data as part of a multi-level survey of children, families, and communities across Los Angeles County, represent one possible source of such data.

These large cohort studies have also traditionally offered important opportunities to acquire more detailed lifestyle and behavioral data for populations of special interest. They have routinely gathered data on variables such as diet, weight, and physical activity, among others, which until recently, were nearly impossible to gather by any other means. Nowadays, these data can be supplemented with two new and novel forms of data.

The first option relies on the outputs of projects that have moved from a variable-based mode of inquiry to one that emphasizes a composite multivariate picture of small geographic reporting units such as census block groups or tracts. Spielman and Singleton [77], for example, recently proposed a series of geodemographic types to describe the populations of small areas as one possible way to circumvent the large margins of error in the ACS. Their geodemographic typology distinguished 10 groups – Hispanic and kids; Wealthy nuclear families; Middle income, single family homes; Native American; Wealthy urbanites; Low income and diverse; Old, wealthy white; Low income minority mix; African-American adversity; and Residential institutions, young people – and was validated using public domain data from the City of Chicago and the U.S. Federal Election Commission. Esri's Tapestry Segmentation takes this approach a step further by first dividing residential areas into 67 distinctive segments based on their socioeconomic and demographic composition and then further classifying the segments into LifeMode and Urbanization groups (see https://www.esri.com/en-us/arcgis/products/tapestry-segmentation/overview for additional details). DeRouen et al. in this volume describe a related approach based on the concept of 'neighborhood archetypes'.

The second option uses Global Positioning Systems (GPS) and various kinds of sensors to link behavior and environmental exposures. Jankowska et al. [37], for example, presented a framework showing how accelerometers could be used with GPS and GIS in physical activity and sedentary behavior studies (Fig. 1.4). Following this framework, the GPS can link objective measures of physical activity

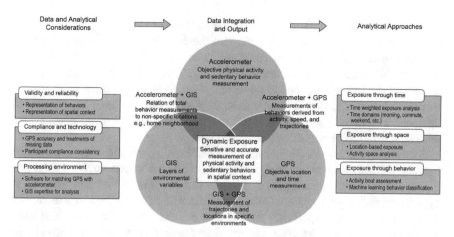

Fig. 1.4 Framework for integration of GPS, accelerometery, and GIS technology to support physical activity and sedentary behavior studies ([37], p. 50)

recorded with the accelerometer to specific locations, and these data can then be represented within the GIS to create detailed contextual measures, such as walkability, park access, and land use mix, which may help in tracing an individual's journey through multiple settings with health-promoting or health-damaging characteristics. These dynamic and fluid approaches offer improved accuracy, sensitivity, and objectivity but are limited by their novelty (the measurements cannot extend very far back in time), technological challenges (short battery life, poor performance in urban canyons and indoors), and the need to develop and share standard operating protocols to guide these kinds of studies. Jankowska et al. [37] and in this volume, for example, documented how these technologies can be used to conceptualize physical activity and sedentary behavior interactions with the environment by tracking exposure through time, space, and behaviors.

The sixth and final class of variables of interest measure the geographic variation in the presence or absence and magnitude of a variety of environmental and/or social risk conditions. These measures can be acquired by spatializing site-specific data: Pastor et al. [59], for example, examined the spatial distribution of toxic air releases and residential demographics in California using 2000 Census data and coeval information from the Federal Toxic Release Inventory for evidence of disproportionate exposure, whereas Tatalovich et al. [85] examined the spatial distribution of ultraviolent radiation and residential demographics using lifetime residential information for evidence of disproportionate exposure in a California case-control melanoma study. There is now the opportunity to acquire estimates of many of the atmospheric risks (PM2.5, O3, UV bands) from satellites circling the Earth (e.g. [7, 86]).

There is also the opportunity to build measures of social risk factors. For example, Abramovitz and Albrecht [1] proposed a Community Loss Index which focuses on the understudied role of place as a source of stress and an aggregator of individual experiences. Building on the relationship between loss and stress, the index attempts to capture collective loss, defined as the chronic exposure by neighborhood residents to multiple resource losses at the same time. Using maps, they analyzed the spatial distribution of six types of loss in New York City and the characteristics of people who live in high- and low-loss neighborhoods. This approach can be contrasted with that of Hodza [30], who around the same time proposed the concept of appreciative GIS to inspire communities to create change based on geographic representations of their strengths and achievements.

Spatiotemporal cluster detection analysis addressing specific disease outcomes can complement area based analyses of associations between environments and health status. These techniques have led to the development of new etiological hypotheses that explain patterns of elevated risk and new epidemiological studies which explore these hypotheses further. For example, Wheeler et al. [89] used spatiotemporal cluster detection analysis and found that the genetic factors and polychlorinated biphenyls (PCBs) exposure, which previous studies had found to be associated with non-Hodgkin Lymphoma (NHL), did not fully explain previously detected areas of elevated risk using a population-based case control study of NHL that included residential histories.

The variability in the associations reported by Wheeler et al. [89] are not uncommon, and we turn our attention next to explore some of the reasons why this happens.

1.4 Methodological Challenges

Many of the studies highlighted thus far have relied on a popular assumption in geographic information science and the health sciences, that the census tract or other census geographies define 'neighborhood' and that census geographic reporting units can be used to measure the effects of social and environmental characteristics on human well-being.

Choosing the census tract, or any of the other administrative units shown in Fig. 1.3, probably does not represent the functional neighborhood or the local social structure and as such creates potential misreporting and error when used to examine the effects of neighborhood on health outcomes [8, 71]. There are three sets of problems with using these administrative units for connecting population, health, and place.

The first is that the units themselves vary tremendously in terms of geographic extent and character, contrary to many people's expectations. Matthews [45], for example, noted that the census tract is officially defined as a compact, recognizable, and homogeneous territorial unit with relatively permanent boundaries, between 2500 and 8000 residents, and an optimum population of about 4000 people but when he checked, he found that the mean population size in the lower 48 states and 2000 census was approximately 4300 and a quarter of all census tracts had either fewer than 2500 or greater than 8000 residents. Similarly, California's 8038 census tracts have land areas that differ by five orders of magnitude and populations that range from 0 to 37,452, with mean 4635, and standard deviation 1974 (2012–2016 ACS estimates).

The second problem is the spatial heterogeneity found within many of the individual census tracts and other administrative units. Several methods have been proposed for handling these effects. The most popular is dasymetric mapping which provides a methodology that disaggregates data contained in a choropleth map to a set of smaller polygons using one or more ancillary data layers [48, 49]. Many applications start with a census tracts portrayed in a choropleth map and then use parcel data and address points to produce fine-resolution population maps which may or may not reduce the heterogeneity within the census tracts or other map units [43, 44, 55, 93]. The LandScan™ database, for example, provides ambient population (averaged over 24 h) for the globe at a 1 km spatial resolution annually using the best available demographic (census) and geographic data along with remote sensing imagery analysis techniques within a multivariate dasymetric modeling framework to disaggregate census counts within administrative boundaries [18].

Other approaches have been proposed to achieve similar outcomes. Mu et al. [54], for example, have proposed an alternative approach to obtain regions of comparable population by decomposing areas of large population (to gain more spatial variability and less internal heterogeneity) and merging areas of small population (to mask privacy of data). These authors proposed a mixed level regionalization method based on the Peano curve algorithm and scale-space clustering that accounts for spatial connectivity and compactness, attribute homogeneity, and exogenous criteria such as minimum (and approximately equal) population or disease counts.

What is clear, irrespective of the approach used, is that continued collaboration between geographers, spatial demographers and health researchers is sorely needed to further develop applications of these approaches to health.

Another approach is to abandon the administrative reporting units altogether and to use buffers to construct egocentric neighborhoods for subjects of interest. Some studies have used the road network but others have used specific shapes to delineate these neighborhoods. Oliver et al. [56], for example, compared circular and network buffers to examine the influence of land use on walking for leisure and errands but the better choice is probably problem-specific since estimation of near-roadway traffic pollutants would probably use neither of the aforementioned options. Strominger et al. [80] constructed seven mutually exclusive built environment (BE) domains (housing damage, property disorder, territoriality, vacancy, public nuisances, crime, and tenancy) using four different index construction methods that differentially accounted for number of parcels and parcel area. The seven indices were constructed at the census block level and two alternative spatial scales – the primary adjacency community specified by constructing a first order adjacency matrix, and a secondary adjacency community that extended the former by additionally including secondary neighbors – which the authors argued would better depict the larger neighborhood context experienced by local residents. The results showed that the impact of construction method on BE measures was index and spatial scale specific and as a consequence, the authors thought that researchers would be well-advised to conduct sensitivity analysis using different construction methods to ensure that associations between the BE and health outcomes are not artifacts of methodological decisions (e.g. [34]).

This, it turns out, is one of the grand challenges for nearly all work that seeks to deploy geospatial tools and data to improve our understanding of the connections between population, health and place.

One suggested way around some of these problems relies on the delineation of natural and meaningful neighborhoods which better represent the functional neighborhood spaces of individuals because they contain the appropriate physical and social amenities [68]. However, the likelihood that natural neighborhoods will be delineated using different criteria (i.e. based on the homogeneity in population and housing characteristics in some instances and on the spatial heterogeneity in the built and social environments in other cases) and the difficulty of connecting population-level census, local administrative, and health facility data with these units pose major challenges. Bell et al. [4] endeavored to sidestep some of these issues by choosing the existing neighborhood boundaries in a study that explored whether neighborhood of residence affected access to primary health care in Mississauga, Ontario. Many large metropolitan regions and cities, including New York and Los Angeles, have delineated neighborhoods and used these units to support governance and the delivery of municipal services.

The implication is that the aforementioned forms of neighborhood capture the locations frequented by the individuals or population of interest. This may or may not be valid, given the results of Matthews [45] and Matthews and Yang [46], who have used surveys to show how individuals in large metropolitan areas (i.e. Boston and Chicago) are much more mobile than we might think. The results for 10 families drawn from a single neighborhood in Boston, MA reproduced in Table 1.4, for

Table 1.4 Residential, adjacent, and non-adjacent activity domains (rank-ordered by percent of activities in nonadjacent tracts; highest to lowest) for 10 families in Boston, MA over 7 days ([45], p. 45)

Domain	N	Tracts		
		Residential	Adjacent	Non-adjacent
Social services	22	4.55	9.09	86.36
Work	11	9.09	9.09	81.82
Nonfood shopping	22	4.55	18.18	77.27
Childcare	15	0	26.67	73.33
Health services	45	6.67	20.00	73.33
Education	26	7.69	19.23	73.08
Social network	18	22.22	5.56	72.22
Other services	12	0	33.33	66.67
Food shopping	37	5.41	29.73	64.86
Recreation	14	0	42.86	57.14
Total	222	6.31	21.17	72.52

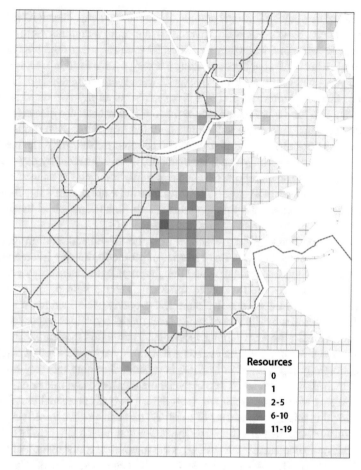

Fig. 1.5 The gridded surface showing the resource sites used by 10 families residing in a single Boston, MA neighborhood over 7 days ([45], p. 44)

example, show the residential, adjacent, and non-adjacent activity domains rank-ordered from highest to lowest by percent of activities in non-adjacent tracts over 7 days. These 10 families utilized 222 unique places (excluding their residences) and the spatial patterning of these 222 places was represented in a map by Matthews [45] using square grid cells that measured 500 m on a side (Fig. 1.5). The most remarkable result here is that just 6% of the activities occurred in the same census tract as home and nearly 73% occurred beyond the home census tract and those census tracts that were immediately adjacent to the home census tract.

This mobility may have some second-order effects, as illustrated in some work using the 2000 U.S. Census and the Los Angeles Family and Neighborhood Study (LAFANS) by Inagami et al. [32], which showed how non-neighborhood exposures may suppress neighborhood effects on self-rated health.

The role of time adds additional complexity to the accurate characterization of an individual's neighborhood as well. This may occur as an individual's life evolves – as happens, for example, when they transition from childhood to adulthood and then old age and because of what happens along the way. I have lived in Los Angeles for nearly 25 years and yet many of my weekends were spent in Bakersfield, Lancaster, Palmdale, Oxnard, Palmdale, and San Bernardino when my two children played club soccer. This kind of transition means that our interest and use of specific neighborhoods (i.e. local amenities) will evolve over the life course even if our place of residence does not change. Similarly, the places themselves, may change over a variety of time scales – Hollywood, for example, is very different by day and night with repercussions for specific activities people might engage in as well as public safety, and many places will have trajectories that show urban renewal and/or urban decay which extends over many decades and affects both the people of the place and those who move towards or away from these places [14].

Robertson and Feick [65] have shown how the aforementioned problems and several new ones noted below point to a series of problems drawing inferences when trying to relate individual level data and the geographical contexts they are associated with in health (as well as other domains). Their article points to multiple sources and forms of uncertainty which, if not properly accounted for, may lead to poor inferences and why the rise of multi-level modeling, which apportions variations in individual outcomes among individual factors and contextual influences, does not solve these problems and in some instances, may make them worse.

Their typology reproduced in Fig. 1.6 is organized around the gray box in the middle which shows the relationship between the measured and true or experienced spatial contexts when using point and areal data. The true contextual unit (TCU) of the individual in this schema is a set of locations that encapsulate the effect or exposure of some environmental variable on the individual, which is typically unknown, and the measured contextual unit (MCU) is the measured representation of the TCU in a given study ([65], p. 460). The mismatch between the MCU and TCU can lead to one or more types of inferential errors.

The remainder of Fig. 1.6 therefore summarizes the roles of five different types of inferential errors which may emerge when using spatial data. Four have been written about extensively and will be covered briefly here. The first two are the most general. The ecological fallacy occurs when erroneous inferences are made about individuals using relationships estimated at the group level [66, 82], whereas the atomistic fallacy occurs when erroneous inferences are made about groups of individuals based on individual level data (e.g. when measurements are taken from a non-representative population sample) for example [16]. The third is the Modifiable Unit Area Problem or MAUP which has perplexed geographers for decades (e.g. [10, 21, 57, 67]). This problem refers to the variation in the outcomes of analysis that occurs when the configuration and/or scaling of the areal unit boundaries are changed (as would happen moving from census tracts to census block groups for example).

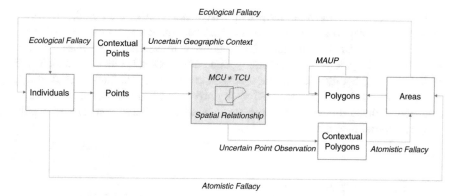

Fig. 1.6 Typology of geographical analysis problems related to inferential errors with geospatial data ([65], p. 459)

The fourth problem is the Uncertain Geographic Context or UGCoP which describes how uncertainties in the measurement of the true causally relevant spatial context can contaminate inferences at the individual level [17, 39, 41]. This may occur due to the arbitrary nature of the areal unit boundaries (as happens when we use census tracts, census block groups, or ZIP codes for example) and/or because the inferences will likely vary with individuals due to gender, age, occupation, or SES for example.

Robertson and Feick [65] also introduce a fifth possible problem, the Uncertain Point Distribution Problem (UPOP), which will likely grow in terms of importance in health studies in the coming years. The UPOP occurs when stationary and/or mobile measurements of individual-level variables (i.e. health status, happiness, stress, perceptions of neighborhood safety) [52] are made via their spatial locations and used to infer group-level differences or relationships. They are likely to grow in both frequency and magnitude due to the rise of volunteered and ambient geographic information [11] as well as sensor (GPS traces, ecological momentary assessments, and various types of personal sensors) [6, 9, 20, 72, 79, 81, 88] and transactional data (transit cards, loyalty cards) [64, 95], and the increased need for geocoding to transform addresses and other kinds of geographic references into geographic coordinates [23, 40]. Robertson and Feick [65] offer a very detailed and forward-looking description of these developments and why the classical issues of representativeness, spatial uncertainty and sampling error and therefore, geographic inference are all relevant here.

The ramifications of these issues for health studies are enormous since two representativeness questions (i.e. problems) accompany most individual tracking data: (1) how representative the sample points are of an individual's true spatial context (which will likely vary if they are indoors or outdoors and/or mobile for example);

and (2) how representative an individual's true context is of the population which
the study is aiming to characterize (given that many tracking studies use small samples and/or specific individuals such as those who regularly use mass transit).
Robertson and Feick [65], for example, point out that most health studies today are
platial in nature but they seldom measure and therefore cannot know if some effect
(i.e. a reduction in stress attributed to the presence of green space) would have
occurred without this exposure and that the measurements can therefore only
crudely approximate the true context.

1.5   Future Opportunities

Many authors have argued for the greater use of spatial perspectives across the
entire human disease and health spectrum, from the basic science of disease
causation to health disparities across space and among different racial and socioeconomic groups, and the impact of health interventions at a global scale during the
past decade (e.g. [2, 51, 63, 70]). In addition, Auchinloss et al. [2] went so far as to
identify three emerging areas – the adoption of spatial methods to understand better
how place-based features affect health; the integration of spatial methods, digital
media and social networks to facilitate spatiotemporal research; and spatial simulation – that they thought would drive greater deployment of spatial methods in health
studies in the future.

This chapter focused on the adoption of spatial methods to understand better how
place-based features affect health, but it is important to note that progress has been
made across the other two as well [see Janies et al. [35, 36], Mennis and Mason
[50], and Bian et al. [5] for some recent, noteworthy examples].

This chapter made three major arguments about what needs to be done to support
the adoption and use of spatial methods to better understand how place-based
features affect health.

The first was the emergence of geographic information science as a separate field
of study focused on all of the ways in which location can be used to gather, organize,
analyze, model, and visualize information. This growth has been matched by the
phenomenal growth in the numbers and variety of geospatial tools and datasets that
can be used for place-based health studies. There are now many proprietary as well
as free and open source software platforms and more changes can be expected
across all of these platforms in the years ahead given that the rate and magnitude of
the changes in information technology show no signs of slowing down. These
advances, which include cloud computing, cyberinfrastructure, interoperability and
software-as-a-service, will encourage the development of new analytical tools and
increase the heft of health applications moving forward.

The second was the need to situate these geospatial tools and data within a
framework that supports: (1) a "relational" view of place in which place is
conceptualized as a process – a fluid dynamic field of constantly interacting
elements, within and beyond itself – rather than as an entity; (2) focusing on the

biological plausibility of associations to help discover causal inferences regarding the impact of place on health; and (3) the need for the chosen place-based exposures to precede the effects on health (and sometimes by many years or even decades given the latencies connected with various types of cancers and behaviors). The genetic geographic information science framework recently proposed by Jacquez et al. [33] is but one example of a framework that supports all three of these requirements.

The third argument concerned a series of interrelated methodological challenges which threaten to propagate uncertainty and error and stall advances in our understanding of place-based health effects if ignored. The first part of this discussion focused on the ways in which a person's neighborhood or activity space has been defined and how the role of time may add additional complexity to the accurate characterization of these spaces as well. The second and in many ways more substantial part of this discussion was organized around the typology of geographical analysis problems related to inferential errors with geospatial data recently proposed by Robertson and Feick [65]. Five frequently encountered problems – the ecological fallacy, the atomistic fallacy, the modifiable areal unit problem, the Uncertain Geographic Context problem, and the Uncertain Point Distribution Problems – were introduced and positioned around the periphery of this typology to show the potential relationships between the measured and true or experienced spatial contexts when using point and areal data or a variety of areal aggregations (as often happens in multi-level modeling). The fundamental problem is that the true contextual unit of the individual in this schema is a set of locations that encapsulate the effect or exposure of some environmental variable on the individual, which is typically unknown, and the measured contextual unit is often a relatively poorly measured representation of the true contextual unit in a given study and/or setting.

This state of affairs means that the role and impact of both existing and new geospatial tools and data will be blunted until we can find better ways of using geospatial tools and data to represent the true contextual units of individuals. There are some exciting new technologies (GIS, GPS, ecological momentary assessment, and various kinds of personal sensors) but there potential is not likely to be realized unless we can produce scholars and working professionals who have been broadly trained in the population, health and spatial sciences, and who are comfortable working at the intersection of all three of these fields. The recent efforts to incorporate social determinants of health into electronic records to promote patient and population health (e.g. [3, 27, 31]) provide a sense of urgency so long as the use of these so-called "community vital signs" is not organized around a robust set of causal inferences and plausible biological and behavioral pathways.

Acknowledgements This work was supported by grants UL1TR001855 and UL1TR000130 from the National Center for Advancing Translational Science (NCATS) and grant 5P30ES007048 from the National Institute of Environmental Health Sciences Center of the U.S. National Institutes of Health. The content is solely the responsibility of the author and does not necessarily represent the official views of the National Institutes of Health.

References

1. Abramovitz M, Albrecht J. The community loss index: a new social indicator. Soc Serv Rev. 2013;87:677–724.
2. Auchinloss AH, Gebreab SY, Mair C, et al. A review of spatial methods in epidemiology, 2000–2010. Annu Rev Public Health. 2012;33:107–22.
3. Bazeman AW, Cottrell EK, Gold R, et al. "Community vital signs": incorporating geocoded social determinants into electronic records to promote patient and population health. J Am Med Inform Assoc. 2016;23:407–12.
4. Bell S, Wilson K, Bissonnette L, et al. Access to primary health care: does neighborhood of residence matter? Annals Am Assoc Geogr. 2013;103(1):85–105.
5. Bian L, Huang Y, Mao L, et al. Modeling individual vulnerability to communicable diseases: a framework and design. Ann Assoc Am Geogr. 2012;102(5):1016–25.
6. Boruff BJ, Nathan A, Nijënstein S. Using GPS technology to (re)-examine operational definitions of "neighbourhood" in place-based health research. Int J Health Geogr. 2012;11:22.
7. Cadet JM, Bencherif H, Portafaix T, et al. Comparison of ground-based and satellite-derived solar UV index levels at six South African sites. Int J Environ Res Public Health. 2017;14(11):1384.
8. Chaix B. Geographic life environments and coronary heart disease: a literature review, theoretical contributions, methodological updates, and a research agenda. Annu Rev Public Health. 2009;30(1):81–105.
9. Chaix B, Méline J, Duncan S, et al. GPS tracking in neighborhood and health studies: a step forward for environmental exposure assessment, a step backward for causal inference? Health Place. 2013;21(Suppl. C):46–51.
10. Clark WAV, Avery KL. The effects of data aggregation in statistical analysis. Geogr Anal. 1976;8(4):428–38.
11. Crooks A, Croitoru A, Stefanidis A, et al. Earthquake: twitter as a distributed sensor system. Trans GIS. 2013;17(1):124–47.
12. Cummins S, Curtis S, Diez-Roux AV, et al. Understanding and representing 'place' in health research: a relational approach. Soc Sci Med. 2007;65:1825–38.
13. Daniel M, Moore S, Kestens Y. Framing the biosocial pathways underlying associations between place and cardiometabolic disease. Health Place. 2008;14:117–32.
14. Delmelle EC. Mapping the DNA of urban neighborhoods: clustering longitudinal sequences of neighborhood socioeconomic change. Ann Am Assoc Geogr. 2016;106(1):36–56.
15. Delmelle EC, Thill JC, Furuseth O, et al. Trajectories of multidimensional of neighborhood quality of life change. Urban Stud. 2013;50:923–41.
16. Diez Roux AV. A glossary for multilevel analysis. J Epidemiol Community Health. 2002;56(8):588–94.
17. Diez Roux AV, Mair C. Neighborhoods and health. Ann NY Acad Sci. 2010;1186(1):125–45.
18. Dobson J, Bright E, Coleman P, et al. A global population database for estimating populations at risk. Photogramm Eng Remote Sens. 2000;66(7):849–57.
19. Duckham M, Goodchild MF, Worboys M. Foundations of geographic information science. Boca Raton: CRC Press; 2004.
20. Dunton GF. Ecological momentary assessment in physical activity research. Exerc Sport Sci Rev. 2017;45(1):48–54.
21. Flowerdew R, Manley DJ, Sabel CE. Neighbourhood effects on health: does it matter where you draw the boundaries? Soc Sci Med. 2008;66(6):1241–55.
22. Gehlert S, Mininger C, Cipriano-Steffens TM. Placing biology in breast cancer disparities research. In: Burton LM, et al., editors. Communities, neighborhoods and health: expanding the boundaries of place. Berlin: Springer; 2011. p. 57–72.
23. Goldberg DW, Wilson JP, Knoblock CA, et al. An effective and efficient approach for manually improving geocoded data. Int J Health Geogr. 2008;7:60.
24. Goodchild MF. Geographical information science. Int J Geogr Inf Sys. 1992;6(1):31–45.

25. Goodchild MF. Geographic information systems and science: today and tomorrow. Ann GIS. 2009;15(1):3–9.
26. Goovaerts P. Geostatistical analysis of health data with different levels of spatial aggregation. Spat Spatio Temporal Epidemiol. 2012;3:83–92.
27. Gottlieb TKJ, Manchanda R, et al. Moving electronic health records upstream: Incorporating social determinants of health. Am J Prev Med. 2015;48(2):215–8.
28. Grubesic TH, Wei R, Murray AT. Spatial clustering overview and comparison: accuracy, sensitivity, and computational expense. Ann Am Assoc Geogr. 2014;104(6):1134–55.
29. Heinrich K, Huber C, Rinner C. Making area-based composite indices comparable across time: the role of standardization and outlier removal. URISA J. 2017;27(2):37–49.
30. Hodza P. Appreciative GIS and strength-based community change. Trans GIS. 2014;18(2):270–85.
31. Hughes LS, Phillips RL Jr, DeVoe JE, et al. Community vital signs: taking the pulse of the community while caring for patients. J Am Board Fam Med. 2016;29:419–22.
32. Inagami S, Cohen DA, Finch BK. Non-residential neighborhood exposures suppress neighborhood effects of self-rated health. Soc Sci Med. 2007;65:1779–91.
33. Jacquez GM, Sabel CE, Shi C. Genetic GIScience: toward a place-based synthesis of the genome, exposome, and behavome. Ann Assoc Am Geogr. 2015;105(3):454–72.
34. James P, Berrigan D, Hart JE, et al. Effects of buffer size and shape on associations between the built environment and energy balance. Health Place. 2014;27:162–70.
35. Janies DA, Treseder T, Alexandrov B, et al. The Supramap project: linking pathogen genomes with geography to fight emergent infectious diseases. Cladistics. 2011;27:61–8.
36. Janies DA, Pomeroy LW, Aaronson JM, et al. Analysis and visualization of H7 influenza using genomic, evolutionary, and geographic information is a modular web service. Cladistics. 2012;28:483–8.
37. Jankowska MM, Schipperjin J, Kerr J. A framework for using GPS data in physical activity and sedentary behavior studies. Exerc Sport Sci Rev. 2015;43(1):48–56.
38. Kemp SP. Place, history, memory: thinking time within place. In: Burton LM, et al., editors. Communities, neighborhoods and health: expanding the boundaries of place. Berlin: Springer; 2011. p. 3–19.
39. Kestens Y, Wasfi R, Naud A, et al. "Contextualizing context": reconciling environmental exposures, social networks, and location preferences in health research. Curr Environ Health Rep. 2017;4(1):51–60.
40. Krieger N, Waterman P, Lemieux K, et al. On the wrong side of the tracts? Evaluating the accuracy of geocoding in public health research. Am J Public Health. 2001;91(7):1114–6.
41. Kwan MP. The uncertain geographic context problem. Ann Am Assoc Geogr. 2012;102(5):958–68.
42. Lee TM. Defining neighborhood for health research in Arizona (Unpublished MS thesis). University Southern California, Los Angeles; 2019.
43. Leyk S, Nagle NN, Buttenfield BP. Maximum entropy dasymetric modeling for demographic small area estimation. Geogr Anal. 2013;45:285–306.
44. Maantay JA, Maroko AR, Herrmann C. Mapping population density in the urban environment: the Cadastral-Based Expert Dasymetric System (CEDS). Cartogr Geogr Inf Sci. 2007;34:77–102.
45. Matthews SA. Spatial polygamy and the heterogeneity of place: studying people and place via egocentric methods. In: Burton LM, et al., editors. Communities, neighborhoods and health: expanding the boundaries of place. Berlin: Springer; 2011. p. 35–55.
46. Matthews SA, Yang TC. Spatial polygamy and contextual exposures (SPACEs): promoting activity space approaches in research on place and health. Am Behav Sci. 2013;57(8):1057–81.
47. Meade M. The geography of life and death: deeper, broader, and much more complex. Ann Assoc Am Geogr. 2012;102:1219–27.
48. Mennis J. Generating surface models of population using dasymetric mapping. Prof Geogr. 2003;55:31–42.

49. Mennis J. Dasymetric mapping for estimating population in small areas. Geogr Compass. 2009;3:727–45.
50. Mennis J, Mason MJ. People, places, and adolescent substance use: integrating activity space and social network data for analyzing health behavior. Ann Assoc Am Geogr. 2011;101(2):272–91.
51. Mennis J, Yoo EHE. Geographic information science and the analysis of place and health. Trans GIS. 2018;22(3):842–54.
52. Mitchell L, Frank MR, Harris KD, et al. The geography of happiness: connecting twitter sentiment and expression, demographics, and objective characteristics of place. PLoS One. 2013;8(5):e64417.
53. Mitchell R, Dorling D, Shaw M. Inequalities in life and death: what if Britain were more equal? Bristol: Policy Press; 2000.
54. Mu L, Wang F, Chem VW, et al. A place-oriented, mixed-level regionalization method for constructing geographic areas in health data dissemination and analysis. Ann Am Assoc Geogr. 2015;105(1):48–66.
55. Nagle NN, Buttenfield BP, Leyk S, et al. Dasymetric modeling and uncertainty. Ann Assoc Am Geogr. 2014;104(1):80–95.
56. Oliver LN, Schuurman N, Hall AW. Comparing circular and network buffers to examine the influence of land use on walking for leisure and errands. Int J Health Geogr. 2007;6(1):41.
57. Openshaw S. The modifiable areal unit problem. Norwich: Geo Books; 1983.
58. Owens A. Neighborhoods on the rise: a typology of neighborhoods experiencing socioeconomic ascent. City Community. 2012;11:345–69.
59. Pastor M, Sadd JL, Morello-Frosch R. Waiting to inhale: the demographics of toxic air release facilities in 21st-Century California. Soc Sci Q. 2004;85(2):420–40.
60. Peña DG. Structural violence, historical trauma, and public health: the environmental justice critique of contemporary risk science and practice. In: Burton LM, et al., editors. Communities, neighborhoods and health: expanding the boundaries of place. Berlin: Springer; 2011. p. 203–18.
61. Popay J, Williams G, Thomas C, et al. Theorizing inequalities in health: the place of lay knowledge. In: Hofrichter R, editor. Health and social justice: politics, ideology, and inequity in the distribution of disease. New York: Jossey-Bass; 2003. p. 385–409.
62. Pred A. Place as historically contingent process: structuration and the time-geography of becoming places. Ann Assoc Am Geogr. 1984;74(2):279–97.
63. Richardson DB, Volkow ND, Kwan MP, et al. Spatial turn in health research. Science. 2013;339:1390–2.
64. Robertson C, Feick R. Bumps and bruises in the digital skins of cities: unevenly distributed user-generated content across US urban areas. Cartogr Geogr Inf Sci. 2016;43(4):283–300.
65. Robertson C, Feick R. Inference and analysis across spatial supports in the big data era: uncertain point observations and geographic contexts. Trans GIS. 2018;22(2):455–76.
66. Robinson WS. Ecological correlations and the behavior of individuals. Am Sociol Rev. 1950;15(3):351–7.
67. Root ED. Moving neighborhoods and health research forward: using geographic methods to examine the role of spatial scale in neighborhood effects on health. Ann Am Assoc Geogr. 2012;102(5):986–95.
68. Ross NA, Tremblay S, Graham K. Neighborhood influences on health in Montréal, Canada. Soc Sci Med. 2004;59(7):1485–94.
69. Sastry N, Ghosh-Dastidar B, Adams JL, et al. The design of a multilevel survey of children, families, and communities: the Los Angeles family and neighborhood survey. Soc Sci Res. 2006;35:1000–24.
70. Schootman M, Gomez SL, Henry KA, et al. Geospatial approaches to cancer control and population sciences. Cancer Epidemiol Biomark Prev. 2017;26(4):472–5.
71. Sharkey P, Faber JW. Where, when, why, and for whom do residential contexts matter? Moving away from the dichotomous understanding of neighborhood effects. Ann Rev Sociol. 2014;40:559–79.

72. Shaughnessy K, Reyes R, Shankardass K, et al. Using geo-located social media for ecological momentary assessments of emotion: innovative opportunities in psychology science and practice. Can Psychol. 2018;59(1):47–53.
73. Shi X, Alford-Teaster J, Onega T, et al. Spatial access and local demand for major cancer care facilities in the United States. Ann Am Assoc Geogr. 2012;102(5):1125–34.
74. Skupin A, Hagelman R. Visualizing demographic trajectories with self-organizing maps. GeoInformatica. 2005;9:159–79.
75. Snow J. Snow on cholera. London: Oxford Univ Press; 1936.
76. Spencer MS, Garratt A, Hockman E, et al. Environmental justice and the Well-being of poor children of color. In: Burton LM, et al., editors. Communities, neighborhoods and health: expanding the boundaries of place. Berlin: Springer; 2011. p. 219–33.
77. Spielman SE, Singleton A. Studying neighborhoods using uncertain data form the American community survey: a contextual approach. Ann Am Assoc Geogr. 2015;105(5):1003–25.
78. Stamp LD. The geography of life and death. Ithaca: Cornell University Press; 1964.
79. Steinle S, Reis S, Sabel CE, et al. Personal exposure monitoring of PM2.5 in indoor and outdoor microenvironments. Sci Total Environ. 2015;508:383–94.
80. Strominger J, Anthopolos R, Miranda ML. Implications of construction method and spatial scale on measures of the built environment. Int J Health Geogr. 2016;15, 15
81. Su JG, Jerrett M, Meng YY, et al. Integrating smart-phone based momentary location tracking with fixed site air quality monitoring for personal exposure assessment. Sci Total Environ. 2015;506–507:518–26.
82. Subramanian SV, Jones K, Kaddour A, et al. Revisiting Robinson: the perils of individualistic and ecologic fallacy. Int J Epidemiol. 2009;38(2):342–60.
83. Sui D, Elwood S, Goodchild MF. Crowdsourcing geographic knowledge: Volunteered Geographic Information (VGI) in theory and practice. Berlin: Springer; 2012.
84. Sutherland I. John Graunt: a tercentenary tribute. J R Stat Soc Ser A Stat Soc. 1963;126:536–7.
85. Tatalovich Z, Wilson JP, Mack T, et al. The objective assessment of lifetime cumulative ultraviolet exposure for determining melanoma risk. J Photochem Photobiol B. 2006;85(3):198–204.
86. van Donkelaar A, Martin RV, Spurr RJ, et al. High-resolution satellite-derived PM2.5 from optimal estimation and geographically weighted regression over North America. Environ Sci Technol. 2015;49(17):10482–91.
87. VoPham T. GIS&T and epidemiology. In: Wilson JP, editor. Geographic information science & technology body of knowledge. Washington, DC: University Consortium Geogr Inf Sci; 2018.
88. Wan N, Lin Kan G, Wilson G. Addressing location uncertainties in GPS-based activity monitoring: a methodological framework. Trans GIS. 2017;21(4):764–81.
89. Wheeler DC, Ward MH, Waller LA. Spatial-temporal analysis of cancer risk in epidemiologic studies with residential histories. Ann Am Assoc Geogr. 2012;102(5):1049–57.
90. Wild CP. Complementing the genome with an "exposome": the outstanding challenge of environmental exposure measurement in molecular epidemiology. Cancer Epidemiol Biomark Prev. 2005;14(8):1847–50.
91. Wild CP. The exposome: from concept to utility. Int J Epidemiol. 2012;41:24–32.
92. Wilson JP, editor. The geographic information science & technology body of knowledge. Washington, DC: University Consortium Geographic Information Science; 2018.
93. Zandbergen PA. Dasymetric mapping using high resolution address point datasets. Trans GIS. 2011;15(s1):5–27.
94. Zhang X, Pérez-Stable EJ, Bourne PE, et al. Big data science: opportunities and challenges to address minority health and health disparities in the 21st Century. Ethn Dis. 2017;27(2):95–106.
95. Zhong C, Manley E, Müller S, et al. Measuring variability of mobility patterns from multiday smart-card data. J Comput Sci. 2015;9:125–30.

Chapter 2
Analyzing Cancer and Breast Cancer in Space and Time

Geoffrey M. Jacquez

Abstract This chapter introduces concepts central to the space-time analysis of cancer and breast cancer in space and time. By "space" we mean geographic location; by time we mean when specific events occurred. We deal with cancer at both the individual- and population-level, and are concerned with quantifying individual exposures through space and time, and the assessment of space-time patterns in cancer outcomes in groups of individuals and in populations. We begin by setting the stage with a discussion of the complexity of the problem, and consider factors including carcinogenesis, models of cancer progression, cancer latency, biological vulnerability, temporal orientation in space-time cancer analysis, and human mobility. Next, specific methods for space-time pattern recognition for mobile individuals are summarized, followed by specific examples for pancreatic, breast and bladder cancers. Sources of error are discussed, with an emphasis on actual exposure measurement for individuals in comparison to model-based estimates. It is suggested that model- and GIS-based estimates substantially underestimate actual exposures, resulting in exposure misclassification and under-estimation of cancer burdens attributable to environmental exposures. Next, future research directions that leverage advances in the mutational signatures for cancers and improved measurement technologies for quantifying the cancer exposome over the life course are identified. The chapter concludes with critical challenges and barriers in the realization of a genome+, exposome, behavome synthesis for cancer prevention and a more complete causal understanding.

Keywords Breast cancer · Space-time · Spatiotemporal · Progression · Latency · Carcinogenesis · Model · Exposure estimation · Prevention

G. M. Jacquez (✉)
BioMedware, Inc., and The University of Michigan, Ann Arbor, MI, USA
e-mail: jacquez@biomedware.com

© Springer Nature Switzerland AG 2019
D. Berrigan, N. A. Berger (eds.), *Geospatial Approaches to Energy Balance and Breast Cancer*, Energy Balance and Cancer 15, https://doi.org/10.1007/978-3-030-18408-7_2

2.1 Setting the Stage

Cancer poses a knotty problem in space-time analysis because the causes of cancer are complex, including environmental exposures, genetics, epigenetics and health-related behaviors; carcinogenesis is a multi-step process; and cancer latency, which is the period between initiating events (e.g. initial mutation) and diagnosis can be decades. This section seeks to familiarize the reader with aspects of this complexity. First, it considers cancer as a dynamic space-time system, in the context of both individual- and population-views. A conceptual model of carcinogenesis at the individual-level is presented for pancreatic cancer, and motivates the definition of cancer latency as residence times through states defined by the initiation-promotion paradigm. Next, other aspects of complexity are considered, including residential mobility and latency, biological periods of vulnerability, and temporal orientation in the space-time analysis of cancer.

2.1.1 The Initiation-Promotion Model, and Cancer Latency Distributions

Carcinogenesis is a multi-stage process, and cancer itself may have a multiplicity of causes. Normal cell metabolism produces oxidants known to modify DNA [68], and there are numerous environmental factors that are probable or known causes of human cancers [8, 11, 69].

That carcinogenesis involves a progression through several cellular states leading to cancer was proposed as early as the 1940's. In a review, Foulds provides a definition of cancer progression as a multistage process with non-reversible states [15], and cites the work by Rous and colleagues on the initiation-promotion model in which healthy cells enter the pathway to cancer through an initiating mutation, with subsequent mutations promoting the initiated cell to a full-blown cancer [16]. DNA repair mechanisms can reverse initiated cells back to healthy cells [66], and this may occur for promoted cells as well. Nonetheless, commonly accepted models of carcinogenesis often treat at least one of the promotion events as non-reversible. Carcinogenesis thus is a progression from normal cells to metastatic cancer, as illustrated for pancreatic cancer in Fig. 2.1.

This may be modeled as a multi-step process comprised of compartments corresponding to healthy, initiated, promoted, *in situ*, and metastatic cancer (Fig. 2.2). The progression to cancer begins with mutations in a healthy cell's DNA that leads to accelerated cell proliferation. Expansion of clones of cancerous cells along and additional mutations progress to pancreatic intraepithelial neoplasia (PanIN) in duration T_1 (Fig. 2.1). Cell states in Fig. 2.1 correspond to compartments in Fig. 2.2. For example, normal duct epithelial cells in Fig. 2.1 are the population of normal cells in compartment q_1. Founder cells from a PanIN lesion start the parental clone that initiates an infiltrating carcinoma with the irreversible flow k_{32} from q_2 to q_3.

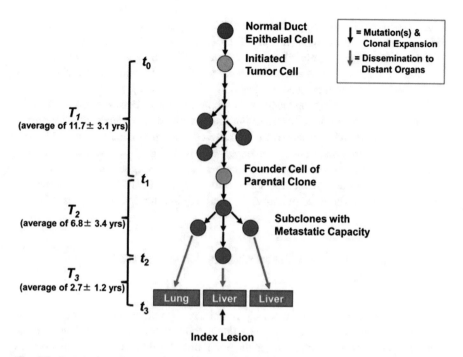

Fig. 2.1 Progression of pancreatic cancer. Normal epithelial cells undergo genetic mutation to become initiated cancer cells. Promotion events and clonal expansion produce a founder cell of the index pancreatic cancer clone, eventually leading to metastatic and dissemination to distant organs. Times shown are the durations in each cancer stage, referred to later as *residence times*. Adapted from Yachida, Jones et al. (2010)

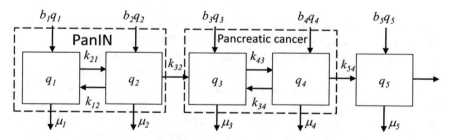

Fig. 2.2 Compartmental model of the PanIN pancreatic cancer pathway. Compartment q_1 is normal pancreatic cells. Normal cells divide and produce normal daughter cells, this is b_1q_1. Compartment q_2 is cells with one strand of damaged DNA. The input $k_{21}q_1$ is the inflow of new damaged cells. DNA repair is the backflow to healthy cells $k_{12}q_2$. The DNA is split into one strand each of damaged and normal DNA, these are copied and the resulting cells with a damaged strand flow into q_2 with rate b_2q_2. Subsequent mutations result in an irreversible promotion event to pancreatic cancer cell and descendants in state q_3. Additional DNA damage occurs ($k_{43}q_3$) giving rise to cells with metastatic capacity (q_4). Spread of these beyond the primary site produce metastases (q_5) that occur at rate $k_{54}q_4$. Cell death is $\mu_1, \dots \mu_5$

The residence time in compartments q_3 and q_4 as reported by Yachida et al. is T_2 [90]. Irreversible flow k_{54} is the proliferation and spread of metastases to other organs occurring in interval T_3. Average times in each compartment are $T_1 = 11.7$ years, $T_2 = 6.8$ years, and $T_3 = 2.7$ years. These empirical residence times were estimated from tumor histology and tumor genetics [9].

The modeling of carcinogenesis as a compartmental system is convenient, since the distributions of residence times of individual cells as they transit from healthy to cancerous states can be directly estimated from the compartmental system [34]. *The residence times for carcinogenic models of the form in* Fig. 2.1 *provide distributions of cancer latencies needed to quantify cancers as dynamic space-time systems.* This is of significant importance in the space-time analysis of cancer as it addresses the "when" portion of the when-what-where triad required for space-time analysis.

2.1.2   Conceptual Models of Cancer for Individuals and Populations

There are conceptual models that help illuminate the relative importance of different putative causes of cancer. For individuals, the construct of the genome+, exposome and behavome is useful [34]; at the population-level Meade's triangle provides a convenient framework [48]. These inform cancer risk modeling, which seeks to quantify risks using information on biological, environmental and behavioral factors. Conceptual models are an important first step in the space-time analysis of cancer as they guide how one generates hypotheses and frames research questions.

2.1.2.1   Individual-Level: Genome+, Exposome and Behavome

Figure 2.3 is a representation of a place-based synthesis of an individual's biology (the genome+), exposome, and behavome [35]. This paradigm recognizes that individual-level health is the result of a person's biology (including their genome, proteome, metabalome, transcriptome *etc.*), health-related exposures over the life course (their exposome), and health-related behaviors (their behavome, including exercise, diet, risk-taking and so on). The latter two are place-based, and along with the genome+, are determinants of individual health. The relative importance of the genome+, exposome and behavome can vary dramatically from one type of cancer to another. The role of biology and behavior in determining an individuals' cancer risk have been recognized for some time (historical examples include scrotal cancer in London chimney sweeps, as described by surgeon Percivall Pott in 1779); and substantial strides are being made in cancer genomics [83]. The cancer exposome [26, 38, 59] is a newer construct that builds on Wild's seminal description of the exposome as health-related exposures over the individual life course [88, 89].

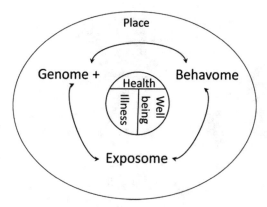

Fig. 2.3 Three determinants of an individual's health, both in terms of illness and well-being, are biology, termed the genome+; the exposome, defined as the totality of exposures over the life course [88]; and the behavome, which is the totality of an individual's health-related behaviors over the life course. These act through place, defined as the geographic, environmental, social, and societal milieus experienced over a person's life course. From Jacquez et al. 2015

Figure 2.3 may be used in space-time analysis to frame the relative importance of known and hypothesized causes of cancer in terms of individual biology, exposure and behaviors. Should these be place-based and vary through time, a space-time analysis may be warranted. If not, a space-time analysis might not be that informative. The genome+, for example oncogene expression, varies over the life course, and is influenced by individual exposures and behaviors. A notable example is the epigenome, where a parent's exposures can influence gene expression in their offspring [39]. As a rule of thumb, individual exposures and behaviors are often associated with specific places and times, motivating the use of space-time analysis of cancer risks at both the individual- and population-levels.

2.1.2.2   Population Level: Meade's Triangle

It is difficult and currently not practical to accurately and routinely measure a person's genome+, exposome, and behavome. However, we can sometimes estimate group-level risks and exposure profiles for local populations, using characteristics of people in that place (Population), their health behaviors (Behavior), and the environmental characteristics of that place (Habitat) (Fig. 2.4). This information can then be used to construct space-time models of population-level cancer risks through time.

Cancer risk models can be used in an inferential framework (e.g. cluster analysis), to identify when and where statistically significant excess cancer risks may be found [86]. Background cancer risk may be accounted for using neutral models of the space-time pattern expected in the absence of the hypothesized cluster process

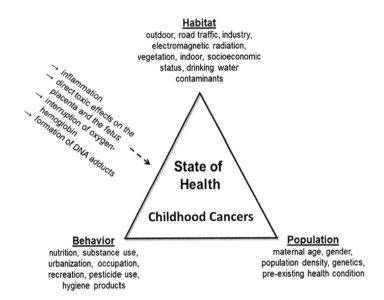

Fig. 2.4 Meade's triangle of human ecology for maternal exposures and childhood cancers: dashed arrow indicates hypothesized mechanisms. Modified from [60]

[22, 23]. The underlying premise is that one might expect cancer risks in populations to be structured in space and time even in the absence of a cluster-generating process. Hence, if one hypothesizes that benzene emissions from an industrial facility are contributing to leukemias in surrounding areas, one would also need to account for clustering that would be attributable to known covariates, such as age. If older individuals live near the plant, this could result in higher leukemia risk in those areas that is not attributable to benzene exposure.

$$r_{it} = f\left(H_{it}, B_{it}, P_{it}\right) + \varepsilon_{it} \qquad (2.1)$$

When more detailed information on risk factors is available space-time models may be used, including stochastic, geostatistical and Bayesian approaches. Here, cancer risk (e.g. predicted cancer rate) in specific populations at specific times is the dependent variable (r_{it}), and risk factors at those times and locations are the predictors Eq. ((2.1). Predictors in the framework of Meade's triangle are vectors of variables describing habitat (H_{it}), behavioral (B_{it}) and population factors (P_{it}). An error term for each local population through time (ε_{it}) is the difference between the observed and predicted risk, and may indicate the action of a risk factor (e.g. environmental exposure, health behavior, covariate) not fully accounted for or included among the predictors.

2.1.3 Additional Complexity: Human Mobility, Latency, Periods of Vulnerability, Temporal Orientation

The spatial and space-time analysis of cancer is a difficult problem with layers of complexity that should be accounted for in any study design. Others have described the complexity of the problem and impacts on scientific inference [30, 67], here we focus on human mobility, latency, biological periods of vulnerability, and the temporal orientation used in analysis.

2.1.3.1 Human Mobility and Latency

The latency between cancer initiation and diagnosis can be long (~21 years for the pancreatic cancer example). Residential mobility varies from one country to another, within populations, by age, socio-economic status and population [6]. Recent research has focused on the use of surveys and commercial sources to reconstruct residential histories and to assess the impacts of errors in residential histories on exposure misclassification [13, 27, 81, 87] When cancer latency is long relative to duration of residential occupancy a space-time disconnect occurs between place of residence at diagnosis and when cancer initiation took place [27, 36, 63, 84]. If not accounted for, this can lead to false findings of "no effect" in studies that explore relationships between exposures at place of residence and cancer outcomes.

Recent years have seen an increasing ability to quantify environmental exposures as individuals move throughout their day, driven, in part, by an increased awareness of the cancer exposome [38, 46, 88]. The integration of detailed data on human mobility and place-related exposures is an enormous opportunity and poses a considerable challenge in the space-time analysis of cancers.

2.1.3.2 Biological Periods of Vulnerability

Life course epidemiology recognizes that individual risk of adverse health outcomes, such as breast cancer, can depend on the stage of development and biological status of the individual [7, 28, 42]. Because of the multifactorial nature of the causes of cancer, and because cancer risk factors can vary by age (smoking, for example, often begins in high school), cancer risks can be a complex function of the intersection of biological periods of vulnerability, age-based risk behaviors and space-time locations associated with specific place-based exposures.

2.1.3.3 Temporal Orientation

One approach to handling complexity is the use of alternative temporal orientations to assess the space-time nexus of causal exposures and age-based periods of vulnerability [54]. "Temporal orientation" refers to how time is assessed in a space-time analysis. Most often, the calendar year or duration since an arbitrary time point (e.g. years prior to diagnosis/recruitment, and calendar year) is used. Alternatively, an age-based temporal orientation (e.g. participant's age) may be used to gain insights into periods of biological vulnerability, latency periods, and the timing of causative exposures [52].

A visualization using a calendar year orientation might show the locations of cases and controls through time using year, month and day as the time measure. A visualization using age orientation would show the locations of cases and controls by age, usually from 1 year of age up to 80 years of age. A space-time cluster analysis using the calendar year orientation would yield locations and dates when cases clustered relative to controls; an analysis using age orientation would yield where cases clustered at similar ages.

As an example, consider a population-based study of bladder cancer in Michigan for 411 incident cases in 11 counties from 2000–2004. Details may be found in the original studies, consult [50, 51]. Using space-time Q statistic (described later in Methods), a comparison was conducted of the significance of space-time clustering of bladder cancer cases relative to controls using both calendar year (Fig. 2.5) and age orientations (Fig. 2.6). The analyses were adjusted for arsenic exposure, education, smoking, family history of bladder cancer, occupational exposure to bladder cancer carcinogens, age, gender, and race. Hence any significant clustering might reveal the signature of unidentified risk factors and risk factors not fully accounted for in the case-control study. Although set-based tests that adjusted for multiple testing were not significant, highly significant local clusters at age 33 years were found in and about Flint, Michigan and in Jackson, Michigan (Fig. 2.6). The Jackson City cluster occurred in working-ages and is consistent with occupational causes.

Subsequent focused space-time cluster analysis identified 20 industrial sites engaged in manufacturing activities associated with known or suspected bladder cancer carcinogens as statistically significant cluster foci (Fig. 2.7), potentially giving rise to new causal hypotheses regarding risk factors not taken into account in the original study design [34].

2.2   Methods

There are many methods for the space-time analysis and modeling of cancer and disease risks at the population level (e.g. treating cancer rates through time as the outcome variable), including Bayesian, regression and geostatistical approaches, among others. Here we will focus our attention primarily on a subset of techniques

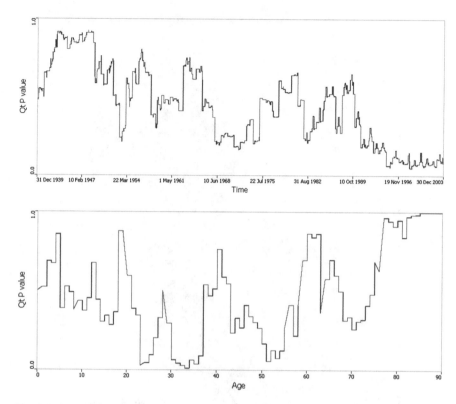

Fig. 2.5 Significance of global space-time clustering of cases using calendar year (top) and age (bottom) temporal orientations. **Top**: Time plot of p(Qt) using year-based measure of time. **Bottom**: Time plot of p(Qt) using age in years. Minima on the time plot indicate periods when global spatial clustering of cases were statistically significant. No periods were statistically significant using year as the temporal orientation (top). Statistically significant clustering of cases occurred at ages 33–35 years (bottom). Adapted from [34]

suited to analyzing case-control, and stage at diagnosis data. We begin with a consideration of how inference may be conducted in a space-time analysis framework.

2.2.1   Disease Inference from Space-Time Analysis

Assume we are interested in increasing our understanding of the causes of cancer and the assessment of the efficacy of cancer control activities. It then can be useful to think about a cancer risk budget, defined here as the allocation of unexplained cancer risk to specific people, places and times. Case-control studies, for example, are effective for determining whether risk factors included in the study design are statistically associated with cancer outcomes. Risk factors not included in the study design give rise to unexplained cancer risks.

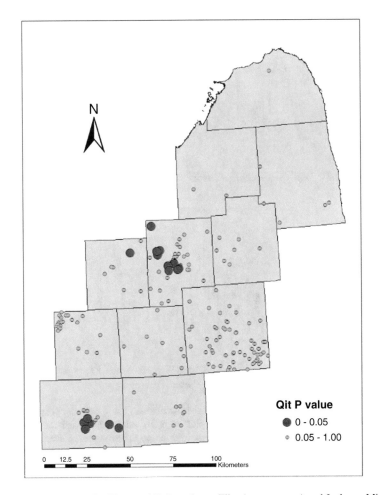

Fig. 2.6 Case clustering for 33 year old's in and near Flint (upper center) and Jackson, Michigan (lower left). Red circles indicate clusters significant at the 0.05 level. Adapted from [34]

When models of the form in Eq. (2.1) are used, unexplained risks will be included in the model residual (ε_{it}) along with other sources of error. Using this construct, Q statistics have been defined for case-control studies to allocate unexplained risk to specific people (e.g. cases), places and times (Table 2.1).

Q-statistics are based on a space-time step function that documents a person's residential mobility over the life course. This is quantified using a matrix representation that measures how geographic nearest neighbor relationships change through time. Q-statistics assess several types of space-time clustering (Table 2.1), for overall global clustering, for spatial and temporally local clustering, for clustering at specific time intervals, and for assessing focused clustering about point sources. These have several desirable properties. The global tests can be decomposed into the local tests such that the sum of the local tests yields the global test statistic. Furthermore, the different tests are sensitive to different aspects of space-time pat-

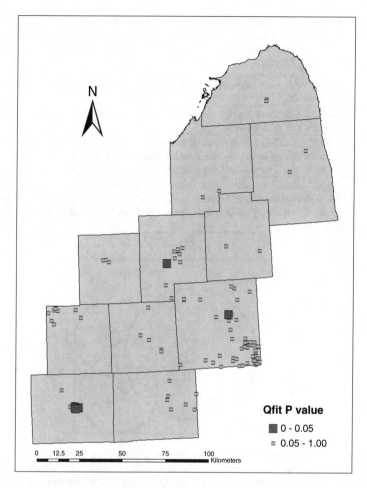

Fig. 2.7 Focused cluster analysis of manufacturing sites statistically significant "foci" of bladder cancer cases. A calendar orientation was used, results for June 1, 1974 are shown. Red squares indicate industrial sites that are the foci of significant case clustering at $p < = 0.05$. The group of statistically significant focused clusters in the southwest are in the city of Jackson, Michigan; in north central is outside Flint, Michigan, and to the east is the site in Oakland County near Detroit. Significant focused clustering was found when all of the industrial sites were considered simultaneously (significant global focused clustering). Adapted from [34]

terns, corresponding to "signatures" that map to alternative cancer etiologies (Fig. 2.8).

That different space-time processes can give rise to different space-time patterns seems self-evident. The term "signatures" captures the notion that inferential and pattern description statistics (such as correlograms, variograms, power spectrum, *etc*) can be used as a diagnostic to relate observed space-time patterns to the processes that gave rise to them [14, 79]. An inferential framework thus relates the "signature" of space-time statistics Q_{it}, Q_i and Q_t to types of disease processes (Table 2.2).

Table 2.1 Definition of Q-statistics for budgeting unexplained risks in case-control studies to specific people (cases), places and times. Interpretation of Q-statistics can help generate hypotheses regarding the locations and timing of causative exposures. Adapted from [33, 34]

Notation	Description
Q_T	"Q sub T" quantifies total clustering of the cases, relative to controls, over the entire study duration.
Q_{it}	"Q sub i t" quantifies whether there is an excess of cases, relative to controls, about the location of the ith case at time t.
Q_i	"Q sub i" quantifies whether there is an excess of cases, relative to controls, about the residential history of the ith case. This has been referred to as the life course statistic because it considers the locations and times where case i resided.
Q_t	"Q sub t" quantifies whether there is an excess of cases, relative to controls when all of the cases are considered together, at time t. This is similar to Cuzick and Edwards spatial only clustering statistic T_k [12] and quantifies spatial clustering of all of the cases at time t.

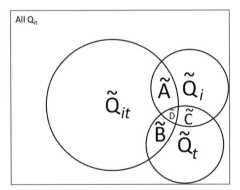

Fig. 2.8 Space-time patterns that can be identified using Q-statistics. Circles are sets of Q statistics that are statistically significant. $\tilde{Q}_{it}$ is that set of participants that had a statistically significant excess of other cases about them at time t. The set $\tilde{Q}_i$ is those participants that had a statistically significant of other cases about them over their residential histories (*e.g.* the life course statistic). $\tilde{Q}_t$ is those participants who were members of large-scale spatial clusters at time t. The intersection of these sets are $\tilde{A}, \tilde{B}, \tilde{C}, \tilde{D}$ and can yield insights leading to hypotheses regarding space-time patterns in the occurrence of cancer cases (refer to Table 2.2). When Q-statistics have been adjusted for the risk factors and covariates found significant in the case-control study, these sets identify where, when and to whom to allocate unexplained. From [78]

2.3   Examples

Q-statistics have been evaluated in simulation studies [78] and applied to testicular cancers [77], diabetes and leukemia [75], non-Hodgkins lymphoma [5], and breast cancer [32, 62], among others. We now consider two examples: a case control study of breast cancer in Denmark, and breast cancer stage at diagnosis in Michigan.

Table 2.2 Cancer etiologies that may explain observed space-time patterns in case occurrence. Modified from [78]

Set	Description	Pattern	Example etiology
$\tilde{Q}_{it}$	Local case-time clustering	Cases (i) that at times t have a significant number of nearest neighbors that are cases	Increased cancer risk for individuals residing in local areas over a defined time period. Duration of elevated risk must be sufficiently long relative to the duration of time individuals live in the affected areas (e.g. exposure time must be sufficient to induce disease response).
$\tilde{Q}_i$	Clustering over the life course	Cases (i) who, over the study period, have a significant number of nearest neighbors that are cases	Neighbors of case i have increased cancer risk and risk is elevated over the life course of case i. An example is behaviors that increase cancer risk for others nearby such as second-hand smoke. May also arise when groups with elevated risk tend to move or remain together over their life course (e.g. familial groups with common genetic and/ or behavioral risk factors).
$\tilde{Q}_t$	Temporal case clustering	Large-scale spatial clustering of cases at time t. Clustering of cases relative to controls is significant at time t when all cases and controls are considered.	Chronic disease with an underlying infectious etiology (e.g. viral hypothesis of cancer) that impacts a large portion of the study participants; Disease risk mediated by environmental exposures that vary across the study area such that risk is elevated for a large number of study participants. Duration of elevated risk must be sufficiently long relative to the duration of time individuals live in the affected areas (e.g. exposure time must be sufficient to induce disease response).
$\tilde{A}$	$\tilde{Q}_{it} \cap \tilde{Q}_i$	Locations and times when cases with significant clustering over their life course are members of a geographically localized cluster. Includes both ephemeral and persistent clusters.	Local areas of persistent elevated risk that are sustained for a sufficient period of time that (1) disease risk is increased for individuals residing in the local area and (2) the duration of residence of cases in the area is of sufficient length to result in a significant Q_i statistic.
$\tilde{B}$	$\tilde{Q}_{it} \cap \tilde{Q}_t$	Local clusters of cases that occur over a large portion of the study area at time t.	Large scale exposures that occur at a specific time(s) t. An example would be leukemia in response to the Chernobyl and Hiroshima incidents.
$\tilde{C}$	$\tilde{Q}_t \cap \tilde{Q}_i$	Cases that have clustering over their life course and are part of large-scale spatial clusters at times t. Includes cases whose Q_{it} are not statistically significant, and some whose Q_{it} are statistically significant.	Large scale exposures that occur at a specific time(s) t with some of the resulting cases that (i) move together through life course or (ii) continue to reside in the affected area over most of the study period.

(continued)

Table 2.2 (continued)

Set	Description	Pattern	Example etiology
$\tilde{D}$	$\tilde{Q}_{it} \cap \tilde{Q}_i \cap \tilde{Q}_t$	Cases that have clustering over their life course, are part of large scale clusters at time t and whose local clusters Q_{it} are all statistically significant.	Etiology is similar to set $\tilde{C}$, but is restricted to include only those individuals that are centers of significant local clustering of cases at times t. For infection, this may be indicative of index cases; for chronic diseases this may indicate individuals who are within local pockets of the largest exposure.

2.3.1 Breast Cancer in Denmark Using Residential Histories

Consider a study of incident breast cancer cases in Denmark that accounted for several known risk factors and residential mobility. Globally, there are over one million new cases of breast cancer annually, making it the most common female cancer [37]. In the last decade industrialized countries have experienced a rapid increase in breast cancer incidence, with higher incidence rates than most Asian and African countries. From 1960 to 2010 in Denmark the incidence rate (age-standardized) more than doubled, from 46.1 per 100.000 person-years to 102.5, respectively.

As noted elsewhere in this book, risk factors for breast cancer include ionizing radiation, alcohol intake, estrogens, reproductive status, hormone replacement therapy, and night-shift work, among others. Socioeconomic status and genetic mutations such as the BRC genotype are also established risk factors ([8, 28, 58]). However, twins and other studies found approximately 30% of breast cancer risk to be due to heritable and genetic factors, suggesting that environment over the life course (the breast cancer exposome) may play a significant role in breast cancer etiology [55, 57].

The example under consideration is a case-control study that used 33 years of residential histories to assess whether space-time excesses of unexplained breast cancer risk exist in Denmark, and, if they do, where they are and when they occurred [62]. As noted earlier, such a finding of significant unexplained risk might suggest the role of an as yet unidentified environmental risk factor (refer to Table 2.2).

The case-control study enrolled 3138 female breast cancer cases from the Danish Cancer Registry, which is a population-wide registry. To be eligible, cases had to be diagnosed in 2003. Two independent control groups (N = 3138 women each) representative of the demographic characteristics of the cases were constructed from the Denmark Civil Registration System. The Denmark Civil Registration System records lifetime residential histories, and residential addresses for the cases and controls from 1971 to 2003 were used and geo-coded. Logistic analyses were used to identify statistically significant risk factors that included reproductive factors (child birth, number of children, age at first birth), aggregate educational level in household area, and aggregated income in the household area. These risk factors were then accounted for in space-time analyses (termed "adjusted" in the results, below) that identified space-time clusters of breast cancer risk. Analyses were also accomplished without adjustment for the risk factors (termed "unadjusted"). These analyses were carried out for both control groups individually and with the control groups combined.

The unadjusted analyses found an area of excess breast cancer risk in the northern suburbs of Copenhagen that persisted from 1971 to 2003 and was consistent across both control groups (Fig. 2.9a). After adjustment the cluster area was significant only for the combined control groups, was smaller in size and of shorter duration, from 1971–1993 (Fig. 2.9b). Additional spatial-only analyses using SatScan [44] identified breast cancer clusters in 1987 and 1997 (Fig. 2.9c, d).

It is worth noting that although this population-based study was based on incident cases across all of Denmark, statistically significant excess breast cancer risk was found only in Copenhagen and Odense, and was confirmed by both Q- and SatScan analyses. The Q-analyses were based on 33 years of residential histories, and prior to adjustment areas of excess risk were found using two control groups. After adjustment for reproductive factors and aggregated income and educational level the excess risk areas became smaller, less persistent, and were observed for the combined control groups only. However, that the risk factors in this study are limited, and known factors that vary geographically and across local populations (e.g. alcohol consumption, HRT use, ionizing radiation, *etc*) were not accounted for. An external exposure such as environmental pollutants cannot be excluded as a contributing cause.

This example is notable because of its use of space-time analyses to localized excess breast cancer risk to specific groups, times and places. Strengths in the study design include a population-wide case enrollment and control selection; the use of two control groups that matched the demographic characteristics of the cases; and the employment of two analytical techniques (Q-statistics and SatScan) that independently confirmed the study findings. The study would have benefited from a more robust quantification of known risk factors, especially at the individual level (rather than aggregated from local census area data). Without this, one cannot exclude the action of known risk factors as plausible explanation of the findings of space-time excesses of breast cancer risk.

2.3.2 Breast Cancer Stage at Diagnosis in Michigan

The identification of local populations that would benefit from increased access to breast cancer screening is an important first step in the allocation of screening resources. This leads directly to breast cancer treatment delivery early in cancer progression, and to better treatment outcomes. Spatial analysis of breast cancer stage at diagnosis can identify clusters of breast cancer at different stages in relation to health care availability, demography and spatially varying risk factors. Data on stage at diagnosis may be available for place of residence (e.g. "individual-level"),

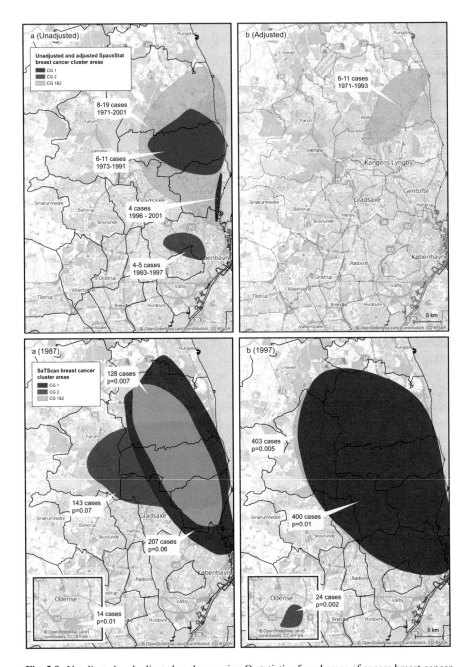

Fig. 2.9 Unadjusted and adjusted analyses using Q-statistics found areas of excess breast cancer risk in the Copenhangen-Odense area of Denmark (upper row, 9a left, 9b right). SatScan spatial only analyses (bottom row) found case clustering using residential addresses of the cases and controls in 1987 (lower left, 9c) and 1997 (lower right, 9d). "CG" indicates control groups used and corresponding color coding

and also for cases grouped, for example, by zip codes, census tracts and census blocks (e.g. "aggregated data"). Analyses using stage of diagnosis have identified stage-based clusters for breast, prostate, and colorectal cancers and have revealed relationships between residing near screening facilities and early stage diagnosis [1, 24, 70, 74, 82]. Important questions arise regarding the geographic scale of analysis, also called the Modifiable Areal Unit Problem (MAUP) by geographers. Are the results of analyses dependent on the geographic scale of the data? Can researchers use residential addresses for individual-level data with equal validity as data aggregated by zip codes or census tract and blocks?

A study designed to develop protocols for the spatial analysis of stage at diagnosis data addressed these questions and analyzed 67,136 incident cases in Michigan for the period 1994–2002 [53]. Of these, the SEER General Summary Stage classification defined 67% as early stage, 22% late stage, and 10% unknown. Several geographic resolutions were used for analyses, including individual place of residence, census block groups, census tracts and legislative districts. Results for two popular methods, Cuzick and Edwards test (appropriate for individual-level data) and the spatial scan statistic were compared and contrasted [12, 29, 43, 45].

The analyses using individual-level data comprised of place of residence at time of diagnosis revealed spatial clusters of early stage diagnoses not found using data aggregated by census block, census tracts, and legislative districts. When comparing analysis methods, Cuzick and Edwards' test found clusters not detected by the SaTScan spatial scan technique. Overall, spatial analyses of individual-level data were more reliable than those conducted using aggregated data. Further, Cuzick-Edwards' test was more sensitive than the widely used SaTScan spatial scan statistic, with acceptable Type I error.

This example is of interest because it seeks to evaluate a protocol for the analysis of stage at diagnosis data that can be employed routinely with cancer registry data. It assessed the importance of scale of analysis and demonstrated that individual place of residence data is superior to aggregated data, and that the preferred technique is Cuzick and Edwards nearest neighbor test. To generalize these results, it seems likely that higher resolution data will often be capable of detecting space-time patterns that would otherwise be missed using aggregated data.

2.4 Sources of Error

In addition to usually-noted sources of error that include under-reporting and misdiagnosis, space-time analyses have additional sources of error related to the recording of the location and timing of cancer and cancer-related events. These include location and temporal uncertainty; the use of location as an exposure surrogate; and systematic underestimation of exposures in location-based models such as Geographic Information Systems (GIS).

2.4.1 Location and Temporal Uncertainty

There is a rich and growing literature on location uncertainty and error, which can be thought of as the mis-measurement of the locations where health-related events were recorded. For example, geocoding – that process of transforming a text-base address such as "9880 Jerome Road, Jerome, MI" into a spatial coordinate such as longitude and latitude – is a known source of location error [31, 91]. Geocoding error has been demonstrated to impact model-based estimates of health-environment relationships [25] and varies systematically with frequently important covariates such as urbanicity and extent rural. Location error is always present regardless of the measurement technique, and is found in cell phone location traces, as well as satellite geopositioning systems. What matters is the resolution and accuracy of the measurement technique in the context of the space-time system being analyzed. Street address geocoding to plus or minus 50 meters is more than adequate for most space-time health analyses above the neighborhood level. While this certainly seems attainable [20], studies have reported geocoding location errors as high as 19 km in rural areas [2, 41, 64, 73]. Rooftop geocoding and E911 locations have been demonstrated to have higher accuracy than geocoded addresses, but these are not always available [71]. Careful inspection and editing ("manual intervention") of geocodes has been demonstrated to be cost effective and results in substantial improvements in accuracy over raw geocodes [47]. Regardless of the geocoding approach employed, a sound study design should include validated residential coordinates to assess the accuracy of alternative methods and to allow assessment of actual geocoding error.

2.4.2 Human Mobility and Location as an Exposure Surrogate

Although near real-time location data on individuals is increasingly available from remote sensing and cell-phone technologies, this information is seldom coupled with measurement of ambient environmental conditions and compounds relevant to cancer. In some instances, the location and timing of cancer-health related events is used to generate model-based exposure estimates (as described in the next section) or used directly as a surrogate of an unmeasured, or even unknown exposure. Many exposures linked to cancers occur outside of the home, but at this writing many spatial and spatio-temporal analyses of cancer rely on place-of-residence to georeference locations of health events. When might place of residence reasonably be used to georeference cancer outcomes and correlates? When human mobility is considered, the potential mismatch between locations where causative exposures may have occurred, an individual's biological windows of vulnerability to such exposures, and the long latencies of many cancers can be problematic.

For what cancers might causative exposures occur in the home? Lung cancers can be attributable to household radon exposures. In addition, combustion byproducts from cooking and household heating can include carcinogens such as polycyclic aromatic hydrocarbons. Exposures to second-hand tobacco smoke can be substantial in enclosed settings such as homes and vehicles. Place-of-residence as an exposure surrogate might be reasonable when the latency period is short and the subject tends to spend a good portion of the day at home; childhood cancers may fit these requirements. For cancers with long latencies, human mobility, especially when commuting and time outside of the residence must be taken into account, poses a substantial analytical challenge to space-time analysis. The assumption of immobile individuals that is implicit when place-of-residence at time of diagnosis is used in spatial analyses is often too simplistic to be acceptable. In particular, findings of geographic cancer clusters can be difficult to interpret when place of residence is used to represent locations of individuals.

Researchers have used space-time information systems to undertake the space-time modeling of individual-level exposures accounting for residential mobility. For example, Meliker et al. considered arsenic exposure as a risk factor in bladder cancers [49, 51]. They reconstructed individual arsenic exposures based on assumptions regarding occupational exposure and the ingestion of arsenic in foods and drinking water. Taking into account residential mobility over the life course appears to provide a more robust quantitative foundation for exposure reconstruction that is not possible when a single location (e.g. place of residence at diagnosis or death) is used to represent an individual's location.

2.4.3 Systematic Exposure Underestimation in GIS-Based Models?

Exposure misclassification leads to bias towards the null finding of "no effect" [72], potentially leading to false findings of no association between putative exposures and cancer. Models that use measured emissions from exposure sources (e.g. point and non-point sources of carcinogenic air pollutants) to estimate exposures at locations such as place of residence are widely used in studies of cancer. Examples of such models include geostatistical, Bayesian, and regression forms where the model inputs consist of contaminant concentrations at specific locations and times, and the outputs are estimated contaminant concentrations at "ungauged" locations that lacked measurement instruments. While estimation error is present such that the estimates at the ungauged locations do not exactly match the true, but not observed, values, it is often assumed that these errors are not biased. However, several studies suggest a systematic bias is present, such that the often underestimate the true values. This is an important issue because it suggests that exposure misclassification may often be present, and effect under-estimation may be large [65].

A study in California compared exposure model estimates for air-born human carcinogens to values measured at air quality monitoring stations [17]. The objective was to identify that model whose estimates corresponded best to actual air monitoring data. That model would then be used in follow-up epidemiologic studies of breast cancer [18]. The correspondence between 12 hazardous air pollutants measured by the California Air Resources Board's air quality monitoring program and modeled annual ambient concentrations from the US Environmental Protection Agency's National Air Toxics Assessment (NATA) database was assessed for 1996, 1999, 2002, and 2005. Although the correspondence in some years was better than others, the modeled estimates consistently underestimated the monitored data. And because the comparison was accomplished at fixed monitoring stations, the role of human mobility and the differences between indoor and outdoor exposures was not accounted for.

The Detroit Exposure and Aerosol Research Study compared NATA model estimates for benzene to those obtained at a community scale, integrating 24 h exposures in both indoor and outdoor settings [19]. They found the NATA estimates usually to be only one half of the actual measured breathing zone concentrations. The measurements for personal concentrations were higher likely due to indoor sources not accounted for in the NATA estimates. Overall, static ambient air toxics observation networks that provide measurements of hazardous air pollutants of relevance to cancer (e.g. benzene, toluene, ethylbenzene, and 1,3-butadiene, formaldehyde, halogenated and semivolatile organic compounds, metals, ethylene dichloride and methylene) have a limited ability to assess exposures over multiple spatial and temporal scales that are of direct relevance in epidemiological studies of cancer [80]. Finally, results from measurement studies using wearable environmental sensors have found that while an individual's personal exposure profile (e.g. exposure measurements over a day or week) tend to be similar, there is often order of magnitude difference in exposure profiles from one individual to another. These person to person differences in exposure profiles occur even when the individuals live in the same neighborhood or household.

The discussion in this section has two implications. First, model-based estimates of individual level exposures that seek to interpolate measurements from static monitoring networks (e.g. NATA and other GIS-based models) are of limited utility because they are incapable of capturing the person to person variability in exposures seen in wearable measurement studies. Second, cancer studies that have employed such models may be biased towards findings of no effect. This is a cautionary tale in space time exposure assessment for cancers – there is a substantial opportunity for improvements in exposure assessment over the life course.

2.5 Conclusions and Future Directions

Consider future research directions using the themes posed at the beginning of this chapter; the genome+, exposome and behavome. Each of these poses future research directions that could illuminate the causes of cancers at both the individual and population levels. Here we will focus on two unique opportunities: Improvements and advances in measurement and modelling; and data and knowledge integration across the genome+, exposome and behavome to advance our understanding of the causes of cancer.

2.5.1 Measurement and Modelling

As noted earlier in the section on sources of error, the timing of causative exposures over the life course can be crucial in carcinogenesis, and cancer latency and human mobility add complexities to the problem. Exposure underestimation may likely be a systematic bias, highlighting the need for both improved measurement and modeling of exposures and the settings in which they occur. Significant advances are being made in wearable environmental sensors, both in terms of near real time measurement of ambient environment for exposure assessment [56] and in the protection of patient privacy when using location-enabled devices [21]. Wearable sensors promise a paradigm shift in data collection and exposure reconstruction, from government sponsored sensor networks, which are coarse in coverage and fixed in locations, to wearable sensors which resolve the space-time paths of individuals as they go about their day. This will provide measurement of exposures in the settings where and when they occur – home, work, commuting, school yard – potentially solving the bias in exposure assessment discussed earlier [10]. New geostatistical and Bayesian space-time models for inferring individual exposures will be needed for systems where:

- some of the individuals are wearing sensors;
- some of these sensors are inoperative or turned off at different, often unpredictable intervals;
- some individuals are not wearing sensors;
- stationary monitoring networks are in operation;
- vehicles and other appliances may also provide sensing data; and
- where additional data may be coming in from remote sensing platforms such as satellites.

This still leaves the important problem of exposure reconstruction over the life course, which will necessitate data and knowledge integration over the exposome, genome+ and behavome.

2.5.2 Integration Across the Genome+, Exposome and Behavome

Given the long latency for many cancers, and the substantial uncertainties regarding the timing of causative exposures in relation to biological periods of vulnerability, exposure reconstruction over the life course is a crucial but difficult problem. There are several ways to approach the problem. A top-down approach might associate differences in cancer risk across local populations with differences in potential exposures, and from there seek to identify associated life course behaviors (behavomes). A bottom-up approach might would seek to link the cancer genome to changes in DNA, and the causes of the observed mutations. Here we sketch out a possible bottom-up approach to illustrate how it might work.

2.5.2.1 Bottom-up: From Cancer Genomes to Cancer Behavomes

While the genetic basis of carcinogenesis, and the roll of somatic mutations is firmly established, relatively little is known about the mutations and mutational processes that lead to cancers. To date over 20 mutational signatures associated with cancers have been identified. Recall that DNA is a double helix where the rungs are base-pairs comprised of pairs of the nucleobases guanine (G), cytosine (C), adenine (A) and thymine (T).

The Watson-Crick base pairs are AT, TA, GC and CG. The genome is comprised of sequences of these base pairs. Mutations occur when the sequence is disrupted, such that a location occupied by one nucleobase or base pair is replaced by another. A mutational signature then is the frequency histogram of the substitutions that comprise the mutations in a given cancer genome (for example, see Fig. 2.10a, upper left).

Certain signatures are associated with the age of the patient at time of diagnosis, suggesting mutagenic exposures over the life course played a causal role; others are of unknown origin. Some of these signatures are common across cancers, including the APOBEC cytidine deaminases family [3, 4]. Others are found only for certain cancers. Several mutagenic signatures for breast cancer have been identified [61].

While research on mutational signatures is in its infancy, it appears mutational signatures can efficiently identify the mutational processes underpinning cancer [92]. In addition, work has begun on a catalog that links mutagenic signatures to cancer genomes (Fig. 2.10b). On the horizon is a *platial catalog of mutagenic signatures*, that links the behaviors and settings associated with the exposures that produce the mutagenic signatures. It has been suggested that a platial approach is better suited to cancer control than the spatial approach often used in space-time cancer research [40], a need that would be met by the platial catalog of mutagenic signatures. A first step in the development of the platial catalog would be the development of mathematical models to formalize relationships between mutational features of a signature and the probability of mutational processes and exposures that cause them. Recent research has specified models that provide the quantitative link between exposures and mutational signatures (Fig. 2.10).

This expresses the mutational catalog of a cancer genome as a mapping from a given cancer genome to a finite alphabet of mutation types, while accounting for errors that arise in sequencing and measurement (Alexandrov, Nik-Zainal et al. 2013). The platial mutagenic catalog would take this a step further by linking spe-

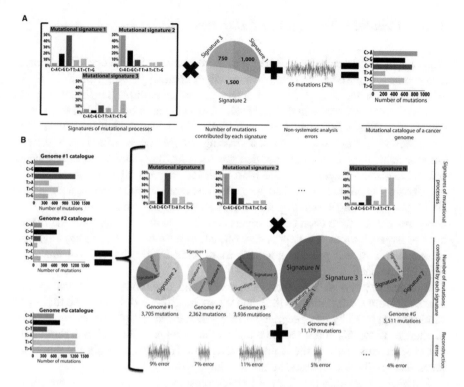

Fig. 2.10 Schematic of a possible mathematical modeling approach for mutagenic signatures and the mutational processes that give rise to them. Such models promise to provide a quantitative framework for linking exposures over the life course to the mutational signatures associated with specific cancers. (A) Three mutational signatures (upper left) are multiplied by the number of mutations contributed by each signature and their analytical errors, giving rise to the frequency distribution of mutations (upper right). This is the *mutational catalog* of a cancer. (B) The mutational catalogs of a set of G cancer genomes (lower left) is modeled as the result of the signatures of mutational processes, the number of mutations contributed by each mutational process, plus analytical errors. Adapted from (Alexandrov, Nik-Zainal et al. 2013)

cific behaviors (e.g. smoking, commuting etc.) and environments with mutagenic signatures of cancer genomes. This woulc allow us to address questions such as: Where do the different mutagenic signatures for cancers occur? Do they vary across populations? Across age groups? Are there disparities in platial mutagenic signatures? Can we identify health related behaviors that give rise to specific mutagenic signatures? The promise in extending space-time analysis of cancer and the cancer genome to platial mutagenic signatures is the ability to causally link cancer outcomes to their genetic bases and the environments and behaviors that give rise to carcinogenesis itself. This is a new frontier with the ultimate promise of identifying the exposures and behaviors that ultimately lead to cancer.

2.5.3   Critical Challenges and Barriers

This Chapter has described a vision of how more complete knowledge of the -omes, the genome+, exposome and behavome — will dramatically strengthen causal analysis and guide technology-focused interventions at multiple levels leading to improved individual and population health. This goal could fail should clearer evidence about causes not arise from such higher dimensional analyses, suggesting that a reductionist approach focused on teasing out specific contributions of different aspects of the -omes might provide greater scientific yield. Yet past advances across the scientific spectrum have been achieved by pursuing both of these avenues, beginning with reductionist approaches and then incorporating higher dimensional analyses using systems approaches as knowledge of the system components burgeons. Should the vision of the -omes described in this chapter have the broad brushes largely correct, it may provide a suitable descriptor of what the large system components are, and provide guidance as to what higher dimensional analyses should be pursued.

Substantial physical, environmental, social, and economic dislocations appear imminent from climate change [85], and it may be difficult or impossible for interventions suggested by this integrated -omes vision to "keep up' with the rapid pace of change. If so, this could reduce the potential benefits of the vision described in this chapter, especially in the realm of prevention. However, it might not diminish potential contributions in causal understanding.

Might it be possible that the genome+, exposome and behavome do not sufficiently capture salient drivers of human health? Is the role of mental health and affect sufficiently captured by the behavome rubric, or should it be featured more prominently, perhaps as the "emotiome" or "affectome" (see for example [76])? This might be described as the sum total of emotions experienced over time that impact human health outcomes. A revision and perhaps expansion of the high-level model posed in Fig. 2.3 might then be indicated, but this would not necessarily diminish the contributions of a higher-level vision in terms of advancing cancer prevention and causal understanding.

As noted earlier, substantial challenges persist in both exposome and behavome measurement. For example, activity spaces in exposure assessment have not realized the promise that seemed so apparent when they were originally proposed. Is this a failure of the activity space approach or is it part of a natural cycle of technology adoption such as the Gartner "hype cycle? The hype cycle illustrates level of interest and stage of development in the technology life cycle. In the *Innovation Trigger* a potential technology breakthrough with proof-of-concept narratives stimulates interest. This leads to the *Peak of Inflated Expectations* in which early versions of the technology may exist, along with some success. During the following *Trough of Disillusionment*: interest wanes as expectations are not met and early implementations fail. Should the technology survive this trough, it enters the *Slope of Enlightenment*. Here, instances where the technologies benefits become more widely understood. Second- and third-generation versions of the technology appear and adoption increases. During the *Plateau of Productivity* mainstream adoption occurs and the full benefits of the technology are realized. From this perspective, activity spaces in exposure assessment are likely in trough of disillusionment, where it will remain unless and until benefits of the approach in exposure assessment are realized.

What is the hype cycle for the genome+, exposome and behavome? Overall, the genome+ is most highly developed and is on the Plateau of Productivity, contributing substantially to our understanding of the genetic and biological bases of breast cancer. The exposome is near the Peak of Inflated Expectations, perhaps turning down into the Trough of Disillusionment. The limitations of exposome measurement, and retrospective exposome reconstruction for chronic disease, are increasingly recognized and solutions are not always clear. So, while global positioning systems and location-enabled smart phone technologies are highly functional, the environmental data layers that could contribute to exposure estimation are not very granular. And at present, there are few personal exposure monitors that are inexpensive, accurate, and that have been implemented on a population level. It seems likely, however, with rapid advances in wearable technologies, Big Data, and the Internet of Things (IOT) that a rapid path through the trough will lead to the slope of enlightenment by 2021. The role of human behaviors in mediating exposures and as an expression and mediator of the genome+ is nascent, placing the behavome at the innovation trigger stage. And the vision of a place-based genome+, exposome, behavome synthesis is at the pre-innovation trigger stage. It may take the development of systems models and approaches to accomplishing this synthesis to provide that trigger.

References

1. Abe T, Martin IB, Roche LM. Clusters of census tracts with high proportions of men with distant-stage prostate cancer incidence in New Jersey, 1995–1999. Am J Prev Med. 2006;30(2 Suppl):S60–6.
2. Abe T, Stinchcomb D. Geocoding practices in cancer registries. In: Rushton G, Armstrong MP, Gittler J, et al., editors. Geocoding health data. Boca Raton: CRC Press; 2008. p. 111–25.
3. Alexandrov LB, Nik-Zainal S, Wedge DC, Aparicio SAJR, Behjati S, Biankin AV, Bignell GR, Bolli N, Borg A, Børresen-Dale A-L, Boyault S, Burkhardt B, Butler AP, Caldas C, Davies HR, Desmedt C, Eils R, Eyfjörd JE, Foekens JA, Greaves M, Hosoda F, Hutter B, Ilicic T, Imbeaud S, Imielinski M, Jäger N, Jones DTW, Jones D, Knappskog S, Kool M, Lakhani SR, López-Otín C, Martin S, Munshi NC, Nakamura H, Northcott PA, Pajic M, Papaemmanuil E, Paradiso A, Pearson JV, Puente XS, Raine K, Ramakrishna M, Richardson AL, Richter J, Rosenstiel P, Schlesner M, Schumacher TN, Span PN, Teague JW, Totoki Y, Tutt ANJ, Valdés-Mas R, van Buuren MM, van't Veer L, Vincent-Salomon A, Waddell N, Yates LR, Genome IAPC, Consortium IBC, Consortium IM-S, PedBrain I, Zucman-Rossi J, Futreal PA, McDermott U, Lichter P, Meyerson M, Grimmond SM, Siebert R, Campo E, Shibata T, Pfister SM, Campbell PJ, Stratton MR. Signatures of mutational processes in human cancer. Nature. 2013a;500:415.
4. Alexandrov LB, Nik-Zainal S, Wedge DC, Campbell PJ, Stratton MR. Deciphering signatures of mutational processes operative in human cancer. Cell Rep. 2013b;3(1):246–59.

5. Baastrup Nordsborg R, Meliker JR, Kjaer Ersboll A, Jacquez GM, Raaschou-Nielsen O. Space-time clustering of non-hodgkin lymphoma using residential histories in a Danish case-control study. PLoS One. 2013;8(4):e60800.

6. Bell ML, Banerjee G, Pereira G. Residential mobility of pregnant women and implications for assessment of spatially-varying environmental exposures. J Expo Sci Environ Epidemiol. 2018;28(5):470–80.

7. Ben-Shlomo Y, Kuh D. A life course approach to chronic disease epidemiology: conceptual models, empirical challenges and interdisciplinary perspectives. Int J Epidemiol. 2002;31(2):285–93.

8. Blackadar CB. Historical review of the causes of cancer. World J Clin Oncol. 2016;7(1):54–86.

9. Campbell PJ, Yachida S, Mudie LJ, Stephens PJ, Pleasance ED, Stebbings LA, Morsberger LA, Latimer C, McLaren S, Lin M-L, McBride DJ, Varela I, Nik-Zainal SA, Leroy C, Jia M, Menzies A, Butler AP, Teague JW, Griffin CA, Burton J, Swerdlow H, Quail MA, Stratton MR, Iacobuzio-Donahue C, Futreal PA. The patterns and dynamics of genomic instability in metastatic pancreatic cancer. Nature. 2010;467(7319):1109–13.

10. Chaix B. Mobile sensing in environmental health and neighborhood research. Annu Rev Public Health. 2018;39(1):367–84.

11. Cogliano VJ, Baan R, Straif K, Grosse Y, Lauby-Secretan B, El Ghissassi F, Bouvard V, Benbrahim-Tallaa L, Guha N, Freeman C, Galichet L, Wild CP. Preventable exposures associated with human cancers. J Natl Cancer Inst. 2011;103(24):1827–39.

12. Cuzick J, Edwards R. Spatial clustering for inhomogeneous populations. J R Stat Soc Ser B. 1990;52(1):73–104.

13. Danysh HE, Mitchell LE, Zhang K, Scheurer ME, Lupo PJ. Differences in environmental exposure assignment due to residential mobility among children with a central nervous system tumor: Texas, 1995–2009. J Expo Sci Environ Epidemiol. 2015;27:41.

14. Diniz-Filho JAF, Bini LM. Thirty-five years of spatial autocorrelation analysis in population genetics: an essay in honour of Robert Sokal (1926–2012). Biol J Linn Soc. 2012;107(4):721–36.

15. Foulds LJCR. The experimental study of tumor progression: a review. Cancer Res. 1954;14(5):327–39.

16. Friedewald WF, Rous PJJOEM. The initiating and promoting elements in tumor production: an analysis of the effects of tar, benzpyrene, and methylcholanthrene on rabbit skin. 1944;80(2):101–26.

17. Garcia E, Hurley S, Nelson DO, Gunier RB, Hertz A, Reynolds P. Evaluation of the agreement between modeled and monitored ambient hazardous air pollutants in California. Int J Environ Health Res. 2014;24(4):363–77.

18. Garcia E, Hurley S, Nelson DO, Hertz A, Reynolds PJEH. Hazardous air pollutants and breast cancer risk in California teachers: a cohort study. Environ Health. 2015;14(1):14.

19. George BJ, Schultz BD, Palma T, Vette AF, Whitaker DA, Williams RW. An evaluation of EPA's National-Scale Air Toxics Assessment (NATA): comparison with benzene measurements in Detroit, Michigan. Atmos Environ. 2011;45(19):3301–8.

20. Goldberg D. A geocoding best practices guide. Springfield: North American Association of Central Cancer Registries; 2008.

21. Goldenholz DM, Goldenholz SR, Krishnamurthy KB, Halamka J, Karp B, Tyburski M, Wendler D, Moss R, Preston KL, Theodore W. Using mobile location data in biomedical research while preserving privacy. J Am Med Inform Assoc. 2018;25(10):1402–6.

22. Goovaerts P, Jacquez GM. Accounting for regional background and population size in the detection of spatial clusters and outliers using geostatistical filtering and spatial neutral models: the case of lung cancer in Long Island, New York. Int J Health Geogr. 2004;3(1):14.

23. Goovaerts P, Jacquez GM. Detection of temporal changes in the spatial distribution of cancer rates using local Moran's I and geostatistically simulated spatial neutral models. J Geogr Syst. 2005;7(1):137–59.

24. Gregorio DI, Kulldorff M, Barry L, Samocuik H, Zarfos K. Geographical differences in primary therapy for early-stage breast cancer. Ann Surg Oncol. 2001;8(10):844–9.

25. Griffith DA, Millones M, Vincent M, Johnson DL, Hunt A. Impacts of positional error on spatial regression analysis: a case study of address locations in syracuse, New York. Trans GIS. 2007;11(5):655–79.
26. Herceg ZJM. Characterizing the epigenome and exposome in evaluating environmental exposures and cancer risk. Mutagenesis. 2014;29(6):500.
27. Hurley S, Andrew H, Nelson David O, Layefsky M, Von Behren J, Bernstein L, Deapen D, Reynolds P. Practice of epidemiology tracing a path to the past: exploring the use of commercial credit reporting data to construct residential histories for epidemiologic studies of environmental exposures. Am J Epidemiol. 2017;185(3)
28. Hertz-Picciotto I, Adams-Campbell L, Devine P, Eaton D, Hammond S, Helzlsouer K, Hiatt R, Hughes-Halbert C, Hunter D, Kramer B, Langholz B, Reynolds P, Tsuji J, Walker C, Zeise L. Breast cancer and the environment: a life course approach. Washington, DC: Institute of Medicine; 2011.
29. Jacquez GM. Cuzick and Edwards' test when exact locations are unknown. Am J Epidemiol. 1994;140(1):58–64.
30. Jacquez GM. Current practices in the spatial analysis of cancer: flies in the ointment. Int J Health Geogr. 2004;3(1):22.
31. Jacquez GM. A research agenda: does geocoding positional error matter in health GIS studies? Spat Spatio Temporal Epidemiol. 2012;3(1):7–16.
32. Jacquez GM, Barlow J, Rommel R, Kaufmann A, Rienti M Jr, AvRuskin G, Rasul J. Residential mobility and breast cancer in Marin County, California, USA. Int J Environ Res Public Health. 2014;11(1):271–95.
33. Jacquez GM, Kaufmann A, Meliker J, Goovaerts P, AvRuskin G, Nriagu J. Global, local and focused geographic clustering for case-control data with residential histories. Environ Health. 2005;4(1):4.
34. Jacquez GM, Sabel CE, Shi C. Genetic GIScience: toward a place-based synthesis of the genome, exposome, and behavome. Ann Assoc Am Geogr. 2015a;105(3):454–72.
35. Jacquez GM, Shi C, Meliker JR. Local bladder cancer clusters in Southeastern michigan accounting for risk factors, covariates and residential mobility. PLoS One. 2015b;10(4):e0124516.
36. Jelleyman T, Spencer N. Residential mobility in childhood and health outcomes: a systematic review. J Epidemiol Community Health. 2008;62(7):584–92.
37. Jemal A, Bray F, Center MM, Ferlay J, Ward E, Forman D. Global cancer statistics. CA Cancer J Clin. 2011;61(2):69–90.
38. Juarez PD, Matthews-Juarez P. Applying an Exposome-wide (ExWAS) approach to cancer research. Front Oncol. 2018;8:313.
39. Kanwal R, Gupta K, Gupta S. Cancer epigenetics: an introduction. Methods Mol Biol. 2015;1238:3–25.
40. Korycinski RW, Tennant BL, Cawley MA, Bloodgood B, Oh AY, Berrigan DJCC. Geospatial approaches to cancer control and population sciences at the United States cancer centers. Cancer Causes Control. 2018;29(3):371–7.
41. Krieger N, Waterman P, Lemieux K, Zierler S, Hogan J. On the wrong side of the tracts? Evaluating the accuracy of geocoding in public health research. Am J Public Health. 2001;91:1114–6.
42. Kuh D, Ben-Shlomo Y. A life course approach to chronic disease epidemiology: tracing the origins of ill-health from early to later life. Oxford: Oxford University Press; 1997.
43. Kulldorff M. A spatial scan statistic. Commun Stat. 1997;26:1481–96.
44. Kulldorff M, SaTScan v4.0: software for the spatial and space-time scan statistics., Information Management Services, 2004.
45. Kulldorff M, Nagarwalla N. Spatial disease clusters: detection and inference. Stat Med. 1995;14(8):799–810.
46. Loh M, Sarigiannis D, Gotti A, Karakitsios S, Pronk A, Kuijpers E, Annesi-Maesano I, Baiz N, Madureira J, Oliveira Fernandes E, Jerrett M, Cherrie J. How sensors might help define the external exposome. Int J Environ Res Public Health. 2017;14(4):434.

47. McDonald YJ, Schwind M, Goldberg DW, Lampley A, Wheeler CM. An analysis of the process and results of manual geocode correction. Geospat Health. 2017;12(1):526.
48. Meade MS. Medical geography as human ecology: the dimension of population movement. Geogr Rev. 1977;67:379–93.
49. Meliker J, Goovaerts P, Jacquez G, Nriagu J. Incorporating individual-level distributions of exposure error in epidemiologic analyses: an example using arsenic in drinking water and bladder cancer. Ann Epidemiol. 2011;. (in Press)
50. Meliker J, Slotnick M, AvRuskin G, Schottenfeld D, Jacquez G, Wilson M, Goovaerts P, Franzblau A, Nriagu J. Lifetime exposure to arsenic in drinking water and bladder cancer: a population-based case-control study in michigan. Cancer Causes Control. 2010a;21:745–57.
51. Meliker JR, Goovaerts P, Jacquez GM, Nriagu JO. Incorporating individual-level distributions of exposure error in epidemiologic analyses: an example using arsenic in drinking water and bladder cancer. Ann Epidemiol. 2010b;20(10):750–8.
52. Meliker JR, Jacquez GM. Space-time clustering of case-control data with residential histories: insights into empirical induction periods, age-specific susceptibility, and calendar year-specific effects. Stoch Environ Res Risk Assess. 2007;21(5):625–34.
53. Meliker JR, Jacquez GM, Goovaerts P, Copeland G, Yassine M. Spatial cluster analysis of early stage breast cancer: a method for public health practice using cancer registry data. Cancer Causes Control. 2009;20(7):1061–9.
54. Meliker JR, Sloan CD. Spatio-temporal epidemiology: principles and opportunities. Spat Spatio Temporal Epidemiol. 2011;2(1):1–9.
55. Möller S, Mucci LA, Harris JR, Scheike T, Holst K, Halekoh U, Adami H-O, Czene K, Christensen K, Holm NVJCE, Biomarkers P. The heritability of breast cancer among women in the Nordic twin study of cancer. Cancer Epidemiol Biomark Prev. 2016;25(1):145–50.
56. Morawska L, Thai PK, Liu X, Asumadu-Sakyi A, Ayoko G, Bartonova A, Bedini A, Chai F, Christensen B, Dunbabin M, Gao J, Hagler GSW, Jayaratne R, Kumar P, Lau AKH, Louie PKK, Mazaheri M, Ning Z, Motta N, Mullins B, Rahman MM, Ristovski Z, Shafiei M, Tjondronegoro D, Westerdahl D, Williams R. Applications of low-cost sensing technologies for air quality monitoring and exposure assessment: how far have they gone? Environ Int. 2018;116:286–99.
57. Mucci LA, Hjelmborg JB, Harris JR, Czene K, Havelick DJ, Scheike T, Graff RE, Holst K, Möller S, Unger RHJJ. Familial risk and heritability of cancer among twins in Nordic countries. JAMA. 2016;315(1):68–76.
58. Neilson HK, Farris MS, Stone CR, Vaska MM, Brenner DR, Friedenreich CM. Moderate-vigorous recreational physical activity and breast cancer risk, stratified by menopause status: a systematic review and meta-analysis. Menopause. 2017;24(3):322–44.
59. Neveu V, A Moussy, H Rouaix, R Wedekind, A Pon, C Knox, DS Wishart and AJNAR Scalbert. Exposome-explorer: a manually-curated database on biomarkers of exposure to dietary and environmental factors. gkw980, (2016).
60. Nielsen CC, Amrhein CG, Osornio-Vargas AR. Mapping outdoor habitat and abnormally small newborns to develop an ambient health hazard index. Int J Health Geogr. 2017;16(1):43.
61. Nik-Zainal S, Morganella S. Mutational signatures in breast cancer: the problem at the DNA level. Clin Cancer Res. 2017;23(11):2617–29.
62. Nordsborg RB, Meliker JR, Ersbøll AK, Jacquez GM, Poulsen AH, Raaschou-Nielsen O. Space-time clusters of breast cancer using residential histories: a Danish case–control study. BMC Cancer. 2014;14(1):255.
63. Nuckols J, Airola M, Colt J, Johnson A, Schwenn M, Waddell R, Karagas M, Silverman D, Ward MH. The impact of residential mobility on exposure assessment in cancer epidemiology. Epidemiology. 2009;20(6):S259–60.. 210.1097/1001.ede.0000362867.0000379502.0000362820
64. Oliver WN, Matthews K, Siadaty M, Hauck F, Pickle L. Geographic bias relating to geocoding error in epidemiologic studies. Int J Health Geogr. 2005;4(29):29.
65. Payne-Sturges DC, Burke TA, Breysse P, Diener-West M, Buckley TJ. Personal exposure meets risk assessment: a comparison of measured and modeled exposures and risks in an urban community. Environ Health Perspect. 2004;112(5):589–98.

66. Peltomäki P. Role of DNA mismatch repair defects in the pathogenesis of human cancer. J Clin Oncol Off J Am Soc Clin Oncol. 2003;21(6):1174–9.
67. Pickle LW, Waller LA, Lawson AB. Current practices in cancer spatial data analysis: a call for guidance. Int J Health Geogr. 2005;4(1):3.
68. Poulsen HE, Prieme H, Loft S. Role of oxidative DNA damage in cancer initiation and promotion. Eur. J. Cancer Prev. 1998;7(1):9–16.
69. Prüss-Üstün A, Neira M. Preventing disease through healthy environments: a global assessment of the burden of disease from environmental risks. Geneva: World Health Organization; 2016.
70. Roche LM, Skinner R, Weinstein RB. Use of a geographic information system to identify and characterize areas with high proportions of distant stage breast cancer. J Public Health Manag Pract. 2002;8(2):26–32.
71. Roongpiboonsopit D, Karimi HA. Quality assessment of online street and rooftop geocoding services. Cartogr Geogr Inf Sci. 2010;37:301–18.
72. Rothmann K, Greenland S. Modern epidemiology. Philadelphia: Lippincott-Raven; 1998.
73. Rushton G, Armstrong M, Gittler J, Greene B, Pavlik C, West M, Zimmerman D. Geocoding in cancer research – A review. Am J Prev Med. 2006;30(2):S16–24.
74. Rushton G, Peleg I, Banerjee A, Smith G, West M. Analyzing geographic patterns of disease incidence: rates of late-stage colorectal cancer in iowa. J Med Syst. 2004;28:223–36.
75. Schmiedel S, Jacquez GM, Blettner M, Schuz J. Spatial clustering of leukemia and type 1 diabetes in children in Denmark. Cancer Causes Control. 2011;22(6):849–57.
76. Siddharthan, A., N. Cherbuin, P. J. Eslinger, K. Kozlowska, N. A. Murphy and Leroy Lowe (2018). WordNet-feelings: a linguistic categorisation of human feelings.
77. Sloan CD, Baastrup-Norstrom R, Jacquez GM, Landrigan PJ, Raaschou-Nielsen O, Meliker JR. Space-time analysis of testicular cancer clusters using residential histories: a case-control study in Denmark. PLoS ONE. 2013;. In Press
78. Sloan CD, Jacquez GM, Gallagher CM, Ward MH, Raaschou-Nielsen O, Nordsborg RB, Meliker JR. Performance of cancer cluster Q-statistics for case-control residential histories. Spat Spatio Temporal Epidemiol. 2012;3(4):297–310.
79. Sokal RR, Wartenberg DE. A test of spatial autocorrelation analysis using an isolation-by-distance model. Genetics. 1983;105(1):219–37.
80. Strum M, Scheffe R. National review of ambient air toxics observations. J Air Waste Manage Assoc. 2016;66(2):120–33.
81. Symanski E, Tee Lewis PG, Chen T-Y, Chan W, Lai D, Ma X. Air toxics and early childhood acute lymphocytic leukemia in Texas, a population based case control study. Environ Health. 2016;15(1):70.
82. Thomas A, Carlin BP. Late detection of breast and colorectal cancer in Minnesota counties: an application of spatial smoothing and clustering. Stat Med. 2003;22(1):113–27.
83. Tomczak K, Czerwińska P, Wiznerowicz M. The Cancer Genome Atlas (TCGA): an immeasurable source of knowledge. Contemp Oncol. 2015;19(1A):A68.
84. Tunstall H, Pickett KE, Dorling D. Residential histories and contemporary mortality geography: using data linkage to develop a data set describing mobility between birth and death. J Epidemiol Community Health. 2010;64:A56–7.
85. USGCRP, R. In: Avery CW, Easterling DR, Kunkel KE, Lewis KLM, Maycock TK, Stewart BC, editors. Impacts, risks, and adaptation in the United States: fourth national climate assessment, Volume II. Washington, DC: U.S. Global Change Research Program; 2018.
86. Waller LA, Jacquez GM. Disease models implicit in statistical tests of disease clustering. Epidemiology. 1995;6(6):584–90.
87. Wheeler DC, Wang A. Assessment of residential history generation using a public-record database. Int J Environ Res Public Health. 2015;12(9):11670–82.
88. Wild C. Complementing the genome with an "exposome": the outstanding challenge of environmental exposure measurement in molecular epidemiology. Cancer Epidemiol Biomark Prev. 2005;14(8):1847–50.

89. Wild CP. The exposome: from concept to utility. Int J Epidemiol. 2012;41(1):24–32.
90. Yachida S, Jones S, Bozic I, Antal T, Leary R, Fu B, Kamiyama M, Hruban RH, Eshleman JR, Nowak MA, Velculescu VE, Kinzler KW, Vogelstein B, Iacobuzio-Donahue CA. Distant metastasis occurs late during the genetic evolution of pancreatic cancer. Nature. 2010;467(7319):1114–7.
91. Zandbergen PA, Hart TC, Lenzer KE, Camponovo ME. Error propagation models to examine the effects of geocoding quality on spatial analysis of individual-level datasets. Spat Spat Temporal Epidemiol. 2011;. (In Review)
92. Zhou N, Yuan Y, Long X, Wu C, Bao J. Mutational signatures efficiently identify different mutational processes underlying cancers with similar somatic mutation spectra. Mutat Res Fundam Mol Mech Mutagen. 2017;806:27–30.

Chapter 3
Creating Maps and Mapping Systems for Cancer Control and Prevention

Zaria Tatalovich and David G. Stinchcomb

Abstract Mapping public health data provides valuable insights into geography of diseases. Maps and mapping systems can also be a useful practical tool for public health planning; the identification of areas of elevated cancer incidence or mortality can inform optimal spatial allocation of resources as well as targeted interventions aimed at cancer prevention and control. This chapter addresses the role of mapping in cancer research and the utility of mapping systems for cancer control activities through a series of examples and best practices. The chapter is organized into three sections. The introductory section briefly traces the evolution from paper maps to modern digital maps and cancer atlases, highlighting their value for understanding the geography of cancer. The second section discusses the relevance of mapping in cancer research and provides examples from recent literature where maps have been used to aid cancer research and inform interventions. The third section focuses on modern cancer mapping systems, their development, design considerations, functionality, and application through a series of examples demonstrating their value for informing cancer control activities.

Keywords Cancer · Mapping · Cancer disparities · Cancer atlas

3.1 The Evolution of Health Maps and Cancer Atlases

Mapping health data has a long and well documented history with numerous examples of excellent mapping work [42, 55, 83]. The evolution of mapping health data can be traced back to early examples of maps of English cholera epidemic during

Z. Tatalovich (✉)
Surveillance Research Program, Division of Cancer Control and Population Sciences, National Cancer Institute, Bethesda, MD, USA
e-mail: tatalovichzp@mail.nih.gov

D. G. Stinchcomb
Westat, Inc., Rockville, MD, USA

© Springer Nature Switzerland AG 2019
D. Berrigan, N. A. Berger (eds.), *Geospatial Approaches to Energy Balance and Breast Cancer*, Energy Balance and Cancer 15, https://doi.org/10.1007/978-3-030-18408-7_3

the period from the 1830s through 1860s, of which John Snow's cholera maps of London [76] are the most famous for providing insight into the causes of disease. Since the early nineteenth century when maps were hand drawn, to the modern times of digital mapping, medical maps have provided insight into geography of cancer and many other diseases[1]. In the mid-twentieth century, the evolving field of Geographic Information Science (GIS) introduced a strong foundation for the development of systems with the power of holding large amounts of geographic information [17] and increased ability for mapping of cancer and other diseases [32].

Cancer Atlases (a collection of cancer maps) have been an important aid for cancer control in the U.S. and worldwide. Many cancer atlases have been published in the past several decades, with the goal to inform public health professionals about the status of cancer and to inspire questions about cancer etiology. In the U.S., Pickle [63] published a noteworthy critical overview of mortality atlases and their significance for informing action to reduce cancer burden. Another notable overview of cancer atlases developed in various countries of the world has been published by D'Onofrio et al. [26]. These reviews provided ample evidence and arguments that cancer atlases may reveal previously undiscovered geographic patterns in cancer data, stimulate hypothesis about cancer etiology, and inform interventions and planning for optimal resource allocation in areas with elevated cancer rates.

Early U.S. cancer atlases include: [50, 51], Pickle et al. [65–67]. Riggan et al. [70], Devesa [28]. These atlases incorporated static printed map images offering ample visual detail for pattern recognition, but without any ability to interact with the content. The 1999 National Cancer Institute (NCI) atlas was accompanied by a website that allowed user interaction to produce historical customized maps of cancer mortality over a 45 year period [63]. With the advancement of computer systems and digital mapping, opportunities for interactive mapping increased, and the new online atlases and mapping systems started to emerge. The following are examples of web-based digital atlases offering user interaction in terms of map display, data download, and visualization via charts, graphs, and Tables.

- NCI Cancer Atlas [58]: Contains most recent 5 years of cancer incidence data linked with maps, graphs, and tables. The atlas also contains historical mortality data since 1973 by state, registry, county, and state economic area, from the original 1999 atlas [28]
- State Cancer Profiles [79]: Incorporates most recent 5 years of incidence and mortality data by state and county with linked maps, graphs and tables by U.S. state and county
- United States Cancer Statistics Data Visualization Tool [84]: Provides incidence and mortality data with maps, graphs and tables by U.S. state
- Cancer in North America (CiNA) [18]: Uses most recent 5 years of incidence data for US and Canada by state/province

---

[1] Mapping systems are tools that combine geospatial data access and query capabilities with geovisualization

The functionality of these types of digital atlases along with other mapping systems will be covered in greater detail later. The next section focuses on the use of maps in cancer research offering a series of examples where mapping has aided research and provided valuable insights into the geography of cancer related information.

3.2 Mapping for Cancer Control: Significance and Research Examples

Maps and mapping systems can be a useful practical tool for public health planning; the identification of areas of elevated cancer incidence or mortality can inform optimal spatial allocation of resources as well as localized targeted interventions aimed at cancer prevention and control. Cancer researchers and public health professionals often rely on the information gathered from maps to develop and test hypotheses about the observed spatial relationships and patterns in cancer-related data. Mapping in cancer research typically involves combining cancer data with other area-based information relevant to cancer risk such as: socio-demographic and economic factors, environmental risk factors, location of health services, residences of people, barriers to health access, distances to general practice, hospital or clinic, to name a few. The following are useful resources for understanding best practices for mapping cancer related data:

- Brewer [14] Designing better maps: a guide for GIS users
- Brewer [15] Basic mapping principles for visualizing cancer data using GIS
- Bell et al. [8] Current practices in spatial analysis of cancer data: mapping health statistics to inform policymakers and the public
- Pickle and Carr [64] Visualizing Data Patterns with Micromaps

Mapping and spatial analysis has proved helpful for cancer control in several research areas:

- Cancer Disparities – mapping geographic distribution of cancer rates among different population subgroups across different geographic areas and over time [2, 9, 20, 36, 37], Tatalovich et al. [81]
- Healthcare services – mapping access, availability, quality, and utilization of healthcare services to understand how well target populations are being served [5, 33, 52, 55, 85, 86]
- Neighborhood context– mapping characteristics of social and built environment, risk related behaviors, and the presence and concentrations of adverse environmental agents to reveal areas in need of intervention [1, 6, 22, 43, 44]

There is a growing body of literature demonstrating the value of maps in each of these cancer research areas. Below we discuss a few examples.

3.2.1 Mapping in Cancer Disparities Research

One key value of mapping cancer disparities is in identifying areas with elevated cancer rates among different population subgroups where interventions could be used to modify factors contributing to the high rates.

Example: Mapping geographic disparities in breast cancer mortality.
Chien et al. [20] sought to identify geographic disparities by race and age using population-based breast cancer mortality in 3109 counties in the contiguous United States, and to use spatial statistics to provide estimated values for unavailable data because of confidentiality and reliability concerns. Within the context of prevailing geographic disparities in different races and ages, the study examined: (1) the magnitude of geographic disparities in breast cancer mortality across the U.S.; (2) where breast cancer mortality was significantly higher or lower; and (3) the magnitude of the breast cancer mortality risk in high-risk counties. The findings show that the relative risk for African American women who lived in high-risk counties was at least 2.5 times higher than for those who lived in lower-risk counties. Thus, this study identified priority counties by age and race that should be targeted for interventions aimed at reducing breast cancer mortality.

Example: Mapping geographic disparities in late-stage breast cancer incidence.
A study by Tatalovich et al. [85] examined geographic disparities in late-stage breast cancer (LSBC) incidence across health service areas (HSAs) [49] of eight states in the United States. Stepwise linear regression was performed, with states treated as random effect, to determine the variables that best explain LSBC incidence for females, ages 40 and older. The independent variables in the analysis represent some of the major factors that were found to contribute to LSBC including:

socio-demographic and economic characteristics, accessibility to health care, availability of screening services and utilization of mammography. Maps were generated to highlight areas that have any combination of high late-stage breast cancer incidence and significantly associated risk factors. The findings suggest that in the eight U.S. states examined, higher rates of late-stage breast cancer are more common in areas with predominantly black population (disparity in race), where English literacy, percentage of population with college degree (disparity in socio-demographic characteristics) and screening availability are low. Identification of areas with higher rates of late-stage breast cancer and factors contributing to them has helped identify where resources might be needed to increase screening for breast cancer and provide greater availability of services that can provide more aggressive treatments.

3.2.2 Mapping in Healthcare Services Research

One important use of mapping in healthcare services research is to identify the healthcare needs of communities and inform access to and utilization of care in medically underserved areas. For example, mapping healthcare facilities and population distribution alongside socioeconomic variables can help identify specific regions that are underserved and determine the best possible placement of new healthcare facilities [52, 55].

Example: Using Mapping to enable community-oriented primary care.
In a study by Bazemore et al. [5], practice maps of the designated medically underserved areas for a clinic were generated to demonstrate variation between federally intended and utilization-derived (actual) service areas. In addition, population penetration maps were generated to depict patterns of utilization. Service area maps revealed previously unrecognized range and overlap of individual clinical services, and wide variation in density of utilization of different clinics in medically underserved areas. Maps provided new information to center leaders and resulted in engagement of administrators and clinicians who were enthusiastic regarding the potential of analytic mapping to help guide strategic planning for further expansion and service.

3.2.3 Mapping Neighborhood Context of Cancer

Mapping and analysis of social, racial, economic, or physical characteristics of neighborhoods and relationships between their features may help us better understand health disparities and what aspects of neighborhood context drives and influences health disparities. This information can further be used to guide community-based interventions.

Example: Using GIS mapping for identifying optimal settings for prevention.
A study by Alcaraz et al. [1] sought to identify community settings most likely to reach individuals from geographically underserved areas and to use this information to inform community-based outreach and intervention planning in St. Louis, Missouri. Computerized breast cancer education kiosks were placed in seven types of community settings: beauty salons, churches, health fairs, neighborhood health centers, laundromats, public libraries and social service agencies. The distance between kiosk users' (n = 7297) home ZIP code centroid and the location where they used the kiosk were measured, mapped, and compared across settings. The study found clear differences in the population reach of different types of settings, with laundromats and libraries reaching the most populations. Secondary analyses found kiosk users in laundromats and libraries to live closer to these two settings than other kiosk locations. Thus, if the objective of a given outreach effort is to reach a localized population, a location in closer proximity to users' residences might be the most optimal setting.

Example: Mapping neighborhood health geo-markers for clinical care decisions.
An article by Beck et al. [6] outlines ways in which geographic data (contextual/ ecological or aggregated individual data, or both) could inform community health assessments and population- or patient-level interventions to address health disparities. The first of the five maps presented depicts all asthma-related emergency visits and hospitalizations in Cincinnati, Ohio, over a 3 year period. The remaining four

layers illustrate specific aspects of the psychosocial, economic, physical, and health service environments that affect the health of neighborhood residents. This example is used to spur the discussion regarding the value of linking place-based data with health systems data to gain understanding of the community health status and guide interventions for populations or patients.

In conclusion, the research examples described in this section have illustrated the utility of maps in informing activities aimed at reducing cancer burden. There is a growing body of research utilizing similar methodology to address the gaps in knowledge in respect to geography of cancer, promising to add precision to our understanding of cancer risk, cancer burden, outcomes, quality of care, etc. [4, 13, 25, 27, 29, 34, 38, 48, 54, 55, 62, 74, 85, 86].

3.3   Online Cancer Mapping Systems

This section describes online cancer-mapping systems, discussing their functionality and design considerations, and illustrating how the unique features of these systems can help inform cancer control activities.

3.3.1   Design Considerations

A number of important considerations should be included in the design of an interactive mapping system for cancer control. The design should follow basic principles of effective data visualization including understanding the needs and capabilities of the intended audience, establishing a clear purpose, keeping visuals clear and simple, minimizing the work required of the user, and establishing an appropriate visual hierarchy [23, 30, 83]. Designers should consult published guidelines for mapping health data [10, 15, 19], as well as research results that describe the process of analyzing complex geospatial datasets within the specific domain of cancer data exploration and analysis [11]. Beyer and colleagues describe five important properties of disease maps that include controlling the population denominator of the disease rates, displaying continuous rates, maximizing geographic detail, adjusting for age differences, and providing appropriate spatial context [10].

The design of interactive cancer mapping systems involves important tradeoffs between geographic scale, time period, and data suppression. In mapping cancer data, respecting patient privacy and confidentiality are key concerns [68]. Most cancer mapping systems suppress data when there are too few cases in a particular geographic area often when the counts are 15 or less. This is done primarily to insure stable rates: a count of 15 or less results in a standard error of the rate that is approximately 25% or more as large as the rate itself [56]. Thus, there is often a tradeoff between the level of geographic aggregation and the amount of suppressed data. This tradeoff is accentuated when mapping data for rare cancer types, smaller population subgroups, and rural areas with sparse populations. Changing the aggregation level from counties to states will likely reduce the amount of suppression but, with the reduced spatial resolution, important differences in local cancer rates may be hidden from view. Likewise, data aggregations can include multiple years of data to reduce suppression but at a loss of temporal resolution. Many online cancer mapping systems show state-level rates for a single year of data but use 5 years of data for county rates.

Choice of a legend classification method and an appropriate map color ramp are also important design considerations. Cartographic research has been conducted to test disease map readability using different legend classification methods [16]. The results of this research have shown that quantile and equal interval classification methods are the most effective. Quantile classification highlights relative rates among groups of areas; equal interval classification keeps areas with similar rates in the same group but can be sensitive to large outliers masking differences in the spatial pattern [78]. A variety of color ramps or color schemes are available for choropleth (shaded area) maps. Different color ramps are available for sequential data, diverging data (from a central value), and qualitative data. For example, the breast cancer incidence map in Fig. 3.1 uses quantile intervals and a diverging color ramp to highlight geographic areas with both high and low rates. Cartographic research has been conducted to establish sets of colors that can be clearly distinguished in map reading activities. The resulting set of color ramp choices are available in a web-based selection tool (http://colorbrewer2.org/) [35, 24].

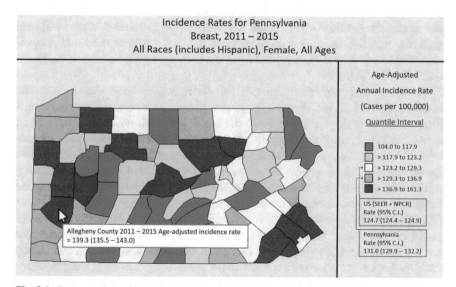

Fig. 3.1 State cancer profiles map of breast cancer incidence rates in Pennsylvania

An interactive online environment offers a significant set of advantages for cancer control mapping. There are a variety of techniques available for the interactive exploration of spatial data [3, 72]. Chief among these is dynamic variable selection – allowing the user to interactively specify the data to be displayed. For cancer mapping systems, this allows users to specify the type of cancer statistic to be displayed (incidence, mortality, survival, prevalence). Most cancer mapping systems provide users with the ability to display data for a specific cancer site. Some cancer mapping systems limit this selection to just the most common cancers. Others group related cancer sites together (for example, combining brain and other central nervous system cancers together). Some cancer mapping systems also allow users to specify particular molecular subtypes such as ER, PR, and HER2 status for breast cancer. Cancer mapping systems can display data for a specific sex, race/ethnicity, age group, or socio-economic indicator. However, the more choices and combinations of these data categories are available, the more areas may be suppressed. Online maps can allow users to zoom in and out and pan to different areas. They can also take advantage of mouse-over actions to display specific information about a particular geographic area such as the specific rate and confidence intervals for the area. Other exploratory spatial data analysis techniques available in an interactive mapping environment include dynamic linking of multiple display frames and brushing. Dynamic linking of multiple display frames allows changes in any one frame to be reflected in the other frames, while brushing allows users to mouse-over a data item in any of the frames and the corresponding data items in the other frames are highlighted [7]. Finally, online cancer maps can take advantage of animation techniques to visualize changes over time [31].

When designing and deploying online cancer mapping systems, the intended purpose and audience should be kept in mind throughout and should drive key design decisions. Initial research into the needs of the intended audience will help guide an overall user-focused design approach. Once a prototype system is available, usability testing will help ensure that the online mapping system meets users' needs [12, 21, 71].

Finally, a number of options are available for conveying uncertainty in an online mapping system [45, 46]. Historically, printed atlases of cancer rates have used some form of hatching or shading to designate areas with high uncertainty [67]. Most online mapping systems use interactive techniques. As mentioned previously, mouse-over actions can allow users the ability to display the confidence intervals. Error bars in dynamically linked graphic frames can also provide this information. Recently, methods have been proposed to consider confidence intervals in the classification method so that areas shown in a common color are more likely to have similar rates [80]. Many online cancer mapping systems either explicitly or implicitly allow users to display ranks of geographic areas. However, these ranks often do not consider uncertainty in the underlying rates. Designers of online mapping systems should consider mechanisms to caution users about interpreting lists of geographic areas sorted by disease rates as a specific rank ordering. The online CI∗Rank tool (https://surveillance.cancer.gov/cirank/) can help designers and users understand the range of possible rankings when confidence intervals are considered [87].

3.3.2   Mapping System Examples

A number of online mapping systems can be and are being used for cancer control and cancer research activities. The purpose and audience of these sites vary as well as the geo-visualization capabilities and the available geospatial data. This section describes a number of examples of these online mapping systems deployed in the U.S. by national and state health agencies. For the most part, geospatial cancer data are displayed at the state and county-level in the U.S., although other sub-state geographic areas are sometimes used. Outside the U.S., examples include the International Agency for Research on Cancer's global interactive maps at the country level (IARC) [40] and the UK Cancer e-Atlas's interactive maps at the National Health Service (NHS) health boundary level [60].

State Cancer Profiles (https://statecancerprofiles.cancer.gov/) [79] is an interactive web site that provides access to cancer statistics, screening rates, risk factor prevalence, and demographic data to allow cancer control planners to focus intervention activities on geographic areas and population subgroups where they are most needed [8]. The web site is a collaboration between the National Cancer Institute (NCI) and Centers for Disease Control and Prevention (CDC) and has been available since 2003. The intended audience is state and local cancer control planners and the features of the web site have been tested extensively with this group. Available cancer statistics include incidence and mortality rates at the state and county-level and prevalence estimates and projections at the state-level by cancer site, sex, race/ethnicity and age group. Generally, only the most recent cancer incidence and mortality data is available, although historic data are used to provide trend information. The web site also provides access to estimates of cancer related knowledge and awareness of cancer prevention strategies from the Health Information National Trends Survey (HINTS) [39]. Based on feedback from user testing, the interactive mapping feature set is relatively limited: only two classification methods are provided (quantiles and equal intervals) and a limited set of color schemes (two sequential schemes and two diverging schemes). The main goal of most users is to get a quick snapshot of geospatial patterns. Hence, the maps themselves are static: the user cannot zoom in or out or pan to different areas. Users are able to mouse-over an area to see the specific rate and confidence interval. The map legend includes information about state and U.S. rates. A sample map is shown in Fig. 3.1. An important feature for users is the ability to capture maps for quick inclusion in reports and presentations so the site allows maps to be easily saved as image files.

The NCI Cancer Atlas (https://gis.cancer.gov/canceratlas/) [58] is a more general and expandable system for the geovisualization of cancer statistics. It is intended for use by public health professionals, cancer control planners and cancer researchers to explore spatial patterns of cancer by cancer type, race/ethnicity, and gender. As of this writing, available cancer statistics include incidence and mortality data at the state and county-levels as well as prevalence estimates at the state-level. Supporting data include screening rates, risk factor prevalence, and demographic data. The mortality data and demographic data are also available by Health Service Area (HSA) and State Economic Areas (SEA). Most data types are available for just the most recent time period. However, historical mortality data are available for 10 year periods from 1970. Unlike State Cancer Profiles, the maps in the NCI Cancer Atlas are fully interactive: users can zoom in and out and pan to different areas. Alaska and Hawaii are shown in separate inset map frames. The map is presented over a base map showing other countries and ocean areas. To facilitate comparison of rates across different maps, there is an option to lock the map legend at its current values. Users are able to mouse-over an area to see the specific rate, confidence interval and total number of cases. See Fig. 3.2 for an example. A unique feature of the NCI Cancer Atlas is the ability to set the geographic area to either a preset or custom group of states. Preset state groupings include the Census regions and divisions as well as states in the "Rust Belt", the "Sun Belt", the "Stroke Belt", etc. An extensive set of map controls are available including options to set the number of classification groups and the classification method; set the color scheme; switch the legend sort order and color ramp order; hide the map title, footnote, and the Alaska and Hawaii inset maps; change the base map; and display state, congressional district, or county borders. Maps can be printed or saved as an image file.

The NCI's Animated Historical Cancer Atlas (https://gis.cancer.gov/atlas/) [57] is an interactive mapping tool that presents maps of cancer mortality data over time as an animated sequence. The intended audience is cancer researchers, public health professionals, cancer advocates, students, and members of the general public who wish to understand and document how spatial patterns of cancer have changed over

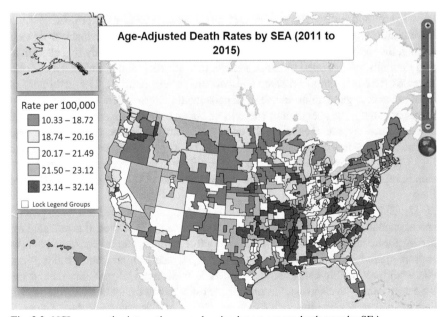

Fig. 3.2 NCI cancer atlas interactive map showing breast cancer death rates by SEA

time. Smoothed age-adjusted mortality rates from 1971 to 2010 in five or 10 year groups are available by cancer site and sex at the HSA level. Maps can be generated for the U.S. as a whole or for individual states. A sequence of static maps are generated for the specified cancer site, sex, and geographic area showing the death rates from 1971 to 2010: eight maps are generated with 5 year intervals or four maps with 10 year intervals. To allow comparison over time, a common set of classification groups is used for all of the maps. A quantile classification method is used across all of the generated maps, assigning colors in one of nine groups such that each group has approximately the same number of HSAs across all of the maps. For an example, see Fig. 3.3. Users can then display the maps in sequence by clicking on the "Animate" button. Individual maps can be saved as an image file or a PDF file. A text view reports the proportion of the HSAs with high, medium, and low rates.

The NCI's Tobacco Policy Viewer (https://gis.cancer.gov/tobaccopolicy/) is an interactive web resource for mapping and download of historical smoke-free policy data in the U.S. [82, 59]. Cancer and tobacco control professionals and advocates can use the NCI Tobacco Policy Viewer to identify gaps in smoke-free policy cover-

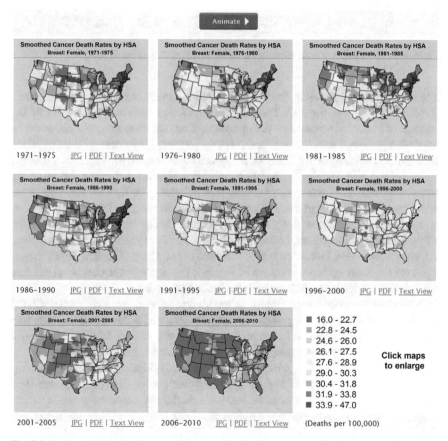

Fig. 3.3 Animated historical cancer atlas maps showing breast cancer death rates over time

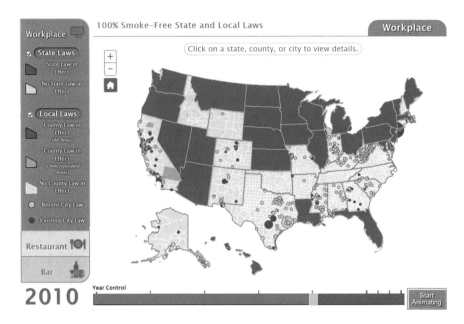

Fig. 3.4 Tobacco policy viewer showing smoke-free workplace policies in 2010

age and to inform planning for education and interventions in the areas of need. Researchers can use the NCI Tobacco Policy Viewer to facilitate analysis of the impacts of historical smoke-free policy coverage on reduction in secondhand-smoke exposures, tobacco use, and tobacco related diseases. Maps present data on when smoke-free policies for workplaces, restaurants and bars have been enacted at the state, county, and city-levels together with information on the percentage of the population who are protected by smoke-free policies. The interactive maps allow zooming and panning and users can control the display of map layers for state laws and local laws (county and city). Mouse-overs provide detailed information for each of the possible multiple smoke-free policy laws in effect at the particular location. An animation control allows users to view the change in smoke-free policy coverage over time. An example is shown in Fig. 3.4. Researchers can download the data for detailed analysis and linkage with health outcomes data.

The Pennsylvania Cancer Atlas (https://www.geovista.psu.edu/grants/ CDC/) provides access to Pennsylvania cancer statistics in a multi-frame format. This web site is a prototype developed at Penn State University intended for cancer control planners, advocates, and researchers who are interested in an in-depth view of cancer rates and the covered population [12, 47]. It displays cancer incidence and mortality data at the county-level with data available for various time periods from 1994 to 2002. An important feature of this web site is the simultaneous presentation of maps, graphs and tables that are dynamically linked together: changes in any one frame are reflected in the other frames and, using brushing, users can mouse-over a data item in any of the frames and the corresponding data items in the other frames

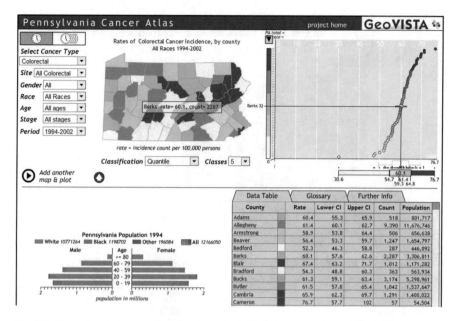

Fig. 3.5 Pennsylvania cancer atlas with dynamically linked map, graph, and data table

are highlighted. See Fig. 3.5 for an example. The geographic area of the map is static – the user cannot zoom in or out or pan to certain areas. There are user controls to set the classification method (quantiles or equal intervals) and the number of classes. The display can be animated to show trend data by year. Another unique feature is the ability to compare two maps and their corresponding data tables.

The CDC's United States Cancer Statistics (USCS) Data Visualizations tool (https://gis.cdc.gov/Cancer/USCS/DataViz.html) is a general visualization tool for USCS data [84]. It is designed to provide information on the most recent cancer incidence and mortality at the national, state, and county-levels for cancer control planners, public health professionals, cancer advocates, and members of the general public. In addition to cancer incidence and mortality data, the tool can display estimates of cancer survival and prevalence as well as supporting demographic data. Static maps of the U.S. by state or of a specific state by county are displayed. The U.S. maps include insets for Alaska and Hawaii and a set of squares representing the smaller states along the East Coast and the District of Columbia. Maps are accompanied by graphs showing the top 10 cancer sites. For an example, see Fig. 3.6. Additional graphs are available to show cancer rates by sex, race/ethnicity, and age group.

There are also a number of state-based examples of online mapping systems for cancer control. The Cancer-rates.info service platform (https://www.cancer-rates.info/) from the Kentucky Cancer Registry at the University of Kentucky provides a means for individual state cancer registries to create web sites that make their data available to cancer control planners and members of the general public [41]. At the

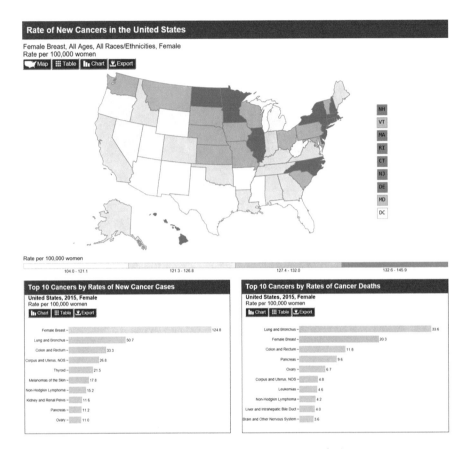

Fig. 3.6 USCS Data visualizations tool with map of incidence rates for breast cancer

time of this writing, registries from Arkansas, California, Connecticut, Georgia, Iowa, Kentucky, Michigan, Mississippi, New Jersey, New Mexico, Seattle-Puget Sound, and Utah are using this platform. Registries can specify what data to make available: years of data, specific cancer sites, race and ethnicity categories, etc. In addition to state and county-levels of geography, data can be aggregated by whatever sub-state geographical regions that are most appropriate for the individual registry. On the Kentucky web site, choices of geographic areas in addition to county include Area Development Districts (an aggregation of counties unique to Kentucky), urban/rural areas, and Appalachia versus Non-Appalachia counties. An example is shown in Fig. 3.7. Other features of the Cancer-rates.info service platform include the ability to compare two maps and the availability of an iOS app for Apple tablets and smart phones.

Another example of a state-based web site that makes cancer data available to cancer control planners and members of the general public is the Missouri Cancer Registry's Instant Atlas Cancer Data Portal (https://instantatlas.umh.edu/IAS/) [53].

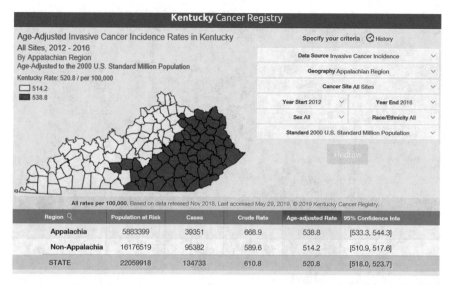

Fig. 3.7 Kentucky data on Cancer-rates. Info with Appalachia and Non-Appalachia rates

Available cancer statistics include incidence, mortality, and breast cancer survival data at the state and county-levels. Supporting data include screening rates, risk factor prevalence, demographic, and socio-economic data. Data are available for just the most recent time period although users can choose between the most recent 5 years, 10 years, and 16 years (1999 to the most recent year). Maps are dynamically linked with graphs and data tables. The maps are fully interactive: users can zoom in and out and pan to different areas. Mouse-overs provide detailed information including confidence intervals. Users can display additional mapping layers including cities and towns, hospitals, etc. The map is presented over a selectable set of base maps. Two layouts are available: one showing data in a single map and one comparing maps of two variables with the associated scatter plot. See Fig. 3.8 for an example of the single map layout.

Rather than a specific web site, our final example is a tool for geovisualization of cancer data called Linked Micromaps (https://gis.cancer.gov/tools/micromaps/) [64]. With it, users can view and compare statistics for multiple variables across geographic areas (for example, states, counties, HSAs, etc.). Rather than displaying a single large map, the display consists of a set of small "micromaps" in a tabular format where each map shows values for up to five geographic areas. Linked Micromaps supports six graph and table display types in addition to the micromaps: bar graphs, box plots, raw data tables, point graphs, point graphs with arrow, and point graphs with confidence intervals. These appear as two additional columns to the right of the micromaps and the rows of data are sorted by the data in one of these two additional columns. For an example of the possible use of Linked Micromaps for cancer control planning, see Fig. 3.9. Here, lung and bronchus cancer incidence rates and confidence intervals for Maryland counties are shown in the middle column and the count of cases are shown

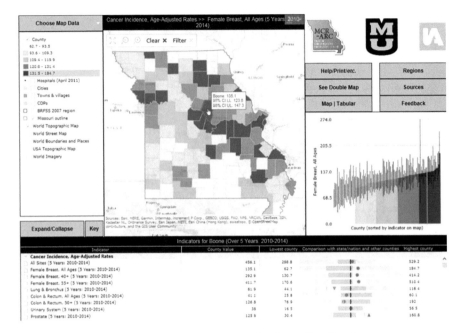

Fig. 3.8 Single map layout from Missouri's InstantAtlas Cancer Data Portal

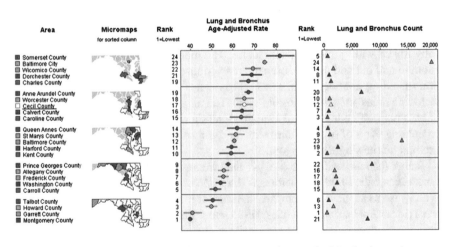

Fig. 3.9 Micromaps example showing lung cancer rates and counts for Maryland counties

in the right column. The data are sorted by descending incidence rate and the micro-maps show the top five counties, the next five counties, etc. A cancer control planner can quickly see both where there are high rates (Somerset, Wicomico, Dorchester, and Charles Counties) as well as large numbers of cases (Baltimore City and Anne Arundel

County). The micromaps help a cancer control planner target groups of neighboring high priority counties that might benefit from a combined intervention program.

3.4 Conclusions

Maps play a central role in cancer control activities to identify areas of need as well as to track progress and evaluate the impact of intervention activities. Mapping tools and methods have proved useful in the areas of health equity and disparities research, healthcare services research, and neighborhood and contextual factor research. In recent years, advancements in the capability and availability on interactive data visualization tools and systems have been utilized to develop and deploy a number of mapping systems for cancer control. These systems share many common features and also provide many unique capabilities.

In the future, we expect the uses of mapping tools and methods for cancer control to continue to develop. In the area of health disparities research, methods to more directly visualize geographic changes in health disparities over time seem within reach. Future mapping methods for health services research will likely include routine consideration of daily travel patterns as well as visualization of both physical and social barriers to access. Availability of tools and methods to define spatial aggregations or zoning systems that meet population size and homogeneity objectives [73, 77] will allow routine reporting and mapping of cancer statistics at a neighborhood level. Such tools could allow dynamic reconfiguration of neighborhood definitions to align with the research goals of a particular study. Interactive data visualization geo-visualization techniques continue to evolve at a rapid pace with the many new open source tools becoming available [61, 69, 75]. With a growing trend to make spatial data available through open web data services, we can expect to see the rapid development of new mapping systems for cancer control based on these open source tools and web data services, perhaps focused on specific cancer control activities and customized for local geographic and cultural needs.

References

1. Alcaraz KI, Kreuter MW, Bryan RP. Use of GIS to identify optimal settings for cancer prevention and control in African American communities. Prev Med. 2009;49(1):54–7. https://doi.org/10.1016/j.ypmed.2009.04.016.
2. Anderson RT, Yang T-C, Matthews SA, Camacho F, Kern T, Mackley HB, Kimmick G, Louis E, Lengerich E, Yao N. Breast cancer screening, area deprivation, and later-stage breast cancer in appalachia: does geography matter? Health Services Research. 2013;49(2):546–67. https://doi.org/10.1111/1475-6773.12108.
3. Anselin L. Interactive techniques and exploratory spatial data analysis. In: Geographical information systems: principles, techniques, management and applications. New York: Wiley; 1999. p. 251–64.

4. Armour BS, Thierry JM, Wolf LA State-Level Differences in Breast and Cervical Cancer Screening by Disability Status: United States, 2008. Women's Health Issues: 2009;12 (6) https://doi.org/10.1016/j.whi.2009.08.006

5. Bazemore A, Phillips RL, Miyoshi T. Harnessing geographic information systems (GIS) to enable community-oriented primary care. J Am Board Fam Med. 2010;23:22–31. https://doi.org/10.3122/jabfm.2010.01.090097.

6. Beck AF, Sandel MT, Ryan PH, Kahn RS. Mapping neighborhood health geomarkers to clinical care decisions to promote equity in child health. Health affairs (Project Hope). 2017;36(6):999–1005. https://doi.org/10.1377/hlthaff.2016.1425.

7. Becker RA, Cleveland WS, Wilks AR. Dynamic graphics for data analysis. Stat Sci. 1987;2:355–95.

8. Bell BS, Hoskins RE, Pickle LW, Wartenberg D. Current practices in spatial analysis of cancer data: mapping health statistics to inform policymakers and the public. Int J Health Geogr. 2006;5:49. https://doi.org/10.1186/1476-072X-5-49.

9. Beyer KM, Tiwari C, Rushton G (2008). Mapping cancer for community engagement. prev chronic dis. Jan; 6(1): A03 http://www.cdc.gov/pcd/issues/2009/jan/08_0029.htm.

10. Beyer KM, Tiwari C, Rushton G. Five essential properties of disease maps. Ann Assoc Am Geogr. 2012;102(5):1067–75. https://doi.org/10.1080/00045608.2012.659940.

11. Bhowmick T, Griffin AL, MacEachren AM, Kluhsman BC, Lengerich EJ. Informing geospatial toolset design: understanding the process of cancer data exploration and analysis. Health Place. 2008a;14(3):576–607. https://doi.org/10.1016/j.healthplace.2007.10.009.

12. Bhowmick T, Robinson AC, Gruver A, MacEachren AM, Lengerich EJ. Distributed usability evaluation of the pennsylvania cancer atlas. Int J Health Geogr. 2008b;7:36. https://doi.org/10.1186/1476-072X-7-36.

13. Boscoe FP, Zhang X. Visualizing the diffusion of digital mammography in New York State. Cancer Epidemiol Biomark Prev. 2017 Apr;26(4):490–4.

14. Brewer CA. Designing better maps: a guide for GIS users. Redlands: ESRI Press; 2005.

15. Brewer CA. Basic mapping principles for visualizing cancer data using geographic information systems (GIS). Am J Prev Med. 2006;30(2):S25–36. https://doi.org/10.1016/j.amepre.2005.09.007.

16. Brewer CA, Pickle LW. Evaluation of methods for classifying epidemiological data on choropleth maps in series. Ann Assoc Am Geogr. 2002;92(4):662–81.

17. Burroughs P, McDonnell R. Principles of geographical information systems. New York: Oxford University Press; 1998.

18. Cancer in North America (CiNA) (2018). Developed by north american association of central cancer registries. Available at: https://www.naaccr.org/cina-public-use-data-set/

19. Centers for Disease Control and Prevention (CDC) (2012). Cartographic Guidelines for Public Health. Available at https://www.cdc.gov/dhdsp/maps/gisx/resources/cartographic_guidelines.pdf.

20. Chien LC, Yu HL, Schootman M. Efficient mapping and geographic disparities in breast cancer mortality at the county-level by race and age in the U.S. Spat Spatiotemporal Epidemiol. 2013;5:27–37. https://doi.org/10.1016/j.sste.2013.03.002.

21. Cinnamon J, Rinner C, Cusimano MD, Marshall S, Bakele T, Hernandez T, Glazier RH, Chipman ML. Evaluating web-based static, animated and interactive maps for injury prevention. Geospat Health. 2009;4(1):3–16. https://doi.org/10.4081/gh.2009.206.

22. Clarke P, Ailshire J, Melendez R, Bader M, Morenoff J. Using Google Earth to conduct a neighborhood audit: reliability of a virtual audit instrument. Health Place. 2010;16(6):1224–9. https://doi.org/10.1016/j.healthplace.2010.08.007.

23. Cleveland WS, McGill ME, editors. Dynamic graphics for statistics. Wadsworth: Pacific Grove; 1988.

24. Color Brewer: Color Advice for Maps; http://colorbrewer2.org/.

25. Conroy SM, Shariff-Marco S, Koo J, et al. Racial/ethnic differences in the impact of neighborhood social and built environment on breast cancer risk: the neighborhoods and breast cancer

study. Cancer Epidemiol Biomark Prev. 2007;26(4):541–52. https://doi.org/10.1158/1055-9965.EPI-16-0935.

26. D' Onofrio A, Mazzetta C, Robertson C, Smans M, Boyle P, Boniol M. Maps and atlases of cancer mortality: a review of a useful tool to trigger new questions. Ecancermedicalscience. 2016;10:670. https://doi.org/10.3332/ecancer.2016.670.

27. DeGuzman PB, Cohn WF, Camacho F, Edwards BL, Sturz VN, Schroen A. Impact of urban neighborhood disadvantage on late stage breast cancer diagnosis in Virginia. J Urban Health. 2017;94(2):199–210. https://doi.org/10.1007/s11524-017-0142-5.

28. Devesa SS. Atlas of cancer mortality in the United States, 1950–94. NIH Publication No. 99–4564: National Cancer Institute, Bethesda; 1999.

29. Doescher MP, Jackson JE. Trends in cervical and breast cancer screening practices among women in rural and urban areas of the United States. J Public Health Manag Pract. 2009;15(3):200–9. https://doi.org/10.1097/PHH.0b013e3181a117da.

30. Evergreen SDH. Presenting data effectively. Los Angeles: Sage Publications; 2014.

31. Greiling DA, Jacquez GM, Kaufmann AM, Rommel RG. Space-time visualization and analysis in the cancer atlas viewer. J Geogr Syst. 2005;7(1):67–84. https://doi.org/10.1007/s10109-005-0150-y.

32. Gromley EK, McLafferty SL. GIS and public health. New York: Guilford Press; 2002.

33. Guagliardo MF. Spatial accessibility of primary care: concepts, methods and challenges. Int J Health Geogr. 2004;3:3.. Available at: http://www.ij-healthgeographics.com/content/3/1/3

34. Gumpertz ML, Pickle LW, Miller BA, et al. Geographic patterns of advanced breast cancer in Los Angeles: associations with biological and sociodemographic factors (United States). Cancer Causes Control. 2006;17:325–39. https://doi.org/10.1007/s10552-005-0513-1.

35. Harrower MA, Brewer CA. ColorBrewer.org: an online tool for selecting color schemes for maps. Cartogr J. 2003;40(1):27–37.

36. Hebert JR, Daguise VG, Adams SA, Puett R, Burch J, Steck S, Bolick-Aldrich SW. Mapping cancer mortality-to-incidence ratios to illustrate racial and sex disparities in high-risk population. Cancer. 2009;115(11):2539–52. https://doi.org/10.1002/cncr.24270.

37. Henry KA, Niu X, Boscoe FP. Geographic disparities in colorectal cancer survival. Int J Health Geogr. 2009;8:48.

38. Henry KA, Sherman R, Farber S, Cockburn M, Goldberg D, Stroup A. The joint effects of census tract poverty and geographic access on late-stage breast cancer diagnosis in 10 US states. Health Place. 2013;21:110–2. https://doi.org/10.1016/j.healthplace.2013.01.007.

39. Hesse BW, Moser RP, Rutten LJ, Kreps GL. The health information national trends survey: research from the baseline. J Health Commun. 2006;11(Suppl 1):vii–xvi.

40. IARC Global Cancer Observatory (2018) The section of cancer surveillance, International agency for research on cancer, Lyon, France. Available at http://gco.iarc.fr/ Accessed 25 Oct 2018.

41. Kentucky Cancer Registry Cancer-rates.info; https://www.cancer-rates.info.

42. Koch T. Cartographies of disease: maps, mapping, and medicine. Redlands: Esri Press; 2016.

43. Kuo T-M, Mobley L, Anselin L. Geographic disparities in late-stage breast cancer diagnosis in California. Health Place. 2011;17(1):327–34. https://doi.org/10.1016/j.healthplace.2010.11.007.

44. Lian M, Struthers J, Schootman M. Comparing GIS-based measures in access to mammography and their validity in predicting neighborhood risk of late-stage breast cancer. PLoS One. 2012;7(8):e43000. https://doi.org/10.1371/journal.pone.0043000.

45. MacEachren AM, Brewer CA, Pickle LW. Visualizing georeferenced data: representing reliability of health statistics. Environ Plan A. 1998;30(9):1547–61.

46. MacEachren AM, Robinson A, Hopper S, Gardner S, Murray R, Gahegan M, Hetzler E. Visualizing geospatial information uncertainty: what we know and what we need to know. Cartogr Geogr Inf Sci. 2005;32(3):139–60. https://doi.org/10.1559/1523040054738936.

47. MacEachren AM, Crawford S, Akella M, Lengerich EJ. Design and implementation of a model, web-based, GIS-enabled cancer atlas. Cartogr J. 2008;45(4):246–60. https://doi.org/10.1179/174327708X347755.
48. MacKinnon JA, Duncan RC, Huang Y, et al. Detecting an association between socioeconomic status and late stage breast cancer using spatial analysis and area-based measures. Cancer Epidemiol Biomarkers Prev. 2007;16(4):756–62. https://doi.org/10.1158/1055-9965.EPI-06-0392.
49. Makuc DM, Haglund B, Ingram DD, et al. Health service areas for the United States. Vital Health Stat. 1991;11(112):1–102.
50. Mason TJ, McKay FW. U.S. cancer mortality by county, 1950–1969. Washington, DC: U.S. Government Printing Office; 1974.
51. Mason TJ, McKay FW, Hoover RN, Blot WJ, Fraumeni JF Jr. Atlas of cancer mortality for U.S. counties, 1950–1969. Bethesda: U.S. Department of Health, Education, and Welfare; 1975.
52. McLafferty SL. GIS and health care. Annu Rev Public Health. 2003;24(1):25–42.
53. Missouri Cancer Registry's Instant Atlas Cancer Data Portal; https://instantatlas.umh.edu/IAS/.
54. Mooney SJ, Joshi S, Cerdá M, Kennedy GJ, Beard JR, Rundle AG. Contextual correlates of physical activity among older adults: a neighborhood environment-wide association study (NE-WAS). Cancer Epidemiol Biomark Prev. 2017;26(4):495–504. https://doi.org/10.1158/1055-9965.EPI-16-0827.
55. Musa GJ, Chiang P-H, Sylk T, et al. Use of GIS mapping as a public health tool—from cholera to cancer. Health Services Insights. 2013;6:111–6. https://doi.org/10.4137/HSI.S10471.
56. National Program Cancer Registries (NPCR) (2014). Suppression of rates and counts. Centers for disease control and prevention, division of cancer prevention and control. Available at http://www.cdc.gov/cancer/npcr/uscs/technical_notes/stat_methods/suppression.htm.
57. NCI Animated Historical Cancer Atlas: U.S. Department of Health and Human Services, National Cancer Institute; https://gis.cancer.gov/atlas/.
58. NCI Cancer Atlas: U.S. Department of Health and Human Services, National Cancer Institute; https://gis.cancer.gov/canceratlas/.
59. NCI Tobacco Policy Viewer: U.S. Department of Health and Human Services, National Cancer Institute; https://gis.cancer.gov/tobaccopolicy/.
60. NCRAS UK Cancer e-Atlas (2018) National cancer registration and analysis service, Public Health England, London. Available at http://www.ncin.org.uk/cancer_information_tools/eatlas/.
61. Neteler M, Bowman MH, Landa M, Metz M. GRASS GIS: a multi-purpose open source GIS. Environ Model Softw. 2012;31:124–30. https://doi.org/10.1016/j.envsoft.2011.11.014.
62. Osypuk TL, Acevedo-Garcia D. Beyond individual neighborhoods: a geography of opportunity perspective for understanding racial/ethnic health disparities. Health Place. 2010;16(6):1113–23. https://doi.org/10.1016/j.healthplace.2010.07.002.
63. Pickle LW. A history and critique of U.S. mortality atlases. Spat Spatiotemporal Epidemiol. 2009;1(1):3–17. https://doi.org/10.1016/j.sste.2009.07.004.
64. Pickle LW, Carr DB. Visualizing health data with micromaps. Spatiotemporal Epidemiol. 2010;1(2–3):143–50.
65. Pickle LW, Mason TJ, Howard N, Hoover RN, Fraumeni JF Jr. Atlas of U.S. cancer mortality among whites, 1950–1980. Washington, DC: U.S. Government Printing Office; 1987.
66. Pickle LW, Mason TJ, Howard N, Hoover RN, Fraumeni JF Jr. Atlas of U.S. cancer mortality among nonwhites, 1950–1980. Washington, DC: U.S. Government Printing Office; 1990.
67. Pickle LW, Mungiole M, Jones GK, White AA. Atlas of United States mortality. Hyattsville: National Center for Health Statistics; 1996.
68. Pickle LW, Szczur M, Lewis DR, Stinchcomb DG. The crossroads of GIS and health information: a workshop on developing a research agenda to improve cancer control. Int J Health Geogr. 2006;5(51):51.
69. Rey SJ. Show me the code: spatial analysis and open source. J Geogr Syst. 2009;11:191–207.

70. Riggan WB, Creason JB, Nelson WC, Manton KG, Woodbury MA, Stallard E et al (1987) U.S. cancer mortality rates and trends, 1950–1979; vol. 4: Maps. U.S. Environmental Protection Agency, Research Triangle Park, NC.
71. Robinson AC, Chen J, Lengerich EJ, Meyer HG, MacEachren AM. Combining usability techniques to design geovisualization tools for epidemiology. Cartogr Geogr Inf Sci. 2005;32(4):243–55. https://doi.org/10.1559/152304005775194700.
72. Robinson AC, Demšar U, Moore B, Buckley A, Jiang B, Field K, Kraak MJ, Camboim SP, Sluter CR. Geospatial big data and cartography: research challenges and opportunities for making maps that matter. Int J Cartogr. 2017;3(sup1):32–60.
73. Sabel CE, Kihal W, Bard D, Weber C. Creation of synthetic homogeneous neighbourhoods using zone design algorithms to explore relationships between asthma and deprivation in Strasbourg, France. Soc Sci Med. 2013;91:110–21. https://doi.org/10.1016/j.socscimed.2012.11.018.
74. Shah TI, Bell S, Wilson K. Spatial accessibility to health care services: identifying underserviced neighbourhoods in Canadian Urban Areas. PLoS One. 2016;11(12):e0168208. https://doi.org/10.1371/journal.pone.0168208.
75. Smith DA. Online interactive thematic mapping: applications and techniques for socio-economic research. Comput Environ Urban Syst. 2016;57:106–17.
76. Snow J. On the mode of communication of cholera., 2nd edn. London: Churchill; 1855. p. 1–162.
77. Spielman SE, Folch DC. Reducing uncertainty in the American community survey through data-driven regionalization. PLoS One. 2015;10(2):e0115626. https://doi.org/10.1371/journal.pone.0115626.
78. State Cancer Profiles (SCP) Interval type. Jointly developed by the NCI and the CDC. 2018. Available at https://statecancerprofiles.cancer.gov/intervaltype.html. Accessed 17 June 2018.
79. State Cancer Profiles: U.S. Department of Health and Human Services, National Cancer Institute and Centers for Disease Control and Prevention; https://statecancerprofiles.cancer.gov.
80. Sun MD, Wong W, Kronenfeld BJ. A classification method for choropleth maps incorporating data reliability information. Prof Geogr. 2014;67:72–83. https://doi.org/10.1080/00330124.2014.888627.
81. Tatalovich Z, Zhu L, Rolin A, Lewis DR, Harlan LC, Winn DM. Geographic disparities in late stage breast cancer incidence: results from eight states in the United States. Int J Health Geogr. 2015;14:31. https://doi.org/10.1186/s12942-015-0025-5.
82. Tatalovich Z, Stinchcomb DG, Lyman JA, Hunt Y, Cucinelli JA. A geo-view into historical patterns of smoke-free policy coverage in the USA. Tobacco Prevention & Cessation. 2017;3:1–11. https://doi.org/10.18332/tpc/80135.
83. Tufte ER. The visual display of quantitative information. Cheshire: Graphic Press; 1983.
84. United States Cancer Statistics Working Group. U.S. Cancer statistics data visualizations tool, based on November 2017 submission data (1999–2015): U.S. department of health and human services, centers for disease control and prevention and national cancer institute: Available at: www.cdc.gov/cancer/dataviz.
85. Wang F, McLafferty S, Escamilla V, Luo L. Late-stage breast cancer diagnosis and health care access in Illinois. PRO. 2008;60(1):54–69. https://doi.org/10.1080/00330120701724087.
86. Wang F, Guo D, McLafferty S. Constructing geographic areas for cancer data analysis: a case study on late-stage breast Cancer risk in Illinois. Appl Geogr. 2012;35(1–2):1–11. https://doi.org/10.1016/j.apgeog.2012.04.005.
87. Zhang S, Luo J, Zhu L, Stinchcomb DG, Campbell D, Carter G, Gilkeson S, Feuer EJ. Confidence intervals for ranks of age-adjusted rates across states or counties. Stat Med. 2014;33(11):1853–66. https://doi.org/10.1002/sim.6071.

Chapter 4
Physical Activity and Exposure in Breast Cancer Survivors Using GPS, GIS and Accelerometry

Marta M. Jankowska, Jiue-An Yang, and Jacqueline Kerr

Abstract Research concerning how the built environment impacts behaviors linked to breast cancer has become of increased interest to public health researchers. Physical activity is a modifiable behavioral factor that can reduce breast cancer risk, cancer recurrence risk, and improve treatment effects by targeting biological mechanisms such as insulin resistance and inflammation. In order to improve population levels of PA, especially in vulnerable groups such as cancer survivors, it is essential to incorporate multiple levels of influence into interventions and analyses, including environmental contexts in which behaviors occur. In order to best measure and intervene on such behaviors, exposure and behavioral sciences have seen a rise in the use of more sensitive and accurate measurement methodologies, primarily using sensors like Global Positioning Systems (GPS) and accelerometers. When coupled with Geographic Information Science data, these three data sources result in dynamic exposure measures that can assess what environments individuals are exposed, where, for how long, and during what behaviors. In this chapter we present three examples of studies that have utilized GPS, accelerometry, and GIS data to better understand cancer risk, disparities, and related behaviors. The goal of the examples is to illustrate decision points that must be made when utilizing GPS data, demonstrate possible processing approaches, and highlight how GPS data can be used in conjunction with GIS and accelerometry to better understand behaviors within specific contexts.

Keywords Physical activity · Spatial energetics · Activity space · Cancer survivors · Breast cancer · Environment

M. M. Jankowska (✉) · J.-A. Yang
Calit2/Qualcomm Institute, University of California San Diego, La Jolla, CA, USA
e-mail: majankowska@ucsd.edu

J. Kerr
Department of Family Medicine and Public Health, University of California San Diego, La Jolla, CA, USA

© Springer Nature Switzerland AG 2019
D. Berrigan, N. A. Berger (eds.), *Geospatial Approaches to Energy Balance and Breast Cancer*, Energy Balance and Cancer 15, https://doi.org/10.1007/978-3-030-18408-7_4

4.1 The Importance of Breast Cancer and Environmental Exposure Research

Behavioral and individual factors such as alcohol use, obesity, and physical inactivity are established risk factors for breast cancer worldwide [5]. Physical activity (PA) is especially of interest as it is a key modifiable behavioral factor that can reduce breast cancer risk, cancer recurrence risk, associated breast cancer risks like obesity, and improve treatment effects by targeting biological mechanisms such as insulin resistance and inflammation [1, 33]. Despite the known benefits of PA for breast cancer prevention, objectively measured PA levels are low (<5%) in many populations, including older adults and survivors [20]. The majority of women do not meet PA guidelines (at least 150 mins of activity a week), yet in a review of 73 studies of breast cancer and physical activity there was a 25% average risk reduction of breast cancer among physically active women compared to the least active women [21]. In order to improve population levels of PA, especially in vulnerable groups such as cancer survivors, it is essential to incorporate multiple levels of influence into interventions and analyses, including environmental contexts in which behaviors occur [31]. Understanding factors that support engagement in healthy lifestyle behaviors, and their relationship to cancer, is critical to understanding disparities in cancer and designing more effective interventions for women at risk for breast cancer.

Literature connecting physical activity behaviors with environmental features is growing, however studies specifically linking health behaviors, environmental context, and breast cancer are rarer. Cross sectional studies of the built environment, PA and obesity show that walkability including connected streets, high density housing and multiple destinations are related to walking for transportation, total PA and obesity [30]. There is also evidence for a relationship between exposure to neighborhood greenspace and cancer-related mortality [13]. Further research is needed to better understand how elements of the built and natural environment specifically affect breast cancer risk, survivorship, and disparities either directly or through behaviors. Such research can help identify key elements of the built environment that facilitate the success of individual behavioral change, identify locations where environmental changes are needed before individual efforts are implemented, and recognize how environments may be fueling underlying cancer disparities [24].

4.2 Using GPS, GIS, and Accelerometry to Study Links Between Environment and Breast Cancer

Exposure and behavioral sciences have seen a rise in research that employs sensors for measuring location, acceleration, and other behaviors and/or biometrics. These methods can also be applied to studies targeting breast cancer and the built environment. It will be important to become more precise in measurement of behavior and environment, because definitions of environment that lack specificity and variability have been tied to contradicting or counterintuitive results, have been shown to underestimate effects, and are questionable in terms of how effectively they can inform interventions [19]. For example, the use of home neighborhoods to measure food access when an individual may do their food purchasing at work or other locations leads to inaccurate measures of food access and reduced effects on food behaviors [12, 14]. Self-reported behavioral data may not have the necessary specificity to discern between PA at certain times of day, locations, or intensities, resulting in reduced ability to evaluate current and changing behaviors, effects of interventions, and relationships between locations, behaviors, and health outcomes [28]. Ethnic differences in self-reported data have not always borne out when objective measures are used [34]. Greater precision of objective measures also means we can discover associations in smaller samples [7]. Thus, behavior sensor data holds much promise for breast cancer research.

For improved exposure data, Global Positioning System (GPS) devices can obtain an accurate representation of a person's movements and trajectories by recording latitude and longitude at varying time intervals (down to the second) while a person engages in their daily routine [18]. Coupled with Geographic Information Systems (GIS), which represent layers of neighborhood and environmental data such as air quality, sidewalk density, poverty, and food stores, GPS is able to create representations of individuals' *actual* daily exposures to environments based on where somebody is and how much time they spend there, as compared to home or neighborhood measures [2, 15]. Accelerometer devices can measure acceleration forces, which can then be extrapolated to obtain objective measures of PA, sedentary behavior, and sleep when worn on the hip and wrist. When coupled with GPS and GIS data, these three data sources result in dynamic exposure measures that can assess what environments individuals are exposed, where, for how long, and during what energy expenditure behaviors [15]. While wearing such sensors can be potentially burdensome for participants, large studies of daily mobility patterns have demonstrated that people are generally habitual, and only one to 2 weeks of sensor data can account for many types of environments to which an individual is exposed [11, 29]. Furthermore, as smartphone use continues to grow even in remote population groups, eventually we will be able to obtain monthly, yearly, and life course metrics of total exposures from unobtrusive mobile data, recognizing privacy challenges of collecting such data. Dynamic exposures that track an individual's actual movement and exposure will enhance our ability to accurately understand and intervene on the relationships between environments, behaviors, and breast cancer risk. The challenge remains how to create meaningful metrics from such vast amounts of data and how to use the information to motivate behavior and policy change.

In this chapter we present three examples of studies that have utilized GPS, accelerometry, and GIS data to better understand cancer risk, disparities, and related behaviors. The goal of the examples is to illustrate decision points that must be made when utilizing GPS data, demonstrate possible processing approaches, and highlight how GPS data can be used in conjunction with GIS and accelerometry to better understand behaviors within specific contexts.

4.3   Examples of Utilizing GPS Data in Cancer-Related Research

The following examples use data from real studies that illustrate how GPS, GIS, and accelerometer can be applied to better understand environmental exposures, plan study recruitment, and assess types of movement patterns. Each study will be described below, however collection of sensor data is replicated between all studies and is briefly described here. GPS and accelerometer data were collected by Qstarz GPS devices (BT-Q1000XT) and a triaxial accelerometer (GT3X+, ActiGraph) attached to a belt worn on the participants' waist. Missing GPS data was imputed using a validated imputation algorithm [22], while accelerometer non-wear time was determined using the Choi algorithm where 90 consecutive minutes of zero activity counts was screened as non-wear [4]. GPS data were joined to the accelerometer data at the minute level using the Personal Activity and Location Measurement System (PALMS) [3]. The PALMS system is an open source tool available for use from the University of Southern Denmark Institute of Sports Science and Clinical Biomechanics. Some R versions of the algorithms from PALMS are also found on GitHub (https://thets.github.io/palmsplusr/) in the PALMS plus R repository developed by Tom Stewart. To ensure adequate representations of participants' days, for all studies a valid day was defined as having a minimum of 600 min of overlapping accelerometer wear time and GPS data. Days below this threshold were dropped from analyses.

4.3.1   Case 1: Measuring Environmental Exposure with GPS Data in an Intervention Cohort

There are numerous spatial analytic techniques that can use GPS data to generate a representation of an individual's environmental exposure. They range from crossing GPS data points with GIS data layers, to generating standard deviation ellipses as a generalized representation of the area an individual traversed [27]. Because each method extracts environmental values from the underlying GIS layers differently, environmental exposure is defined differently by each method – an important factor to consider when selecting an analytic method. This is particularly salient when factoring in time. Some methods treat each GPS point equally in their contribution to the exposure metric (each GPS point is one measure of exposure). This type of approach may be problematic if individuals in the study spend considerable amounts of time in one type of environment, effectively reducing variability and weighting the exposure measure significantly toward where time is spent most, even if a behavior of interest is not occurring in that environment. Other methods completely remove time as a factor in the exposure metric by using GPS data to define a geographic extent, and then measuring environmental attributes within that extent. This approach has its own drawbacks by treating all exposure equal no matter how brief the exposure may have been.

For these reasons it is helpful to generate summarized and/or smoothed representations of space *and* time. Movement trajectories, key locations, and aggregated rasters (or continuous square grid of data values) are examples of how GPS data might be summarized with the inclusion of time. One such methodology is called kernel density estimation (KDE), which is a method for smoothing point patterns into a generalized surface by applying a kernel function with specified search radius to each point in the data set [32]. Smoothed GPS representations like KDE can be further honed by utilizing other sensors that capture salient behaviors, thereby reducing data that does not represent the behavior of interest. In other words, only data pertinent to the behavior or sensor measure of interest might be included in the smoothed location model. In the following example, GPS data from an intervention in cancer survivors is assessed using KDE to measure participants' exposure to walkability during the baseline of the study. We demonstrate how differences in exposure can be assessed based on time (weekend vs. week days), location (assessment of exposure around the home vs. only exposure beyond the home), and behavior (exposure during activity vs. exposure during sedentary behavior).

4.3.1.1   Case 1: Study Description and Data

The Reach for Health (RfH) study (completed in 2015) was a randomized trial in overweight or obese women with a history of early-stage postmenopausal breast cancer assessing how weight loss and/or metformin influenced breast cancer related biomarkers [25, 26]. Study measurements taken at baseline clinic visits included questionnaires, 7 days of wearing accelerometer and GPS sensors, physical measurements, and fasting blood draws. Baseline data were collected from 249 women living in San Diego County with an average age of 62.4 years (SD 7.2), 9.6% were Hispanic, 67.9% were married, and 52.2% were employed.

To calculate walkability for San Diego County, GIS data was downloaded from the San Diego Regional Planning Agency (SANDAG) in dates ranging from 2012–2014 to best match the baseline study period. Walkability was calculated on a 200 × 200 m grid for all of San Diego County using the added z-scores of land use mix, intersection density, and residential density [10]. Analysis was performed in ESRI ArcMap 10.5 and a HIPAA compliant PostgreSQL geodatabase to allow for rapid and secure analysis. ArcMap is a commonly used commercially available mapping software from ESRI Inc., while PostgreSQL is an open source extension of PostSQL database software commonly used for creating spatial databases.

4.3.1.2   Case 1: Methods

In general terms, Kernel Density Estimation (KDE) is a process of applying a smoothing equation function in the shape of a bell curve in a moving window over the space of the GPS points on a map. Instead of a series of points, it results in a continuous density surface raster. Specifically, KDE operates by calculating a kernel function of GPS points over a specified distance at each GPS point, and aggregating those values over a fine raster grid of cells. The raster is populated with values derived from the weighted value of the kernels, increasing in weight as the participant spends more time in each cell. The kernel function can also be weighted by other factors, for example activity intensity measured from the accelerometer. KDE in ArcGIS utilizes a quartic kernel function [32]. Bandwidth of the search radius was set to 200 m to keep density estimates relatively tightly aligned with the original GPS data. If greater smoothing or greater consideration of the surrounding environment is desired, these parameters could be changed to engulf a larger area around the GPS track. The resulting weighted KDE raster is then multiplied by the walkability raster, giving an exposure to walkability measure for each participant. This procedure was completed for the following GPS data sets for each participant: total valid GPS data, weekend GPS data, weekday GPS data, GPS data within 1000 m of the home, GPS data beyond 1000 m of the home, GPS data during active behavior measured by ≥760 counts per minute from the accelerometer, GPS data during less and non-active behavior measured by <760 counts per minute from the accelerometer.

4.3.1.3 Case 1: Results and Observations

Of the 249 participants from the RfH in San Diego, 246 women had adequate GPS and accelerometer data to have at least one valid day of data. To visualize what different definitions of exposure might look like, KDE rasters for 6 of the exposure definition detailed above are demonstrated in Fig. 4.1 (exposure around the home vs. only exposure beyond the home, exposure during activity vs. exposure during sedentary behavior, weekend vs. week days. The figure illustrates exposures for one participant. In Fig. 4.1A and Fig. 4.1B, the point density distributions of the home area compared to the non-home area are seen, clearly demonstrating a significant amount of time being spent in places beyond the home that may be important for exposures to types of environments. In Figs. 4.1C and 4.1D KDEs are calculated for points that are active vs. non-active based on accelerometer counts. Figures 4.1E and 4.1F shows the varied pattern of movement between weekend and weekdays, indicating possible shifts in behaviors between those days.

Table 4.1 shows results from the KDE analysis when multiplying the density of GPS points by walkability values. The table allows us to investigate how exposure to walkability changes when the definition of exposure changes (based on times, locations, or behaviors). For each of the KDE definitions, some participants fall out of the analysis if they do not have valid GPS points that meet the exposure definition, e.g. they did not collect data over a weekend. Of note is a decrease in participants with KDE exposures around the home, which is likely due to loss of signal when inside the home for prolonged periods. The area value denotes the total average area of the KDE for each definition. The table shows the largest KDEs are measured for total and non-active points, and the smallest for active points. Home area is on average 1 km², per our earlier definition of home as a 1 km buffer around a participant's

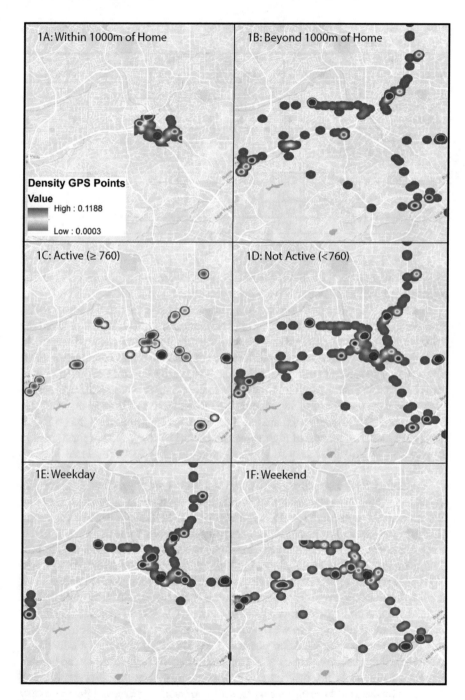

Fig. 4.1 Kernel Density Estimations of GPS and accelerometer derived movement patterns of one participant taking points that belong to (A) within 1000 m of the home, (B) outside 1000 m of the home, (C) active points defined as accelerometer values ≥760, (D) non-active points defined as accelerometer values <760, (E) points collected on weekdays, and (F) points collected on weekends

Table 4.1 Average results of KDE walkability estimates for total, active, non-active, within home, beyond home, weekday, and weekend points

GPS points in KDE	Participants	Area (km²)	Range walkability	Mean walkability (10⁻⁴)	Sum walkability
Total Valid	246	23.34	0.12	3.59	63.57
Active (≥760 counts)	245	2.83	0.01	2.79	7.18
Non-active (<760)	246	23.01	0.11	3.27	56.31
Within 1000 m of home	230	1.03	0.12	36.21	45.72
Beyond 1000 m of home	244	21.97	0.03	1.05	20.49
Weekday	241	18.66	0.09	3.72	45.97
Weekend	227	8.23	0.04	7.18	18.86

address. It is, however, of interest to see how much area of exposure is occurring beyond the 1 km home buffer (on average 23.34 km²).

The walkability measure used for this study was normalized to a scale of 0–10, however the scale does not have a normal distribution and skews heavily toward the lower values of the range. For this reason, walkability scores are low overall. In Table 4.1, range is a measure of the difference between the highest and lowest walkability exposure scores in a single participant. Those differences were then averaged across all participants. Measures with the largest ranges were total, non-active, home, and weekday, all of which include the most amounts of time spent in places. Because the KDE measure increases as more time is spent in a place, these higher ranges are likely a function of high values generated from significant time spent in a place that is walkable, as well as short bouts of time spent in places that are unwalkable.

Walkability scores are shown with mean and summed values. How to summarize an exposure measure (and what that summation means) is another decision point that needs to be considered in this type of analysis. In Table 4.1 mean values are relatively similar across the measures except for the within home measure, which is much higher than the other measures. This may be a function of extended periods of time spent inside of the home generating a significant weighted effect, with limited time spent outside the home but in the neighborhood. If that effect is undesired, a small buffer (~50 m) around the home location could be created and points that are inside the home could be removed from the analysis. Weekend exposure is slightly higher than other measures as well, potentially indicating higher exposure to walkable environments over weekend periods. The sum measure shows a cumulative exposure rather than an average but is going to be heavily influenced by the number of points included in the measure. The most cumulative walkability exposure is measured by the total exposure measure, followed by non-active, and then weekday and home measures. The active measure has the smallest walkability sum value due to the smallest number of points in this measure.

This type of sensitivity analysis of utilizing various definitions for exposure is an important exercise to conduct when settling on a methodological approach for a spatial energetics study. At the core of the analysis is understanding how exposure measures may vary depending on how exposure is defined, and then tailoring the measure to the question at hand. For example, if understanding where breast cancer survivors exercise is of interest, it would be most appropriate to utilize exposure measures during the behavior of interest. If trying to understand disparities in access, it may be more beneficial to include total exposure. If trying to change behavior, perhaps examining differences in weekday vs. weekend exposure and then tailoring messaging around weekend related opportunities may be most suitable. In each of these cases by ascertaining how exposure changes when we consider different times, behaviors, and contexts, we can better develop an analytic procedure that is precise in its definition of a relevant exposure.

4.3.2 Case 2: Increasing Variability in Environmental Exposures Through GPS Data

An issue for many studies that assess environment as related to health outcomes or behaviors is lack of variability in environmental exposure when measured at the home location of the participant, which impairs statistical analysis and resulting conclusions [14]. GPS data may provide an alternative way to increase variability in environmental exposure without the need to increase sample size or add more locations to a study. This is of interest for studies that are not originally planned to include geographic variation, but rather are sampling individuals based on a medical factor such as cancer risk or survivorship. In such cases, attempting to impose geographic and environmental variation on what is likely to already be a limited sample can make study recruitment overly challenging. Instead, addition of GPS data, which will include the variation of environments that people move in throughout their week, may add necessary environmental exposure variability. In the following case study we demonstrate differences in environmental exposure measures based on home location as compared to GPS data for a variety of environmental factors (walkability, greenspace, crime, socio-economic deprivation, socio-economic advantage, and pollution). We also explore how environmental exposure measures differ for various demographic groups (Hispanic vs. non-Hispanic, men vs. women, and middle age vs. retirement age).

4.3.2.1 Case 2: Study Description and Data

The Community of Mine Study (CoM) was completed in 2017 in San Diego County as a cross-sectional observational study intended to better understand the role of environmental exposures in cancer related biomarkers. Participants were randomly sampled from urban census block groups selected to maximize environmental variability in walkability and fast food access (as a proxy for unhealthy eating environments). The study protocol is pending publication [16]. Study measurements included questionnaires, 14 days of wearing accelerometer and GPS sensors, physical measurements, dietary recalls, and fasting blood draws. Data were collected from 602 adults with an average age of 58 years (SD 10), 55% female, 40% Hispanic, and 52% married.

Walkability was calculated as described in Case 1. Greenspace was derived as an NDVI (vegetation) index from composite 2015 Landsat imagery, and calculated at a 200 × 200 m raster. Crime data was obtained from SANDAG; violent crime was aggregated for the years 2010–2013 at the census block group level. Measure of socio-economic deprivation and advantage were derived from 2011–2015 American Community Survey 5-year estimates at the census block group level. SES disadvantage was created through a Principle Components Analysis of variables related to education, unemployment, rented housing, crowding, cost of housing, poverty, use of public assistance programs, lack of car, and use of public health insurance. SES advantage was derived from variables related to house value, employment, higher education, high income, and home ownership. An overall pollution index was provided by the CalEnviroscreen 3.0 tool at the census track level [23].

4.3.2.2 Case 2: Methods

Home-based measures of exposure were derived from circular buffers around participant homes. The majority of studies that examine the relationship between home environment and behaviors utilize a 400 m–2 km buffer around a location to define an individual's environment [6]. A 1600 m (~1 mile) buffer around participants' homes was created, and environmental variables contained in that buffer were calculated for each participant using average values. GPS-based measures of exposure were calculated with KDE methods described in Case 1, using all valid GPS points for the participant's wear time. Z scores were generated for all resulting variables to allow for comparison across variables.

4.3.2.3 Case 2: Results and Observations

Comparison of the range of KDE exposure measures to home buffer measures are shown in Fig. 4.2. Generally, there is greater variability in the KDE measures than the home buffer measures. There is similarity in range for the NDVI (KDE: min −4.30, max 4.12; Home: min −3.29, max 4.09) and Crime measures (KDE: min −0.43, max 8.75; Home: min −0.96, max 8.52). Walkability, pollution, and both SES measures show larger ranges in their values for the KDE measures. By increasing variability in the exposure measure, it may be easier to detect how differences in extent of exposure impact health behaviors or outcomes in a population. It is important to note that in this sample, individuals were recruited based on variability in

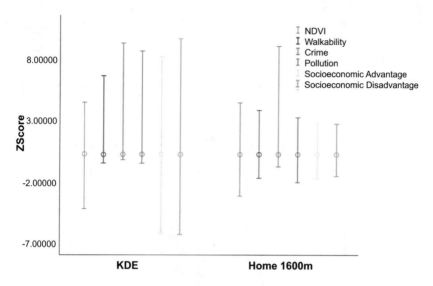

Fig. 4.2 KDE exposure from GPS data compared to home buffer (1600 m) measures of exposure for six environmental attributes: NDVI, walkability, crime, pollution, SES advantage, and SES disadvantage

walkability of their home census block group. Thus, in many studies that do not consider home environment as part of the selection criteria, the variability in environmental exposure around the home is likely to be much smaller. Therefor increasing variation in exposure measure with an overall measure of exposure based on GPS data may improve a study's ability to detect impact of environment on health.

When we break down differences in exposure measures across various demographic groups, further differences arise between home and KDE based exposure measures. In Fig. 4.3, KDE exposures are shown on the left and home exposures are shown on the right of the figure. In the top two graphs age groups are compared for 35–65 years and 66 or over (retirement age). Home exposure ranges do not change substantially between the two age groups, except for crime which has a slightly larger range for the younger age group. However, the KDE exposure shows much larger differences between the groups for almost every exposure variable. This pattern holds true for the other two demographic indicators, sex and Hispanic/not-Hispanic. Home based buffers of exposure show very little difference between each demographic category, while the KDE exposure measures indicate larger ranges. For example, NDVI and walkability for males have larger ranges than for females – a potentially important factor for exploring gender differences in PA or sedentary behaviors. There is a pronounced difference in almost all the KDE exposure variables for Hispanics compared to non-Hispanics, with non-Hispanics showing a greater range in exposures compared to Hispanics. However, this difference is not seen in the home measures, a result which would indicate that there are ethnic differences in movement behaviors in the sample.

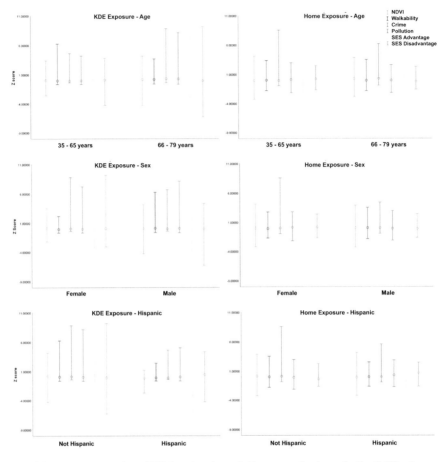

Fig. 4.3 KDE exposure from GPS data (graphs on left) compared to home buffer (1600 m) measures of exposure (graphs on right) for six environmental attributes: NDVI, walkability, crime, pollution, SES advantage, and SES disadvantage. Exposures are compared for three demographic groupings: age (top), gender (middle), and Hispanic/not Hispanic (bottom)

These results could have implications for how gender, ethnic, or age-based difference are statistically estimated in a study. If home measures are under estimating the amount of variability that certain populations experience in exposures, this could have impacts on our understanding of how demographic differences are playing out for environmental effects on cancer risk. The benefit of adding GPS to a study must be weighed in terms of costs and effort involved. Purchasing GPS devices training staff in protocols and data management, finding and consenting willing participants, and processing resulting data are all added effort and cost to a study. Yet, because GPS data generates significantly more variability in environmental exposures, as our analysis indicates the sample size of a study may be able to be reduced when compared to using home environment exposure, which may have considerably less variability. The addition of GPS measures may be particularly important if a study sample is selected to represent a cancer population that has little variability in environments in which they live, which may negatively impact efforts to obtain estimates of neighborhood effects on cancer related health factors.

4.3.3   Case 3: Using GPS and Accelerometer Data to Aid in Machine Learned Algorithms for Assessing Movement

While accelerometers are useful for representing acceleration and total movement counts, they are less ideal for identifying specific types of movement – in particular those associated with travel modes. Environmental changes are designed to impact daily behaviors such as active transportation, so accurate measurement of these modes is important. Intensity based accelerometer cut points are not ideal for identifying car vs. bus travel or running vs. bicycling. Interventions focusing on increasing active travel have been demonstrated to be effective ways of increasing PA and possibly reducing obesity [8]. This type of daily activity behavior has potential to change cancer risk in large population groups. Such methods may be useful for natural experiments where new transportation services, for example, are provided. Accurately measuring active travel modes can be a challenge, as self-report and even travel diaries have been shown to be unreliable and coarse in their measurement (e.g. only possible over a small number of days) [17]. Furthermore, there are demographic disparities in self-reporting on specific behaviors, which may confound results in studies focusing on underserved groups [9].

Machine learned algorithms that use accelerometer and GPS data can offer more precise measures of active travel behavior, as demonstrated in the following case study. Better measures of activity and travel mode will help discern associations between built environments and active travel. Furthermore, greater precision of objective measures means we can discover significant associations in smaller samples. In the following case study, the goal was to train and validate machine-learned algorithms to classify patterns of accelerometer and GPS data to better discriminate types of sedentary behavior, PA, and active travel in participants including those with high breast cancer disease risk. Such techniques are also employed in many commercial wearables and could be incorporated in a mobile phone application. The key, however, is the training process which must be representative, valid and reliable.

4.3.3.1   Case 3: Study Description and Data

Data were drawn from several samples, including women surviving breast cancer and at increased risk for breast cancer. All participants wore hip accelerometers and GPS devices, as previously described. We employed two main methods to establish a 'ground truth' which provides the training data required of a supervised machine learning approach. One method prescribed active travel (AT) trips of a specific type,

Table 4.2 Samples studied for ground truth data in machine learning classification

Sample	N	Average Age	Number Days	Ground Truth
Prescribed adult AT trips	2	–	30	Trip diary
Prescribed child AT activities	36	10	N/A	Observation
Free living cyclists	40	36	169	Annotated images from camera
Free living overweight/obese women	36	55	324	Annotated images from camera

length and sequence. This ensures that all types of travel are included in the training dataset but does not represent the probability of the behavior occurring naturally. A second, more intensive method assessed behaviors by a person worn camera. Annotators reviewed the images and assigned a behavioral code to them using a protocol after reliability was established. Table 4.2 describes the samples studied, which came from a variety of study protocols and ground truth methods. Two adults participated in several prescribed AT trips over the course of 30 days recorded with trip/travel diaries. A total of 36 children participated in one AT trip each while being observed. The remaining samples had cameras with annotation of activities.

4.3.3.2   Case 3: Methods

Random Forest classifiers were employed using a leave one out crossover validation method. This method trains the model on all but one participant, and then tests the model on the remaining participant that was left out, thus no data from a single individual is included in both the training and testing set. Features of the data were created using standard statistical techniques and these were entered into the Random Forest. Hidden Markov Modeling was employed to smooth the data from the annotated image dataset, using the probability that the behavior occurred naturally to help ascertain the correct sequence of behaviors.

4.3.3.3   Case 3: Results and Observations

Figure 4.4 shows the results of the accuracy testing following the machine learning process. The ability of the algorithm to predict the behaviors was compared to the standard accelerometer cut points employed in most studies to date. Clearly, the machine learning algorithms predicted the behaviors with high accuracy, greatly improving upon the cut point approach. Further, this approach had similar accuracy across different population groups. Of note, however, an algorithm, using the same machine learned method, was developed for each dataset. When algorithms are trained on one population and applied to another they lose some accuracy (about 5%). The prescribed training set also resulted in greater accuracy, but this is expected

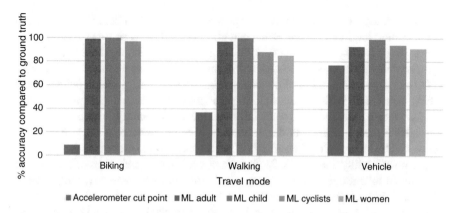

Fig. 4.4 Detection of travel mode by machine learning compared to accelerometer cut-points

because the data were more controlled thus providing less 'noise' that can disrupt the algorithm. The image-based datasets have stronger validity, based in the real world scenarios, but are more burdensome to collect for participants and researchers. Thus, a feasible first step might be a prescribed ground truth. In addition, the algorithm performed better with both GPS and accelerometer data. Challenges to machine learning approaches include the availability and size of the training data set, the number of categories to be predicted, and the similarities of behaviors to each other. For example, distinguishing bus from vehicle travel on heavy traffic roads with many stop lights is difficult.

4.4   Discussion

Sensor-based data is an important tool for the accurate and specific measurement of behaviors that are related to PA, cancer risk, and health outcomes. In the three example cases presented in this chapter, we demonstrate that GPS and accelerometer sensors can provide a range of benefits such as enhancing specificity of exposure measures, increasing variability in exposure in a sample, and providing better estimates of travel related behaviors. It is important to note that data collection and processing is more complex than traditional questionnaires or survey-based methods, and there are multiple decision points throughout the processing framework that must be made when utilizing these approaches. Working in teams that include computation and/or data scientists can aid in easing these difficulties and implementing a data flow that is replicable.

The bulk of this chapter has been devoted to studies that are either observational or cross-sectional in nature. However, the use of sensors such as GPS and accelerometers for cancer related research is also of interest as we move into m-Health interventions that utilize out of the box sensor solutions such as smart phones. Just in Time Adaptive Interventions (JITAIs) employ temporal and spatial cues to prompt behavior change, but little is known about spatial predictors of behaviors and health at the minute level and beyond home neighborhoods. The work we are performing, developing algorithms to detect specific behaviors and matching those behaviors to specific contexts in GIS, is needed to inform the computational models that drive JITAIs. Without such information we are 'guessing' at what decision points, under which rules and with which tailoring variables JITAIs are designed. Micro-randomization trials can elicit some information experimentally, but we risk alienating users by not having data driven models. Health applications need to be able predict when an unhealthy behavior is likely to occur and to prevent such a behavior or prompt a healthy alternative. While there is potential in such approaches, we still have much to learn about identifying meaningful space-time-behavior trajectories. We hope this chapter inspires others to endeavor to uncover such intervention points, but we caution that data should be complimented by relevant behavioral and spatial theories.

References

1. Anzuini F, Battistella A, Izzotti A. Physical activity and cancer prevention: a review of current evidence and biological mechanisms. J Prev Med Hyg. 2011;52:174–80.
2. Berrigan D, Hipp A, Hurvitz PM, et al. Geospatial and contextual approaches to energy balance and health. Ann GIS. 2015;21:157–68. https://doi.org/10.1080/19475683.2015.1019925.
3. Carlson JA, Jankowska MM, Meseck K, et al. Validity of PALMS GPS scoring of active and passive travel compared with sensecam. Med Sci Sports Exerc. 2015;47:662–7. https://doi.org/10.1249/MSS.0000000000000446.
4. Choi L, Ward SC, Schnelle JF, Buchowski MS. Assessment of wear/nonwear time classification algorithms for triaxial accelerometer. Med Sci Sports Exerc. 2012;44:2009–16. https://doi.org/10.1249/MSS.0b013e318258cb36.
5. Danaei G, Vander Hoorn S, Lopez AD, et al. Causes of cancer in the world: comparative risk assessment of nine behavioural and environmental risk factors. Lancet. 2005;366:1784–93. https://doi.org/10.1016/S0140-6736(05)67725-2.
6. Ding D, Gebel K. Built environment, physical activity, and obesity: what have we learned from reviewing the literature? Health Place. 2012;18:100–5. https://doi.org/10.1016/j.healthplace.2011.08.021.
7. Dodge HH, Zhu J, Mattek NC, et al. Use of high-frequency in-home monitoring data may reduce sample sizes needed in clinical trials. PLoS One. 2015;10:e0138095. https://doi.org/10.1371/journal.pone.0138095.
8. Dons E, Rojas-Rueda D, Anaya-Boig E, et al. Transport mode choice and body mass index: cross-sectional and longitudinal evidence from a European-wide study. Environ Int. 2018;119:109–16. https://doi.org/10.1016/j.envint.2018.06.023.
9. Dyrstad SM, Hansen BH, Holme IM, Anderssen SA. Comparison of self-reported versus accelerometer-measured physical activity. Med Sci Sports Exerc. 2014;46:99–106. https://doi.org/10.1249/MSS.0b013e3182a0595f.
10. Frank LD, Sallis JF, Saelens BE, et al. The development of a walkability index: application to the neighborhood quality of life study. Br J Sports Med. 2010;44:924–33. https://doi.org/10.1136/bjsm.2009.058701.
11. González MC, Hidalgo CA, Barabási A-L. Understanding individual human mobility patterns. Nature. 2008;453:779–82. https://doi.org/10.1038/nature06958.

12. Hurvitz PM, Moudon AV, Kang B, et al. Emerging technologies for assessing physical activity behaviors in space and time. Front public Heal. 2014;2(2) https://doi.org/10.3389/fpubh.2014.00002.
13. James P, Hart J, Banay R, Laden F. Exposure to greenness and mortality in a nationwide prospective cohort study of women. Environ Health Perspect. 2016a;124:1344–52. https://doi.org/10.1289/ehp.1510363.
14. James P, Jankowska MM, Marx C, et al. "Spatial Energetics": integrating data from GPS, accelerometry, and GIS to address obesity and inactivity. Am J Prev Med. 2016b;51:792–800.
15. Jankowska MM, Schipperijn J, Kerr J. A framework for using GPS data in physical activity and sedentary behavior studies. Exerc Sport Sci Rev. 2015;43:48–56.
16. Jankowska MM, Sears DD, Natarjan L, et al. Protocol for a cross sectional study of cancer risk, environmental exposures and lifestyle behaviors in a diverse community sample: the community of mine study. BMC Public Health Submitted. 2018;19(1):186.
17. Kelly P, Doherty AR, Hamilton A, et al. Evaluating the feasibility of measuring travel to school using a wearable camera. Am J Prev Med. 2012;43:546–50. https://doi.org/10.1016/j.amepre.2012.07.027.
18. Krenn PJ, Titze S, Oja P, et al. Use of global positioning systems to study physical activity and the environment. a systematic review Am J Prev Med. 2011;41:508–15. https://doi.org/10.1016/j.amepre.2011.06.046.
19. Kwan M. The uncertain geographic context problem. Ann Assoc Am Geogr. 2012;102:958–68. https://doi.org/10.1080/00045608.2012.687349.
20. Lynch BM, Dunstan DW, Healy GN, et al. Objectively measured physical activity and sedentary time of breast cancer survivors, and associations with adiposity: findings from NHANES (2003–2006). Cancer Causes Control. 2010a;21:283–8. https://doi.org/10.1007/s10552-009-9460-6.
21. Lynch BM, Neilson HK, Friedenreich CM. Physical activity and breast cancer prevention. In: Courneya K, Friedenreich C, editors. Physical activity and cancer. Recent Results in Cancer Research. Berlin: Springer; 2010b. p. 13–42.
22. Meseck K, Jankowska MM, Schipperijn J, et al. Is missing geographic positioning system data in accelerometry studies a problem, and is imputation the solution? Geospat Health. 2016;11 https://doi.org/10.4081/gh.2016.403.
23. OEHHA California communities environmental health screening tool, version 2.0. (CalEnviroScreen 2.0) Guidance and Screening Tool 2014.
24. Osypuk TL, Acevedo-Garcia D. Beyond individual neighborhoods: a geography of opportunity perspective for understanding racial/ethnic health disparities. Heal Place. 2010;16:1113–23. https://doi.org/10.1016/j.healthplace.2010.07.002.
25. Patterson RE, Marinac CR, Natarajan L, et al. Recruitment strategies, design, and participant characteristics in a trial of weight-loss and metformin in breast cancer survivors. Contemp Clin Trials. 2016;47:64–71. https://doi.org/10.1016/j.cct.2015.12.009.
26. Patterson RE, Marinac CR, Sears DD, et al. The effects of metformin and weight loss on biomarkers associated with breast cancer outcomes. J Natl Cancer Institute. 2018;2110: 1239–1247. doi: doi.org/https://doi.org/10.1093/jnci/djy040
27. Perchoux C, Chaix B, Cummins S, Kestens Y. Conceptualization and measurement of environmental exposure in epidemiology: accounting for activity space related to daily mobility. Health Place. 2013;21:86–93. https://doi.org/10.1016/j.healthplace.2013.01.005.
28. Prince SA, Adamo KB, Hamel ME, et al. A comparison of direct versus self-report measures for assessing physical activity in adults: a systematic review. Int J Behav Nutr Phys Act. 2008;5:56. https://doi.org/10.1186/1479-5868-5-56.
29. Rainham D, McDowell I, Krewski D, Sawada M. Conceptualizing the healthscape: contributions of time geography, location technologies and spatial ecology to place and health research. Soc Sci Med. 2010;70:668–76. https://doi.org/10.1016/j.socscimed.2009.10.035.
30. Sallis JF, Cerin E, Conway TL, et al. Physical activity in relation to urban environments in 14 cities worldwide: a cross-sectional study. Lancet. 2016;387:2207–17. https://doi.org/10.1016/S0140-6736(15)01284-2.

31. Sallis JF, Owen N, Fisher EB. Ecological models of health behavior. In: Glanz K, Rimer B, Viswanath K, editors. Health behavior and health education: theory, research, and practice. 4th ed edn. Jossey-Bass. San Francisco; 2008. p. 465–85.
32. Silverman B. Density estimation for statistics and data analysis. Chapman Hall. 1986;37:1–22. https://doi.org/10.2307/2347507.
33. Su LJ. Diet, epigenetics, and cancer. Methods Mol Biol. 2012;863:377–93.
34. Troiano RP, Berrigan D, Dodd KW, et al. Physical activity in the United States measured by accelerometer. Med Sci Sports Exerc. 2008;40:181–8. https://doi.org/10.1249/mss.0b013e31815a51b3.

Chapter 5
Towards Systematic Methods in an Era of Big Data: Neighborhood Wide Association Studies

Shannon M. Lynch

Abstract Methodologic challenges related to variable selection exist in neighborhood studies. In the era of "Big Data", this variable selection issue will only continue to grow as neighborhood data become increasingly more complex and integrated with multilevel data. To allow for consistency and comparability of neighborhood variables across studies, systematic approaches for variable selection are needed. Borrowing concepts from empiric methods in biology, a novel neighborhood-wide association study (NWAS) and a neighborhood-environment wide association study (NE-WAS) were recently developed. This chapter introduces key concepts of the NWAS/NE-WAS designs, provides criteria for evaluating these systematic approaches, and discusses the potential impact these empiric methods have on future multilevel interventions.

Keywords Neighborhood wide association study (NWAS) · Neighborhood-environment wide association study (NE-WAS) · Big data · Machine learning · Variable selection

5.1 Introduction

In recent years, there has been a growing interest in evaluating the effect of environment, particularly the social and built environment, on cancer outcomes. The social environment is defined as the socioeconomic circumstances (SES; i.e. poverty, education, employment) of a neighborhood or geographic area where a person lives [1, 2]. The built environment is characterized by man-made, physical structures of a neighborhood, including housing, transportation networks and availability of health-related resources, such as cancer screening facilities [1, 3]. A number of multilevel conceptual frameworks support the study of neighborhood environment and cancer, suggesting that risk factors at the biologic, individual and neighborhood

S. M. Lynch, Ph.D., M.P.H. (✉)
Fox Chase Cancer Center, Philadelphia, PA, USA
e-mail: Shannon.lynch@fccc.edu

© Springer Nature Switzerland AG 2019   99
D. Berrigan, N. A. Berger (eds.), *Geospatial Approaches to Energy Balance and Breast Cancer*, Energy Balance and Cancer 15, https://doi.org/10.1007/978-3-030-18408-7_5

level can each individually and collectively work together to impact cancer outcomes [4] and inform cancer health disparities [5]. According to a recent systematic review, even after adjustments for individual level factors, such as race/ethnicity, social and built environmental measures remain independently associated with a number of cancer types across the cancer control continuum, from risk through survival [1]. However, the strength and direction of these associations vary [1]. While these variations have been partially explained by the differential effect of specific neighborhood factors on cancer etiology across cancer types (i.e. living in higher poverty areas may play more of a role in black women with breast cancer; whereas transportation or access may be more impactful for black men with prostate cancer) [1], understanding how neighborhood exposures lead to cancer development is still being elucidated [4] and is complicated by methodological challenges that exist in the neighborhood literature.

Two of these methodologic challenges relate to variable selection and choice of geographic scale [1, 6]. In most neighborhood and cancer studies in the U.S., secondary data from the U.S. census is used to characterize neighborhood SES and physical environment at the census tract level (average population of 4000) or lower (i.e. block group level; average population of 1000) [1]. Previous studies suggest that when choosing U.S. census administrative boundaries, smaller geographies are preferred, and census tract and census block group data perform similarly in cancer association studies [6]. Thus, this chapter focuses on neighborhood studies conducted at the census tract level.

No clear consensus exists for selecting U.S. census variables to represent neighborhood SES or built environment [1, 6]. Utilizing existing ecosocial theories [7], investigators often chose different single variables from the U.S. census and/or composite variables that combine multiple SES measures (i.e. education, employment, income, poverty, etc) into a single summary score [6]. One study might define poverty as proportion of households below poverty, another as percentage receiving public assistance. This inconsistency in the choice of neighborhood measures has affected comparability and consistency across studies and has made both etiologic inferences and the translation of neighborhood findings into relevant multilevel interventions challenging [8].

5.2   In the Era of Big Data: Application of Systematic Methods

The variable selection issue in neighborhood studies will only continue to grow with advent of the "Big Data" era. Big Data has previously been defined in terms of the "3Vs": high variety, high volume, and high velocity [9]. Variety describes integrating data that were previously collected for other purposes into a single analysis file [10]. In the context of neighborhood studies, an example of variety would be the combination of U.S. Census variables with electronic medical records or cancer registry data. Volume refers to data with large data files, often with tens of thousands (or more) variables and/or observations, where the number of variables could exceed the number of observations. An example of this would be genomic data that contain millions of genetic markers [11, 12]. Velocity refers to a data creation process that is often automated or analyzed by computer algorithms to rapidly scan large data [10]. The majority of Big Data studies have been conducted within the biologic level, focusing on large scale genomic and proteomic studies that look for the association between millions of biomarkers and a disease outcome in datasets with thousands of patients [11, 12]. However, access and open availability of more sources of diverse, area-level data are becoming publicly available. Examples of neighborhood "Big Data" resources in the context of a multilevel conceptual framework are provided in (Fig. 5.1) [13–22].

As complex neighborhood data sets continue to be identified and become integrated with other neighborhood, individual, and biologic level data (Fig. 5.1), studies will increasingly begin to use secondary data sources for hypothesis-generation and to provide new insights into how neighborhood factors interact within and across levels to impact cancer. However, findings from these studies should be interpreted carefully because systematic biases often exist in secondary data due to data collection procedures [10]. Additionally, neighborhood "Big Data" will introduce magnitudes of new variables to study. At the biologic level, agnostic and empiric methods that analyze all available, existing data are often employed to systematically evaluate Big Data [23]. This is a departure from traditional neighborhood approaches that focus on testing the hypothesis that specific neighborhood factors impact cancer outcomes under existing social theories [7]. However, given that variable selection methods have traditionally varied across neighborhood studies [24], an emphasis on empirical assessments and the application of systematic variable selection methods seems warranted.

Empiric and systematic approaches from biology could be applied to neighborhood data. In genome-wide association studies (GWAS), high throughput, agnostic,

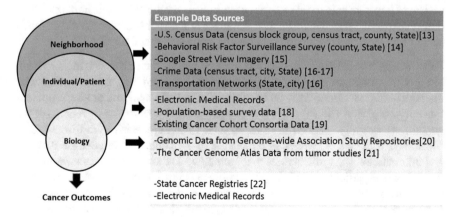

Fig. 5.1 Example multilevel, big data resources

data reduction approaches are used to rapidly scan millions of genetic markers across the whole genome to identify which genetic markers have the strongest associations with cancer and can serve as useful candidates for future clinical and multilevel research studies [23, 25]. Applying agnostic concepts from GWAS, environmental-wide association studies (EWAS) have also been developed to study the effect of exposures (i.e. pesticides) at the individual level in order to inform gene-environment interaction studies [26]. Given that neighborhood datasets are increasingly growing in size and variable selection has been an ongoing challenge, neighborhood research may also benefit from these empiric, agnostic approaches. This is because the systematic nature of agnostic approaches can allow for standardized replication [10, 27], which could improve consistency and comparability of findings across neighborhood studies. Borrowing methods and approaches from GWAS and EWAS, two neighborhood-wide association study approaches (NWAS [8] and NE-WAS, where the "E" stands for environment) have been developed, one with prostate cancer as an outcome (NWAS), and another with physical activity outcomes (NE-WAS) [28]. This chapter will review the overall study design, methods, assumptions/considerations, and limitations of current NE-WAS/NWAS, and conclude with next steps for future research.

5.3   Neighborhood-Wide Association Studies (NWAS/ NE-WAS): Overview and Study Design

Neighborhood-wide association studies (NWAS), also known as neighborhood environment-wide association studies (NE-WAS), have been developed to systematically evaluate and identify the effect of multiple neighborhood-level exposures on disease outcomes and to address gaps in neighborhood research related to empiric assessments and variable selection [24]. The NWAS/NE-WAS study design was influenced by concepts and assumptions of current GWAS. Here we present a review of key concepts in GWAS that have influenced the NWAS design, introduce the NWAS/NE-WAS design, and summarize the published NWAS/NE-WAS according to adapted evaluation criteria originally developed for GWAS.

Key Concepts in GWAS   GWAS is a high throughput, data reduction method from biology that takes an empiric, agnostic approach to studying the role of genetic markers in disease. In GWAS, up to millions of genetic markers, or single nucleotide polymorphisms (SNPs) that serve as surrogate markers for larger regions of the genome, are rapidly scanned in order to look for relationships with disease [29]. Most GWAS in cancer have been conducted in the context of large-scale national and international consortia studies that include up to thousands (and sometimes up to millions) of participants [12, 19]. Nested case-control studies are often conducted with these consortia, where standardized rules for defining binary cancer outcomes (such as risk and later stage disease) are consistently applied to help minimize information bias [19]. Big Data is typically utilized in GWAS to ensure that GWAS are powered to detect small effect estimates (typically risk estimates that are between 1.1–2, when an estimate of 1.0 signals no effect) [30]. This is because SNP markers are common in the general population (usually found at frequencies >5%). Thus, while these SNPs individually contribute to disease, they have a very small total effect on disease [31].

Linkage disequilibrium or LD is a property that describes the degree to which SNPs are correlated with one another [32]. Tag-SNPs selected as markers or independent variables in GWAS are often in LD with SNPs across larger gene regions. When a positive association between a tag-SNP and outcome is found, this could be the result of a direct association, i.e. when the tag-SNP is the true SNP associated with disease, or indirect association, when the tag-SNP is in high LD with the SNP that is truly associated [33]. Because of these two possibilities, a significant tag-SNP association from a GWAS should not be assumed as the causal variant and may require *fine-mapping* studies to map the precise location of the truly associated SNP [34].

Population stratification is another consideration in GWAS. Patterns of LD can be different across race/ethnic groups [35]. In addition to differences in tag-SNPs by race/ethnicity, there are also known differences in disease prevalence due to race/ethnicity [32]. This means in a multi-ethnic sample, SNP associations could be identified due to confounding by race/ethnicity or population stratification [32, 35]. For this reason, most GWAS are conducted within a single race/ethnic group.

The foundation of GWAS *statistical analyses* include a series of single variable statistical tests examining each gene marker or SNP in the dataset independently for an association with disease [32] (Fig. 5.2). This means there are as many statis-

Fig. 5.2 Overview of genome-wide association study (GWAS) statistical analysis and key concepts

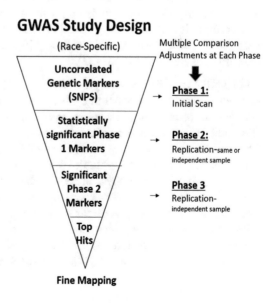

GWAS Study Design
(Race-Specific)

Multiple Comparison Adjustments at Each Phase

Uncorrelated Genetic Markers (SNPS)

Phase 1:
Initial Scan

Statistically significant Phase 1 Markers

Phase 2:
Replication-same or independent sample

Significant Phase 2 Markers

Phase 3
Replication-independent sample

Top Hits

Fine Mapping

tical tests as there are variables, so if there are 1000 SNPs in the dataset, 1000 statistical tests would be conducted. The statistical test selected depends on whether the outcome is continuous or categorical, and regression models such as linear and logistic regression are most often used [32]. A p-value, which is a measure of the probability that an association equal to or greater than the observed association would occur if there was no true association is generated for each test [36]. A smaller p-value suggests that an association is more likely to exist because the chance of seeing an association if a true association does not exist would be very small [36]. While there is debate around the issue of what p-value level should be considered "statistically significant" [37], most disease association studies select a p-value of <0.05 to indicate significance or correlation with a disease outcome. This means that 5% of the time, a disease association is detected when there really is not one (a.k.a. a false positive would be indicated 5% of the time). In a GWAS setting, thousands to millions of statistical tests are conducted, each with this own p-value. In this scenario, the likelihood of finding a false positive result is much higher; therefore, stricter p-values and adjustments for multiple testing are often employed. While a number of multiple testing approaches exist, GWAS analyses typically use a Bonferroni correction, which adjusts p-values by the number of statistical tests used (i.e. 0.05/number of statistical tests or independent variables in the data) [32].

Replication is also used to further address the issue of false positive results (Fig. 5.2). GWAS studies often employ a multi-phase approach, where in the first phase, all SNP or variable associations are assessed, and in subsequent phases, only variables that are significant after adjustments for multiple comparisons are carried forward to the next phase. Each phase can be conducted in the same study population and/or a new study population that is similar in demographics and study ascertainment to the sample population tested in the first phase [29]. Replication of findings across independent study populations that are similar to the study population of origin is a hallmark of GWAS [29]. In a GWAS setting, "top hit" variables, i.e. those SNPs identified as statistically significant, replicated SNPs, are considered to be true positive associations [32].

NWAS/NE-WAS Study Design NWAS/NE-WAS are empiric, data reduction methods derived from GWAS that have similar key concepts to address related to correlation, confounding by race, multiple comparisons, and false positives (Fig. 5.3). There are two publications related to the NWAS, each with different research questions and study populations (Table 5.1), as well as slightly different overall study designs (Fig. 5.3). Briefly, a neighborhood environment-wide (NE-WAS) study utilized physical activity data collected in 2011 from a cohort of older adults (n = 3497) in New York City, where the main outcome was a quantitative total physical activity scale for the elderly (PASE) [28]. Additional outcomes related to physical activity including walking, gardening, etc. were also analyzed, but we just report on the total physical activity score here since the goal is to focus on the overall NE-WAS design [28]. An NWAS study utilized cancer registry data

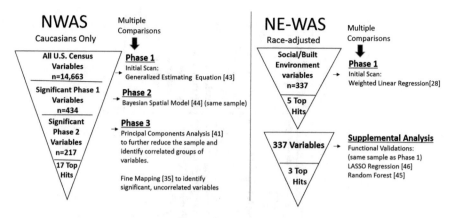

Fig. 5.3 Neighborhood-wide (NWAS) and Neighborhood environment wide (NE-WAS) association study design/study flow

from Pennsylvania (n = 77, 086) from 1995–2005, where the outcome of interest was defined in terms of case/control status. Cases were men diagnosed with >Stage 3 and > Gleason grade 7 incident, primary prostate cancer, and controls were men with <Stage 3 and/or Gleason grade 7 [8]. Most men die with and not of prostate cancer, thus it's more clinically relevant to investigate advanced prostate cancer as an outcome [8].

Both the NE-WAS and NWAS linked outcome data to neighborhood variables from the U.S. Census, but at different geographies. The NE-WAS also included additional neighborhood sources, such as transportation network and crime data, and looked for differences in findings by network buffers (0.25 km and 1.0 km), analyzing a total of 337 neighborhood variables [28]. The NWAS analyzed all available U.S. Census data (n = 14,663) from the Year 2000 Summary Files 1 and 3 at the census tract level [8, 38] to look for association with aggressive prostate cancer. Thus, the NWAS is a more traditional empiric approach because the full data is used and variables are not selected prior to analysis.

Correlation of U.S. Census variables is a well-known methodologic concern in neighborhood analyses. The correlation structure of neighborhood variables is generally known to be strong, convoluted, and difficult to tease apart since these neighborhood variables are inter-related both statistically and etiologically [39]. For instance one can imagine how employment could impact both income and poverty, which are each separate neighborhood domains. While correlation structures are generally known for GWAS SNPs, they are not well-characterized for neighborhood data. Thus, if a neighborhood variable is identified as significant in an analysis, it is difficult to determine whether this is a direct or indirect association, i.e. whether that particular neighborhood variable, or a variable it is highly correlated with, is responsible for the association. In the NWAS, correlation among variables

Table 5.1 Study design and methods overview for neighborhood wide (NWAS) and neighborhood environment-wide association studies (NE-WAS)

	Design	Location	Level of geography	Neighborhood variables	Outcome(s)	Statistical analysis
NWAS [8]	Case-control design	Pennsylvania	Census tract	14,663 Year 2000 U.S. Census Variables	Aggressive prostate Cancer cases (>stage 3 & Gleason 7; n = 6416 cases) vs controls (<stage 3/ Gleason 7; n = 70, 670)	Multiphase, successively more stringent statistical models-odds ratios (OR) reported (Fig. 5.3)
NE-WAS [28]	Cross-sectional	New York City, NY	Network buffer size (0.25 km/1 km)	337 variables from: −2006-2010 U.S. Census American community survey; -street layouts and NY transit reports; −crime data (ESRI; New York state); −park/recreation measures (NYC)	Total physical activity score for the elderly (PASE; n = 3497); (other activity measures not presented here)	Single phase weighted linear regression (correlations reported) (Fig. 5.3)

was accounted for during Phase 3 of the analysis by first running a principal components analysis to identify groups of correlated neighborhood variables [40]. Next a "fine-mapping" approach was applied where the most significant variable (after adjustment for multiple comparisons) within each component was selected as a final study "top hit" or significant variable (Fig. 5.3) [8, 34]. In the NE-WAS, investigating correlation structure of neighborhood predictors was listed as outside the study scope, but was stressed as an important future area of study [28]. At the neighborhood level, there are known differences in cancer disease rates by race/ethnicity and certain race/ethnic groups are more likely to live in neighborhoods with poor built and social environmental characteristics [41]. Thus, to address *confounding by race*, the NWAS, like GWAS was conducted within a single race/ethnic group [8]. In the NE-WAS, race/ethnicity was adjusted for in the statistical model [28].

At the *statistical analysis* phase, both the NE-WAS and NWAS completed an initial scan of all available neighborhood variables, using a Bonferroni correction to minimize false positives. The NE-WAS used weighted linear regression models for analysis in a single phase for each network buffer area [28]; whereas the NWAS used generalized estimating equation (GEE) models that took into account clustering by census tract in Phase 1 [8, 42]. To further minimize false positives and account for the unique geospatial considerations associated with using neighborhood data, in Phase 2 of the NWAS, significant findings from Phase 1 were then tested in the same study population using a more stringent, Bayesian hierarchal logistic regression model that allowed for adjustment of spatial random effects [8, 43] (Fig. 5.3). Final variables were then selected in Phase 3 during fine mapping [8].

Replication in the NWAS/NE-WAS setting is challenging [47] and findings in both studies were not replicated in an independent study population [8]. Use of independent datasets across cities or States to validate findings may mask real differences between neighborhood variables and outcomes because geographic areas and the social and built environmental conditions in those geographies are so different. However, while comparisons across geographical areas may be difficult, they should be undertaken to continue to test the utility of NWAS/NE-WAS approaches. When traditional replication studies are not viable, under certain circumstances, a single discovery phase [44] and other biologic or functional-based approaches may be favored over statistical replication [45]. An example of functional validation study would be the comparison of neighborhood findings across different methodologies within the same study population to determine replication potential.

5.4   NWAS and NE-WAS Results and Discussion

The NWAS and NE-WAS study designs and results have been standardized across the two studies to more generally discuss the findings and utility of these two empiric approaches (Fig. 5.3 and Table 5.2). Starting with close to 15,000 variables,

Table 5.2 Summary of significant variables in the NWAS and NE-WAS by direction of association (+ or -)

NWAS variables associated with aggressive prostate cancer		NE-WAS variables associated with total physical activity score for the elderly	
1. %white alone population for whom poverty status is determined age 6–11 years	+		
2. %white, non-hispanics where poverty status determined aged 18–64 below poverty	+	1. People living in households with incomes below the poverty line	−
3. % male nonfamily households below poverty	+		
4. %male householder living alone (nonfamily household)	+		
5. % renter occupied housing unit built 1939 or earlier with householder aged 15–24 years	+	2. No problems with windows in The New York City Housing and Vacancy survey	+
6. Imputed civilian non-institutionalized population 5 years and older	+		
7. %household income $60 K-74,999	−	3. People living in households with incomes more than twice the poverty level	+
8. %foreign born naturalized citizen at or above poverty level	−		
9. %household income $10 K-19,999 with owner-occupied housing unit value of $10 K-19,999	+		
10. % where the ratio of income to poverty level for persons aged 45–54 years, under 0.50	+	4. People living in households with incomes less than half the poverty level	−
11. Aggregate household income of renter occupied housing units with householders 15–34 that were built 1940–1949	+		
12. %workers 16 years and over taking public transportation, namely trolley or street cars, to work	+	5. People living in households with incomes between half and three-quarters of the poverty level	−
13. %renter occupied housing units with householder aged 55–64 with no vehicle	+		
14. %male protective service occupations: Fire-fighting, prevention, law enforcement workers	−		
15. %males with earnings of $7500–9999 in 1999	+		
16. %male householder over 65 living alone in nonfamily household	+		
17. % 1 unit detached or attached household renters aged 55–64 years	+		

the NWAS identified 17 variables significantly associated with prostate cancer aggressiveness. Like GWAS, the NWAS top hits or variables that remained statistically significant across the 3 phases, generally had small effect sizes, with odd ratios or disease risks ranging from 0.93–1.08 [8]. Previous studies of neighborhood and prostate cancer have found that neighborhoods with poor socioeconomic (SES) circumstances and housing environments [46] are related to high-grade prostate cancer [41], independent of individual-level exposures [47, 48]. The NWAS findings are biologically plausible and support literature in that variables representing both single and combined domains related to social and built environment (Table 5.2) were associated with prostate cancer aggressiveness. These included poverty/income (NWAS variables # 1, 2, 3, 7, 9, 10, 15), employment and/or transportation (NWAS variables #12, 14) housing and/or transportation (#13), renting vs owning a house (#5, 9, 11, 17), and immigration/social support (#4, 8, 16). The difference between NWAS and previous study findings is that the NWAS identified more complex, joint effect variables that, for instance, combined race, age, and poverty information into a single variable; previous studies select variables that generally represent one domain [41]. Thus, given the fine mapping approach identified variables that had the strongest statistical association with disease, after accounting for correlation of neighborhood factors, it is possible that the more complex variables from NWAS could be hypothesis-generating and could be indicative of interactions that may exist among demographic domains that are often considered individually in current neighborhood studies [10]. However, it is also possible that given the size of the neighborhood data, the complexity of the correlation structure of the variables, and the inability to fully adjust for individual level socioeconomic factors, some associations could have been identified due to confounding. Based on previous studies, with large-scale, highly correlated data, there is a greater chance that agnostic approaches could be identifying strongly confounded variables [28]. Further, the NWAS was conducted in White men, and given the association between neighborhood, black race/ethnicity, and prostate, future NWAS in Black men are also warranted [47, 48].

The NE-WAS variables, which were selected based on data availability, include social/built environment variables commonly used in neighborhood studies that often represent single socioeconomic domains [6], i.e. income or housing. Given neighborhood variables in the NE-WAS were pre-selected, it does not take a purely empiric approach, like the NWAS, which utilized all available U.S. Census Data. The NE-WAS identified 5 neighborhood SES variables that were most significantly associated with PASE (Table 5.2). These findings are also biologically plausible given older adults from higher socioeconomic backgrounds are more likely to exercise and both utilize and invest in the neighborhood environment [49]. The NE-WAS included data collected at the individual level, thus, this analysis was able to adjust for additional individual SES factors that could impact associations, including age, income, education, race/ethnicity and home size. Further, the NE-WAS had additional data sources to address the issue of confounding in agnostic investigations by including a negative control, or an outcome not believed to be associated with neighborhood, in order to determine the effect of residual confounding in the study [50]. However, accounting for the correlation structure of the neighborhood data was not a main consideration in the NE-WAS analysis.

Traditional replication of findings in a separate study population was not conducted in either the NWAS or NE-WAS. In the NWAS, a multiphase approach was employed with successively more stringent statistical models to identify associations. As a secondary analysis, in NE-WAS, different geographic buffers were compared in the same study population and found to have comparable results [28]. Additionally, other empiric methods were explored as a functional validation in the NE-WAS study population. Random forest [51] and LASSO regression [52] are empiric, Big Data, machine learning approaches [53]. Random forest identified numerous variables within the same domain (related to mostly to housing), and was thus sensitive to the correlation structure of the data. However, in LASSO regression, which does consider correlation structure during model-building, 2 of the 5 top neighborhood hits from the primary NE-WAS design replicated (NE-WAS variables #4, 5 from Table 5.2) . Interestingly, despite different research questions and study design approaches, both the NE-WAS and NWAS found associations in the expected direction for neighborhoods where household incomes were less than half the poverty level (overall for NE-WAS and for persons aged 45–54 for NWAS) and for people living in households with incomes below the poverty line for NE-WAS (For NWAS: White, Non-Hispanics living below poverty aged 18–64). Although physical activity and older age are both associated with cancer, physical activity is not a known risk factor for prostate cancer [54]. Further, it's premature to speculate what this could mean from a causal standpoint, but from a replication standpoint, these similarities in neighborhood findings across the NWAS and NE-WAS appear promising.

5.5 Future Directions

The NE-WAS and NWAS have the ability to systematically identify neighborhood variables. Thus, these methods can be useful for variable selection in future studies that utilize large-scale built and social environmental data from the U.S. census and other sources. Further, NWAS/NE-WAS have the potential to improve reproducibility across studies by identifying consistent patterns in associations across different study populations [28]. Given the potential utility of these approaches, NWAS/NE-WAS should continue to be developed and tested in the context of other studies. However, systematic, empiric methods in neighborhood research and NWAS/NE-WAS designs are in their infancy and still being refined. Thus, moving forward, we propose that future NWAS/NE-WAS continue to address (and be evaluated according to) the following series of questions. These questions were adapted from existing evaluation criteria for genetic investigations [27, 29], and were derived from lessons-learned during the review of current NWAS/NE-WAS designs.

Evaluation Criteria for future NWAS/NE-WAS studies:

- Are outcomes defined clearly and reliably to allow for translation across clinical, population-based, and community studies? This question is meant to help minimize misclassification and to improve eventual translation of findings across study populations.

- In the context of case and control data, are participants comparable to each other on important characteristics that might be affecting both the neighborhood exposure and the disease?, i.e. Were confounding effects considered, particularly those by race/ethnicity?
- Is the study adequately powered to detect small effect sizes, given neighborhood influences generally have small effects?
- Is the correlation structure of neighborhood variables adequately addressed in the study design?
- Were appropriate quality control and sensitivity analyses conducted and discussed, including assessments of both missing data and potential study bias related to data collection procedures?
- Were corrections made for multiple comparisons?
- Did the study detect associations with previously reported neighborhood variables to support potential biologic plausibility?
- Were the results replicated in an independent study sample or was an appropriate functional validation study (i.e. comparison of different methods in at the same study sample) conducted?

Both the NWAS and NE-WAS designs generally address these criteria (Table 5.3), but additional research is needed to address challenges related to correlation, replication, and functional validation. Replication can be addressed as more studies apply and adapt the NWAS approach to unique datasets. Machine Learning approaches can assist in investigating issues related to multicollinearity and functional validation. Broadly speaking, machine learning models are empiric, Big Data approaches that utilize computer algorithms to systematically identify data patterns that can then be used to select variables that independently, and in conjunction with other variables, best predict disease outcomes [10]. Some machine learning approaches, such as LASSO regression, and principal components can account for data correlation structure. The NWAS applied principal components in Phase 3 of the analysis; however, future NWAS may look into modeling components prior to the initial scan to more aggressively reduce multicollinearity and data complexity, similar to the GWAS design. Additionally, in the NE-WAS, the LASSO machine learning approach, which accounts for correlation among variables when selecting predictors [52], also showed promise as a potential functional validation/replication step. However, it is still not known how well LASSO approaches account for the complex correlation found in neighborhood research. Other machine learning approaches, including multi-dimension reduction type methods [55], may also be explored to provide additional insights into not only correlation structure, but complex interactions between neighborhood variables that might influence study associations and comparisons of findings across studies. This is because part of the challenge in applying empiric methods to neighborhood data is that the mechanisms for how neighborhood factors interact with one another is complex and not well

Table 5.3 Evaluation of NWAS and NE-WAS study deigns

	Outcome clearly defined	Adequate power	Correlation considered	Confounding considered	Quality control	Multiple comparison adjustments	Plausible results?	Replication	Functional validation
NWAS [8]	Yes	Yes, to detect effect sizes or odds ratios of 1.01	Yes; phase 3	Adjusted for age and diagnosis year; stratified by race	Yes; missing data reported	Yes, Bonferroni adjustments	Yes	Not in an independent sample	No, future studies needed
NE-WAS [28]	Yes	Yes, to detect a change of 3.5 total PASE or 10 min of walking/day	Somewhat in functional validation	Adjusted for age, income, education, race, home size; negative confounding explored	Yes; missing data reported	Yes, Bonferroni adjustments	Yes	Not in an independent sample	Yes, utilized machine learning methods in the sample study sample

understood [10]. Thus, it is difficult to interpret the relevance of study findings from empiric approaches, not only from an etiologic standpoint, but also from a statistical standpoint [39], given false positive results are also a concern in an agnostic setting [56]. Given this, the use of simulated datasets, where the correlation structure and "true associations" can be pre-determined, may be useful to provide insights into which methods or combinations of methods, could be standardized in future neighborhood research. Further, NWAS/NE-WAS and other related empiric approaches are meant to be hypothesis-generating and significant findings from these studies should be followed up in more traditional, multilevel studies focused on hypothesis testing and etiologic inference [39]. This is because distinguishing between a highly replicable finding, and a finding with potential clinical or intervention importance is critical to goals of the Precision Medicine Initiative [57, 58].

The Precision Medicine Initiative calls for the consideration of not just a person's genes and lifestyle, but also environment, when making treatment and screening decisions. However, rarely is environment considered in clinical decision-making [57, 58]. This is because the translation of neighborhood findings to the clinic have been complicated by the inconsistencies in neighborhood literature and the differences in variable selection across studies. Understanding which neighborhood factors are most clinically relevant could potentially improve patient care, particularly by identifying those patients who are likely to have a poor cancer outcome because they may be on a disparity-related pathway to disease. This is because neighborhood is a measure of health disparities, and many cancers, including prostate cancer, are heavily affected by differences in SES and access to care [59]. In recognition of the importance of the impact of neighborhood and social determinants of health, the National Academies of Sciences, Engineering, and Medicine have recommended social and behavioral measures that should be incorporated in electronic health records as standards [60], and healthcare systems are increasingly recognizing the need to address neighborhood and social environmental factors to promote health and wellness [61].

Further, given the geospatial nature of neighborhood variables, it is also possible that improvements in variable selection could lead to improvements in community level intervention efforts. This is because neighborhood factors that are most significantly related to a disease outcome could be geospatially mapped to identify target neighborhoods for cancer education or screening interventions, a concept known as precision prevention [57, 58]. As an illustration, percentage of workers in a census tract is a standard variable used to represent employment. NWAS identified percentage of workers taking trolley or street cars to work as a top hit, which is a more specific, combination variable representing employment and transportation. Given the NWAS variable is a more complex measure, and thus rarer in the population, this information could potentially be used to identify fewer target areas for intervention compared to a standard variable. This is particularly useful if intervention resources are limited (Fig. 5.4).

In conclusion, NWAS/NE-WAS are promising new approaches designed to empirically identify neighborhood factors that are most strongly related to disease. While NWAS/NE-WAS should continue to be tested in other study populations, these approaches demonstrate potential to address methodological limitations in

• NWAS Top Hit

%Workers 16 and over public transport to work

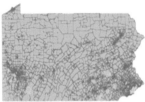

• Standard Variable

% Workers 16 and over

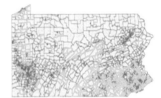

N=66 Census Tracts
(highlighted in blue)

N=472 Census Tracts
(highlighted in blue)

Fig. 5.4 Identification of Census Tracts(black boundaries) above the Pennsylvania State Median for the NWAS and Standard Variable: Example of how NWAS approaches, once replicated or functionally validated, can inform intervention efforts

current neighborhood studies related to systematic variable selection. Further, NWAS/NE-WAS approaches are likely to inform efforts in precision medicine [62], and could have implications for future, multilevel, health disparity studies across a number of cancer sites [8].

References

1. Gomez SL, Shariff-Marco S, DeRouen M, Keegan THM, Yen IH, Mujahid M, et al. The impact of neighborhood social and built environment factors across the cancer continuum: current research, methodological considerations, and future directions. Cancer. 2015;121(14):2314–30.
2. Yen IH, Syme SL. The social environment and health: a discussion of the epidemiologic literature. Annu Rev Public Health. 1999;20(1):287–308.
3. Jackson RJ. The impact of the built environment on health: an emerging field. Am J Public Health. 2003;93(9):1382–4.
4. Lynch SM, Rebbeck TR. Bridging the gap between biologic, individual, and macroenvironmental factors in Cancer: a multilevel approach. Cancer Epidemiol Biomark Prev. 2013; 22(4):485–95.
5. Warnecke RB, Oh A, Breen N, Gehlert S, Paskett E, Tucker KL, et al. Approaching health disparities from a population perspective: the National Institutes of Health centers for population health and health disparities. Am J Public Health. 2008;98(9):1608–15.
6. Krieger N, Chen JT, Waterman PD, Soobader M-J, Subramanian SV, Carson R. Geocoding and monitoring of US socioeconomic inequalities in mortality and Cancer incidence: does the choice of area-based measure and geographic level matter? The public health disparities geocoding project. Am J Epidemiol. 2002;156(5):471–82.
7. Krieger N. Theories for social epidemiology in the 21st century: an ecosocial perspective. Int J Epidemiol. 2001;30(4):668–77.
8. Lynch SM, Mitra N, Ross M, Newcomb C, Dailey K, Jackson T, et al. A Neighborhood-Wide Association Study (NWAS): example of prostate cancer aggressiveness. PLoS One. 2017;12(3):e0174548.

9. Weber GM, Mandl KD, Kohane IS. Finding the missing link for big biomedical data. JAMA. 2014;311(24):2479–80.
10. Mooney SJ, Westreich DJ, El-Sayed AM. Commentary: Epidemiology in the era of big data. Epidemiology. 2015;26(3):390–4.
11. Low S-K, Zembutsu H, Nakamura Y. Breast cancer: the translation of big genomic data to cancer precision medicine. Cancer Sci. 2018;109(3):497–506.
12. Kar SP, Beesley J, Amin Al Olama A, Michailidou K, Tyrer J, Kote-Jarai Z, et al. Genome-wide meta-analyses of breast, ovarian, and prostate Cancer association studies identify multiple new susceptibility loci shared by at least two Cancer types. Cancer Discov. 2016;6(9):1052–67.
13. U.S. Census Data [Internet]. United States Census Bureau. 2010 cited Accessed 11 Sept 2018.
14. Behavioral Risk Factor Surveillance Data [Internet]. Center for disease control. 2010–2017 cited 21 Sept 2018. Available from https://www.cdc.gov/brfss/data_documentation/index.htm.
15. Google Imagery [Internet]. Google, Inc. 2018 cited 11 Oct 2018. Available from https://lp.google-mkto.com/Google-imagery.html.
16. Open Data Philly [Internet]. 2018 cited 11 Oct 2018. Available from https://www.opendata-philly.org/.
17. Crime Data [Internet]. ESRI. 2018 cited 15 Oct 2018. Available from https://doc.arcgis.com/en/esri-demographics/data/crime-indexes.htm.
18. Community Health Database [Internet]. Public health management corporation. 2016 [cited 16 June 2016]. Available from http://chdb.phmc.org/.
19. National Cancer Institute(NCI) Division of Cancer Control and Population Sciences. NCI cohort consortium. Bethesda, MD. 1 Dec 2018. Available from https://epi.grants.cancer.gov/Consortia/cohort.html#proposing.
20. MacArthur JBE, Cerezo M, Gil L, Hall P, Hastings E, Junkins H, McMahon A, Milano A, Morales J, Pendlington Z, Welter D, Burdett T, Hindorff L, Flicek P, Cunningham F, Parkinson H. The new NHGRI-EBI Catalog of published genome-wide association studies (GWAS Catalog). Nucleic Acids Res. 2017;45(Database Issue):D896–901.
21. The Cancer Genome Atlas [Internet]. 2018 [cited 12 Nov 2018]. Available from https://tcga-data.nci.nih.gov/docs/publications/tcga/?
22. Surveillance, Epidemiology, and End Results (SEER) Program [Internet]. National Cancer Institute, DCCPS, Surveillance Research Program. 1973–2015 [cited 1 Dec 2018]. Available from https://seer.cancer.gov/data/.
23. Varghese JS, Easton DF. Genome-wide association studies in common cancers—what have we learnt? Curr Opin Genet Dev. 2010;20(3):201–9.
24. Sampson RJ, Morenoff JD, Gannon-Rowley T. Assessing Neighborhood Effects: social processes and new directions in research. Annu Rev Sociol. 2002;28:443–78.
25. Eeles RA, Kote-Jarai Z, Giles GG, Olama AA, Guy M, Jugurnauth SK, et al. Multiple newly identified loci associated with prostate cancer susceptibility. Nat Genet. 2008;40(3):316–21.
26. Patel CJ, Bhattacharya J, Butte AJ. An Environment-Wide Association Study (EWAS) on type 2 diabetes mellitus. PLoS One. 2010;5(5):e10746.
27. Ioannidis JPA, Loy EY, Poulton R, Chia KS. Researching genetic versus nongenetic determinants of disease: a comparison and proposed unification. Sci Transl Med. 2009;1(7):7ps8.
28. Mooney SJ, Joshi S, Cerdá M, Kennedy GJ, Beard JR, Rundle AG. Contextual correlates of physical activity among older adults: a neighborhood environment-wide association study (NE-WAS). Cancer Epidemiol Biomark Prev. 2017;26(4):495–504.
29. Pearson TA, Manolio TA. How to interpret a genome-wide association study. JAMA. 2008;299(11):1335–44.
30. Hindorff LA, Sethupathy P, Junkins HA, Ramos EM, Mehta JP, Collins FS, et al. Potential etiologic and functional implications of genome-wide association loci for human diseases and traits. Proc Natl Acad Sci USA. 2009;106(23):9362–7.
31. Reich DE, Lander ES. On the allelic spectrum of human disease. Trends Genet. 2001;17(9):502–10.

32. Bush WS, Moore JH. Chapter 11: genome-wide association studies. PLoS Comput Biol. 2012; 8(12):e1002822.
33. Hirschhorn JN, Daly MJ. Genome-wide association studies for common diseases and complex traits. Nat Rev Genet. 2005;6:95–108.
34. Meuwissen TH, Goddard ME. Fine mapping of quantitative trait loci using linkage disequilibria with closely linked marker loci. Genetics. 2000;155(1):421–30.
35. Wang Y, Localio R, Rebbeck TR. Evaluating Bias due to population stratification in epidemiologic studies of gene-gene or gene-environment interactions. Cancer Epidemiol Biomark Prev. 2006;15(1):124–32.
36. Benjamin DJ, Berger JO, Johannesson M, Nosek BA, Wagenmakers EJ, Berk R, et al. Redefine statistical significance. Nat Hum Behav. 2018;2(1):6–10.
37. Chawla DS. "One-size-fits-all" threshold for P values under fire. Nature News [Internet] 2017. Available from https://www.nature.com/news/one-size-fits-all-threshold-for-p-values-under-fire-1.22625#/ref-link-2.
38. Year 2000 US. Census SF1 and SF3 Form variables [Internet] 2014. cited 1 Jan 2014. Available from http://www.socialexplorer.com.
39. Oakes JM. The (mis)estimation of neighborhood effects: causal inference for a practicable social epidemiology. Soc Sci Med. 2004;58(10):1929–52. https://doi.org/10.1016/j.socscimed.2003.08.004.
40. Messer L, Laraia B, Kaufman J, Eyster J, Holzman C, Culhane J, et al. The development of a standard neighborhood deprivation index. J Urban Health. 2006;83(6):1041–62.
41. Diez Roux AV, Mair C. Neighborhoods and health. Ann NY Acad Sci. 2010;1186(1):125–45.
42. Hubbard AE, Ahern J, Fleischer NL, Laan MV, Lippman SA, Jewell N, et al. To GEE or not to GEE: comparing population average and mixed models for estimating the associations between neighborhood risk factors and health. Epidemiology. 2010;21(4):467–74.
43. Ru H, Martino S. Approximate Bayesian inference for latent Gaussian models by using integrated nested Laplace approximations. J R Stat Soc Ser B Stat Methodol. 2008;71(2):319–92.
44. Thomas DC, Casey G, Conti DV, Haile RW, Lewinger JP, Stram DO. Methodological issues in multistage genome-wide association studies. Stat Sci Review J Inst Math Stat. 2009;24(4):414–29.
45. Aslibekyan S, Claas SA, Arnett DK. To replicate or not to replicate: the case of Pharmacogenetic studies: establishing validity of Pharmacogenomic findings: from replication to triangulation. Circ Cardiovasc Genet. 2013;6(4):409–12.
46. Thomson H, Thomas S, Sellstrom E, Petticrew M. Housing improvements for health and associated socio-economic outcomes. Cochrane Database Syst Rev. 2013;
47. Zeigler-Johnson C, Tierney A, Rebbeck TR, Rundle A. Prostate Cancer severity associations with neighborhood deprivation. Prostate Cancer. 2011;2011:1–9.
48. Carpenter W, Howard D, Taylor Y, Ross L, Wobker S, Godley P. Racial differences in PSA screening interval and stage at diagnosis. Cancer Causes Control. 2010;21(7):1071–80.
49. Kamphuis CB. Socioeconomic differences in lack of recreational walking among older adults: the role of neighbourhood and individual factors. Int J Behav Nutr Phys Act. 2009;6(1)
50. Lipsitch M, Tchetgen Tchetgen E, Cohen T. Negative controls: a tool for detecting confounding and bias in observational studies. Epidimiology. 2010;21(3):383–8.
51. Breiman L. Random forests. Mach Learn. 2001;45(1):5–32.
52. Tibshirani R. Regression shrinkage and selection via the lasso. J R Stat Soc Ser B Methodol. 1996;58:267–88.
53. Olson RS, La Cava W, Mustahsan Z, Varik A, Moore JH. Data-driven advice for applying machine learning to bioinformatics problems. Pac Symp Biocomput. 2018;23:192–203.
54. LoConte NK, Gershenwald JE, Thomson CA, Crane TE, Harmon GE, Rechis R. Lifestyle modifications and policy implications for primary and secondary Cancer prevention: diet, exercise, sun safety, and alcohol reduction. Am Soc Clin Oncol Educ Book. 2018;38:88–100.
55. Urbanowicz RJ, Moore JH. ExSTraCS 2.0: description and evaluation of a scalable learning Classifer system. Evol Intel. 2015;8(2.3):89–116.

56. Ioannidis J. This I believe in genetics: discovery can be a nuisance, replication is science, implementation matters. Front Genet. 2013;4:33.
57. Collins FS, Varmus H. A new initiative on precision medicine. N Engl J Med. 2015;372(9):793–5.
58. Rebbeck TR. Precision prevention of Cancer. Cancer Epidemiol Biomark Prev. 2014;23: 2713–5.
59. O'Keefe EB, Meltzer JP. Health Disparities and Cancer: Racial Disparities in Cancer Mortality in the United States, 2000–2010. Frontiers in public health. 2015;3:51.
60. Institute of Medicine (IOM). Capturing social and behavioral domains and measures in electronic health records: Phase 2. Washington, DC: National Academies Press; 2014.
61. Cowley D. New Alliance seeks to promote health and prevent illness by addressing social determinants of health in Ogden, St George Utah 2018. Available from https://intermountain-healthcare.org/news/2018/06/new-alliance-seeks-to-promote-health-and-prevent-illness-by-addressing-social-determinants-of-health-in-ogden-st-george/.
62. Lynch SM, Moore JH. A call for biological data mining approaches in epidemiology. BioData mining. 2016;9(1):1.

Chapter 6
Geospatial Approaches to Environmental Determinants of Breast Cancer in the California Teachers Study

Peggy Reynolds, Susan Hurley, Julie Von Behren, and David O. Nelson

Abstract With the increasing availability of georeferenced data about people and places there are expanded opportunities to assess risk relationships for disease outcomes associated with living in areas impacted by adverse environmental insults. For the most part, particularly for cancer outcomes, estimates of exposures have been based upon a single address and single point in time, and for which traditional epidemiologic methods such as interview may be impractical for assessing earlier residences in large scale studies. Likewise environmental data are often not available for specific time periods of interest or at an appropriate geographic scale for epidemiologic studies. Using an example from the California Teachers Study (CTS), a large statewide prospective study of women, we sought to develop strategies to assess temporal and spatial changes in participant residences, temporal changes in ambient air pollutants, and the intersection between the two in time and space to form a basis for future risk analyses. Key findings suggest the importance of careful attention to data quality, to assumptions about data gaps, and the influence of modeling decisions. Nonetheless, these efforts show promise for future environmental health research.

Keywords Record linkage · GIS · Breast cancer · Residential history · Air pollution

P. Reynolds (✉) · S. Hurley · J. Von Behren
University of California San Francisco, San Francisco, CA, USA
e-mail: peggy.reynolds@ucsf.edu

D. O. Nelson
Cancer Prevention Institute of California, Fremont, CA, USA

© Springer Nature Switzerland AG 2019   119
D. Berrigan, N. A. Berger (eds.), *Geospatial Approaches to Energy Balance and Breast Cancer*, Energy Balance and Cancer 15, https://doi.org/10.1007/978-3-030-18408-7_6

6.1   Section I: Introduction

Where a woman lives is one of the strongest predictors of her breast cancer risk. Breast cancer incidence rates vary several-fold across regions of the world, with rates highest among westernized, urban and industrialized areas and the lowest in rural, developing parts of Asia and Africa [1–8]. Within the U.S. similar, albeit less dramatic, geographic patterns exist with elevated incidence rates in urban compared to rural areas [6, 7]. Although long-recognized, these geographic disparities remain poorly understood. Geographic differences in culturally-based behavioral risk factors (e.g., diet, alcohol consumption, smoking, child bearing and breastfeeding practices, etc.) are likely to play a role [2, 9] but they do not, however, appear to fully-explain regional disparities in breast cancer incidence [6, 7]. These observations have led to interest in the potential role of environmental factors in the disease's etiology [10–12].

Broadly speaking, environmental factors of importance may include both contextual features of the built environment that may indirectly impact breast cancer risk by mediating risk-related behaviors (e.g., neighborhood 'walkability' that might influence physical activity level or neighborhood density of fast-food outlets that could affect diet), as well as elements of the physical environment that may more directly impact risk (e.g., chemical contaminants in ambient air or drinking water, light-at-night). For the purpose of the current chapter, we will focus our discussion on an example for studying the latter. Ascertainment of these types of exposures via traditional epidemiologic methods such as interviews, questionnaires and biomonitoring, often is not feasible in large-scale cohort studies. Such exposures typically are involuntary and invisible, rendering them impossible to self-report. While there may be laboratory methods available to measure biomarkers of exposure for some environmental exposures of interest, often such biomarkers are not reflective of chronic exposures or exposures from earlier in life that may be most etiologically-relevant for cancer. Furthermore, the collection of biological specimens and the conduct of biomarker assays can be prohibitively expensive and time-consuming for large cohort studies. Thus, geospatial methods for exposure assessment offer an attractive alternative approach.

Geospatial approaches to explore environmental determinants of disease typically use geographic information system (GIS) tools to link geographic location (usually residences) of study participants to existing data resources to characterize potential environmental exposures [13–15]. While offering a number of advantages over more traditional epidemiologic methods, these approaches are not without their own set of challenges. Because these methods often rely on data resources that were not collected specifically for the purposes of health research, there are often a number of limitations to their use (Table 6.1).

These common data limitations can be especially problematic in studying cancer, for which chronic long-term exposures are likely to be of importance, and particularly for breast cancer, for which windows of vulnerability to exposures experienced early in life (in utero, puberty, childbearing years) may be especially

Table 6.1 Summary of common limitations to data available for geospatial approaches to explore environmental determinants of breast cancer risk

Data on participant location	Environmental exposure data
Limited to residential location – lack of information on workplace locations or other locations where participants may spend significant time	Limited quantitative information – insufficient information on dose or level of exposure for specific chemicals or agents of interest
Limited temporal coverage – often available at only one point in time (e.g. residence at time of diagnosis or study enrollment), no historical data	Limited temporal coverage – often lacks historical information that might be most etiologically relevant
	Limited geographic coverage – incomplete and missing data
	Insufficient geographic scale – scale may be not be relevant to estimating personal exposures

relevant [16–20]. This chapter describes and discusses a number of approaches we have developed to overcome some of these challenges in our efforts to identify environmental determinants of breast cancer in the California Teachers Study (CTS), a large, on-going prospective cohort study of nearly 134,000 California women [21]. Established in 1995–1996 specifically to study breast cancer, the CTS has proven to be a valuable resource not only for exploring and identifying personal breast cancer risk factors [22–32], but for conducting a number of preliminary analyses of environmental determinants of breast cancer and other disease outcomes [33–39]. These preliminary efforts, however, have generally been hindered by the challenges imposed by the limitations of existing data, as summarized in Table 6.1.

This chapter describes a number of approaches we have developed to overcome some of these challenges in our efforts to identify environmental determinants of breast cancer in the CTS, including:

• Approaches to develop residential histories (Section II)
• Approaches to develop environmental exposure measures (Section III)
• Approaches to integrate residential histories with environmental exposure measures (Section IV)

To illustrate these approaches, we use as an example our efforts to characterize exposures to hazardous air pollutants in our examination of risks for breast cancer in the CTS. Extension of these approaches in other cohort studies could be fruitful, especially in the future, as the availability of electronic publically-available georeferenced exposure data for etiologically relevant time periods grows.

6.2   Section II: Development of Residential Histories

Like most large-scale prospective cohort studies, address information has been collected for CTS members for the purpose of continued follow-up and study contact. In addition to changes in address received from direct contact with CTS participants, these addresses are compiled through a variety of other means, including linkages to US Postal Service change-of-address forms, as well as through routine linkages to major credit reporting companies. While the CTS has compiled a dataset of over 250,000 addresses for its members since its inception in 1995, these data have a number of limitations for the construction of lifetime residential histories. Because addresses are collected and maintained for the primary purpose of contacting CTS members for their continued participation in the study, they are mailing addresses and do not necessarily represent residential locations but may be post office boxes, or addresses for second/vacation homes, or workplaces. Furthermore, the dates associated with the addresses are not necessarily representative of 'move-in' and 'move-out' dates but rather capture a variety of dates, depending on the source of the address update (e.g. the date a participant submitted her US Postal Service change-of-address form, the date the study center received a returned questionnaire from the Post Office indicating the participant had moved, etc.). Although not without limitations, this existing address information collected during the nearly 25 years of the CTS offers a valuable resource for the construction of residential histories from which estimates of chronic exposures from georeferenced environmental data potentially could be based. However, the lack of address information prior to the initiation of the study, represents a major obstacle to characterizing earlier life exposures associated with residential location during potentially important windows of susceptibility that may be most etiologically relevant to breast cancer.

With funding from the National Cancer Institute (NCI), we explored a variety of approaches to augment the existing CTS address information in an effort to build more complete residential histories (see Fig. 6.1). As described in the following sections, these efforts yielded promising, if not somewhat limited, results.

6.2.1   Linkage to Consumer Reporting Data

Consumer reporting companies collect, maintain and sell data on individuals for the purposes of generating reports that help inform financial, employment, insurance, and other decisions about individuals [40]. In the U.S. there are dozens of consumer reporting companies, of which Equifax, Experian, and TransUnion are perhaps the most widely-known. Similar to an earlier analyses conducted by Jacquez and colleagues [14], who to our knowledge, were the first to use consumer reporting data to construct residential histories for participants in a cancer study, we chose to use LexisNexis (a division of RELX, Inc., Dayton, Ohio) [41].

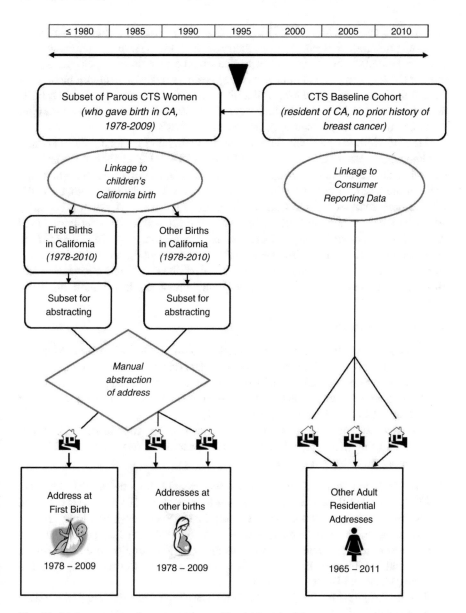

Fig. 6.1 Linkage strategy for constructing residential location history

Among its services, LexisNexis will provide all known addresses for a requested set of individuals for a relatively modest fee. Although the algorithm used by LexisNexis is proprietary, it considers myriad data sources to compile addresses, including: real estate/tax assessor records (current and archived); deed transfers and mortgage records; motor vehicle, boat, and aircraft registrations; driver license records; court filings, including bankruptcy and Uniform Commercial Code (UCC) judgment records and federal and state tax liens, jury verdicts, settlement and arbitrations; professional licenses; voter registrations; social security administration death records from 50 states; marriage and divorce records from selected states; criminal history records and inmate indexes; business records, including incorporation, limited partnership and limited liability companies information, fictitious business names and DBA ("Doing Business As") registrations; and Office of Foreign Asset Control (OFAC) master list of suspected terrorists.

After providing LexisNexis with a data file containing personal identifiers and last known addresses (as of June 2011) for the 133,479 CTS cohort members, we received a dataset containing 358,520 addresses linked to 130,921 CTS participants (98% of the CTS), along with geographic coordinates (latitude/longitude), the earliest and most recent dates associated with these addresses, and match probability scores which show how well the names, dates of birth, and social security numbers matched their corresponding CTS data record. The usefulness of these data for the construction of residential histories for CTS cohort members were the focus of a formal evaluation, the results of which are described in detail elsewhere [13]. Briefly, there were a number of take home messages from these analyses, including:

1. The data are messy!

   • Prior to use, the data need to undergo extensive QA/QC efforts. Although representing a small proportion of the total addresses received, care must be taken to remove duplicate addresses (4%), non-residential addresses (12%), and addresses with illogical or implausible dates such as dates after date of death (2%) or before date of birth (< 1%).
   • Given some of these apparent inaccuracies in dates, caution should be taken when using this approach for research that requires residential location at a highly-precise point in time.

2. The data are reasonably accurate for establishing residential location. Comparisons of the LexisNexis addresses to the known CTS addresses collected prospectively since the start of the study in 1995, demonstrated high rates of concordance, generally around 85% — a finding supported by similar concordance rates reported among a random sample of 1000 participants enrolled in the National Institutes of Health-American Association of Retired Persons (NIH-AARP) Diet and Health Study [15].

3. The data can be effective for establishing historical residential location possibly as far back as 1980.

   • LexisNexis provided nearly 25,000 addresses for the time period prior to the start of the CTS study – a time for which no addresses had been available through the routine activities of the CTS.
   • LexisNexis was able to provide addresses for 81% of the cohort prior to 1990, but only 18% of these were prior to 1980.

4. Effectiveness and accuracy of this approach may vary by age and race/ethnicity, with potential limitations for elderly and very young women, and for Native American and Black women.

Despite these limitations, the results from our efforts, as well as two other studies that used a similar approach [14, 15], suggest that this method may provide a feasible, time efficient, and cost-effective strategy for constructing, or augmenting, residential histories for large-scale epidemiologic cohort studies.

6.2.2   Linkage to Birth Records

Because our desire to build residential histories was driven by a study of breast cancer, we had a particular interest in where women resided during pregnancy – a recognized window of increased vulnerability of breast tissue to environmental insults. Over 95,000 CTS participants have been identified as parous by virtue of reporting a live birth on one of the self-administered questionnaires. In order to determine where these women lived at the time they gave birth, we conducted a probabilistic record linkage to the confidential live birth data files (1966–2009) maintained by the Office of Vital Records at the California Department of Public Health. Although California birth certificates are available dating back to the late 1800's, electronic versions of the confidential birth data files are only available for 1966 and later. Another limitation of this approach is that complete maternal birthdates and full names are not available for all years. In order to address these data gaps, we conducted a number of ancillary linkages to statewide and county marriage data to gather additional information which was then used to optimize the record linkages of the CTS to the California birth records.

Most problematic was the lack of maternal birthdates and full names on California birth certificates for some years prior to 1989. More specifically, from 1982 to 1988 only maternal age (not date of birth) was recorded on California birth certificates. During 1966–1981 the data were further limited by the lack of maternal first name on the California birth records. To overcome these limitations, we used statewide and county marriage files (1960–1985) to gather additional name and date of birth information. These ancillary linkages also helped to address a fundamental challenge in conducting probabilistic record linkages of adult women posed by surname changes due to marriage. The additional name and date-of-birth information gathered through these linkages was then appended to the California birth records in order to optimize the linkage of the CTS women to the births of their children.

Ultimately these efforts resulted in the linkage of over 65,000 parous women in the CTS to the birth of a child. Unfortunately, we were not able to get addresses for all these women (Table 6.2) because full street addresses are only available on California electronic birth files since 1996 (although it is present on the paper/fiche copies for prior years). In order to assess address at the time of birth for births occurring prior to 1996, we contracted with the State of California Department of Public

Table 6.2 Parous women in the California teachers study linked to their children's births.

Birth years	Linked to birth certificate N	Street addresses obtained N (%)
1966–1977[a]	9868	0
1978–1988[a]	25,787	3313 (13%)[b]
1989–1991[a]	6570	1221 (19%)[b]
1992–1995[a]	8744	1472 (17%)[b]
1996–1999	7547	7598 (100%)
2000–2003	4571	4609 (100%)
2004–2006	1538	1545 (100%)
2007–2009	553	557 (100%)
TOTAL	65,178	20,315 (31%)

[a]addresses not available on electronic files
[b]addresses manually abstracted by special request to Vital Records Office for a targeted subset of participants

Health Office of Vital Records to obtain maternal addresses by manual data abstraction from birth certificates for a subset of 6000 births occurring 1978–1995, targeted to maximize the years of interest for our particular exposure, and to ensure sufficient representativeness of cases and controls in our breast cancer study. While we were only able to capture addresses for roughly 20% of the linked births identified during the 1978–1995 time period, we were able to gather 14,309 birth addresses for births occurring between 1996–2009 (for which full residential street addresses are available electronically on the birth files), reflecting nearly 100% completeness in the maternal address field of the California birth records during this latter time period.

Ultimately our efforts to link to California birth records yielded mixed success. On the one hand, they resulted in the identification of over 20,000 residential locations for our study participants at the time they gave birth. This information, not previously available for the CTS, was geocoded, and has been and continues to be, a potential resource for using georeferenced environmental data to explore health risks associated with ambient exposures associated with residential location at a time of potential heightened susceptibility to such exposures (see next section for an example). Thus for breast cancer studies, this method holds some promise. There however were a number of limitations to this approach worth noting, including:

1. We only captured births in California. These initial exploratory efforts to use birth records to augment residential histories were focused on California. Since we do not know how many, and which, of our parous participants gave birth outside California, we do not have reliable denominator estimates and therefore cannot ascertain our linkage success rate nor establish residential location for women who lived outside California when they gave birth. While this limitation was not necessarily prohibitive for the conduct of our nested breast cancer case-control study (currently in progress), care should be taken in applying this approach in epidemiologic studies, with a keen consideration for potential selection biases. Furthermore, epidemiologic studies focused on populations in other

geographic regions, or among highly mobile populations that tend to migrate across state lines, would need to evaluate the completeness and availability of birth data in the regions of interest for their study population.

2. This approach may not be practical for establishing maternal residential location for California births prior to 1996 when the address information is not available electronically. While the process of manual data abstraction of the residential addresses by staff at the California Office of Vital Records was fairly successful, it may not be feasible for large scale studies. Although the California Office of Vital Records was quite supportive of our efforts, there were many bureaucratic hurdles that had to be cleared as the address data are not publically available and needed to be obtained by special request. Additionally, manual data abstraction for large batches of individuals is not ordinarily a part of vital records staff job duties, and thus these efforts had to be scheduled so as not to interfere with their other job duties. Due to these time and cost constraints, we were able to request manual abstraction for only a fraction of the addresses we desired.

3. This approach may become more feasible in the near future. The California Department of Vital Records is working to digitize many of their historic records. As a result, full maternal residential addresses may become more readily available for births prior to 1996. Furthermore, as time passes, the proportion of older women at risk for breast cancer who were of childbearing age for whom digitized birth records are available will grow.

4. Our efforts to use birth records to augment residential histories to pinpoint residential location for the potential window of susceptibility surrounding childbirth were exploratory with a focus on a very specific population with a given age structure. Our experience may not reflect the feasibility of such an approach for populations residing in other geographic regions or in populations with different age structures. Regardless, the addition of over 20,000 additional addresses for nearly 65,000 parous women illustrates the potential value of this approach for the exploration of geographic-based environmental factors as risk factors for breast cancer. Additional efforts to explore similar approaches in other study populations in other geographic regions are warranted.

6.3   Section III: Developing Geospatial Measures of Environmental Exposures

Combining residential history data with spatiotemporal environmental exposure estimates presents its own set of challenges, not the least of which are the spatial and temporal congruity and robustness of exposure assessment metrics or measures. In the context of our developmental residential history profiles we chose to incorporate environmental attribute data optimized for the temporal and geographic coverage of our cohort participants, and for which we had conducted previous studies in the CTS cohort [36, 42, 43].

Given the residential histories developed for CTS participants as described in the previous section, the next task was to use these residential histories to develop estimates of pollutant exposure to the participants as they traveled through space and time. Based on our previous work evaluating CTS participants' breast cancer risk and residential exposure (based on baseline addresses) to a set of hazardous air pollutants, we selected five compounds of interest for our study: acrylamide, arsenic, benzene, cadmium, and diesel [36, 43].

We developed methods to estimate exposure for individual study participants in two basic stages, using the information sources shown in Table 6.3 and described in more detail below. In the first stage, we constructed geospatial annual average concentration surfaces for selected pollutants, based on the EPA's National Air Toxics Assessment (NATA) simulation-based data [44]. For each selected pollutant, these surfaces covered the area of interest, i.e., the entire state of California, as well as

Table 6.3 Some sources and types of information available about air pollutants

	Information source		
	EPA NATA	CARB Ambient Air Toxics Monitoring Network	CARB Air Monitoring Network (not used in this analysis)
Potential compounds of interest	30–100+ HAPs, depending on year	9 HAPs: Acetaldehyde, Benzene, 1–3 Butadiene, Formaldehyde, Methylene Chloride, Perchloroethylene, Styrene, Toluene, Trichloroethylene	6 criteria pollutants: Ozone, Carbon Monoxide, Nitrogen dioxide, Sulfur dioxide, PM10 and PM2.5
Years available	1996, 1999, 2002, 2005	1990 to present	Approx. 1980 to present
Type of data to be used	Predicted annual average from ASPEN simulation (assessment system for population exposure nationwide)	Annual averages (other temporal resolutions available)	Annual averages (other temporal resolutions available)
Spatial resolution	Census tract averages	~ 31 fixed stations	~ 250 fixed stations
Coordinate system	Not applicable	NAD83	NAD83
Good things	Lots of HAPs	Actual measurement values, not simulations	Actual measurement values, not simulations
	Complete coverage of state	Back further in time	Back further in time
Complications	Areal data	Sensors go offline from time to time	Sensors go offline from time to time
	Simulation bias (differs by year)	Not many stations	Different set of compounds than used in NATA

spanned the 30-year time period of interest, which ranged from 1980 through 2009. In the second stage, we produced exposure estimates for participants over time by combining the geographical location information about the times and places of residence that were constructed in the previous section with concentration information from the geospatial surfaces constructed in the first stage. For a given pollutant, two types of estimated exposures to CTS participants were created: (a) an integrated residential exposure estimate, over time and place, as the participants change residences over time; and (b) residential exposures in specific years of interest, such as the year of birth of participants' children, especially first births.

In addition to using solely NATA-based surfaces to generate exposure estimates, we also explored methods for combining the NATA-based surfaces with measurement data from sensors located throughout the state (data from the California Air Resources Board (CARB)). The goal of this exploratory effort was to use the additional CARB data to increase the accuracy and precision of exposure estimates based solely on the NATA data.

6.3.1   Stage 1: Developing Geospatial Annual Pollution Surfaces

Geospatial data sets on pollutant concentrations over time are available from a number of different sources. The main source of interest to us was the Environmental Protection Agency's (EPA's) National-Scale Air Toxics Assessment (NATA) database [44]. In addition, we explored using pollution concentration datasets from the California Air Resources Board (CARB) [45]. Table 6.3 provides a summary of the geospatial pollutant information from those two sources that could be used in creating pollution exposure estimates for the CTS, described below.

The National Air Toxics Assessment (NATA) Data   A simulation-based database called the National Air Toxics Assessment (NATA) is constructed by the EPA approximately once every 3–5 years and is described in detail at https://www.epa.gov/national-air-toxics-assessment. Briefly, the goal of NATA is "to identify those air toxics which are of greatest potential concern in terms of contribution to population risk." Construction of a NATA database proceeds in four basic steps: (1) compiling a National Emissions Inventory; (2) constructing model-based ambient concentration estimates; (3) estimating population exposure; and (4) characterizing the public health risk. Our focus was on exploiting the results from step (2) of this process: a database of ambient concentration estimates. For each pollutant, the resolution of the NATA data for the years that we had available at the time (1999, 2002, and 2005) was at the level of a yearly average value for each year 2000 census tract. (For these analyses we decided not to use the 1996 NATA, partially for reasons cited in Garcia [42]).

Producing Annual NATA Surfaces The major goal here was to create a census tract level NATA surface for each year from 1978 to 2009, using as a foundation the NATA surfaces for 1999, 2002, and 2005. Two steps were necessary to produce annual NATA surfaces from the existing NATA data. The first step, an *interpolation* step, filled in the years between 1999 and 2005 for which there was no pre-existing NATA data (i.e., the years 2000, 2001, 2003, and 2004). This step was conceptually more reliable, as the bounding NATA surfaces, combined with smoothness constraints, served to constrain the new surfaces. The second step, an *extrapolation* step, tried to extend the NATA data to years before and after any NATA data existed. It was more speculative and depended critically on the concordance between the smoothness of the actual unknown data and assumptions made in the extrapolation. Figure 6.2 shows the NATA quantile summaries for the years 1999, 2002, and 2005, when NATA predictions were available. The 5%, 25%, and Median quantiles for acrylamide were missing for the year 2002 as approximately 70% of the NATA acrylamide predictions for that year were zero.

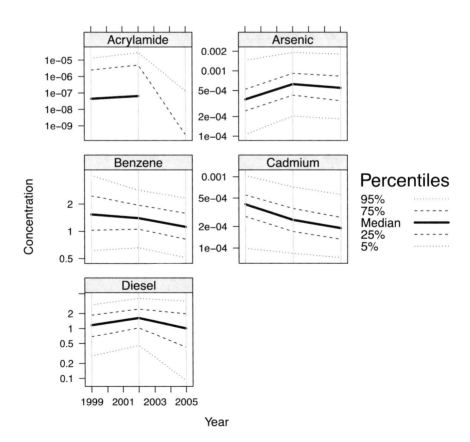

Fig. 6.2 NATA quantiles for the five pollutants of interest for the years for which reliable NATA data were available

For step one (interpolation), Generalized Additive Models (GAMs) were use to create yearly NATA surfaces between 1999 and 2005 for each pollutant of interest. First, the *gam()* function in the **mgcv** package in R (https://CRAN.R-project. org/package=mgcv) was used to fit a smooth spatiotemporal surface to the NATA data for 1999, 2002, and 2005 by regressing the log of the pollutant concentration for a given census tract by year combination on the (x,y) location for the centroid of that census tract and the year. Then, the resulting smooth function of three variables was used to predict the log concentration at the centroid of each census tract for the missing years between 1999 and 2005. In step 2 (extrapolation), the smooth predictions returned by the GAM in step one were then used to drive an exponential smoothing state space model with additive errors and an additive trend provided by the **forecast** package (https://CRAN.R-project.org/ package=forecast) to extrapolate the interpolated fit in order to get yearly estimates back to 1978 and forward to 2009.

At the end of step 2, we had simulation-derived annual surfaces from 1978 to 2009 for each of the desired pollutants, where the predicted value for census tract centroid in that particular year was used as the value for the census tract in that year. These NATA-derived surfaces served as "prior" knowledge about the distribution of NATA pollutants over time. Fig. 6.3 shows the predicted distribution of annual average benzene concentrations over all the census tracts in California for the entire time span from 1978 through 2010.

6.3.2   Stage 2: Using Geospatial Pollution Surfaces to Estimate the Annual Average Exposure at a Location

Once we had generated the annual pollutant surfaces, the next step was to use those surfaces to estimate the average annual exposure of a pollutant for a location and year combination. Given an (x,y) location, the simplest possible exposure estimate was the concentration estimate at the centroid of census tract containing the location, or the concentration estimate at the centroid nearest to the location. A slightly more complex approach was to use geographically-weighted regression to create an estimate based on a weighted average of census tract centroids for nearby census tracts, perhaps augmented by other information about nearby census tracts. In this case, the weights were functions of the distance to each census tract centroid. In order to compute geospatially weighted average exposure estimates for a location, locations were transformed from the WGS84 coordinate system (a geographic coordinate system) to the Albers Equal Area coordinate system (a projected coordinate system) in an attempt to equalize distances over latitudes.

Incorporating Measurement Data from the California Air Resources (CARB)   After completing this initial two-stage process to assign individual exposure based solely on the NATA simulation data, we explored the use of additional measurement data to improve the accuracy and precision of our initial estimates.

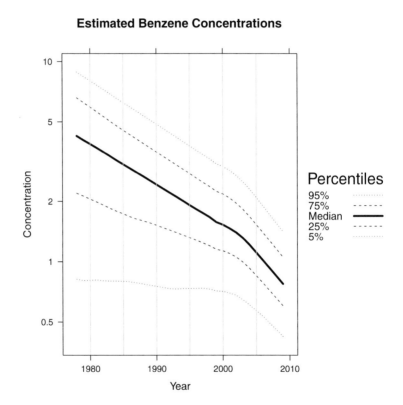

Fig. 6.3 Quantiles of estimated NATA-derived annual benzene concentration predictions from 1978 through 2010

One approach to using more complex methods to estimate an exposure from concentration data involve combining the information derived from NATA surfaces with measurement data from point source sensors, such as the CARB data available in California. The CARB data are maintained by the California Air Resources Board in publicly available databases that go back to 1990, and are described in detail at https://ww2.arb.ca.gov/resources. Figure 6.4a shows the presence of CARB data by sensor and year combination for arsenic, benzene and cadmium. (Acrylamide was eliminated due to lack of data, and diesel due to differences in measurement

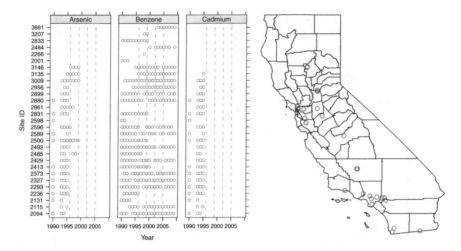

Fig. 6.4 Presence and geographic locations of CARB sensors in California. Acrylamide and Diesel were removed from consideration for technical considerations (lack of data for Acrylamide and units of measurement for Diesel

units.) Note that, with the exception of benzene, there is little overlap between years with CARB data and years with NATA data. Hence, for the purposes of exploiting CARB data, we focused on benzene. Figu re 6.4b shows the location of the benzene sensors throughout the State.

Given that we had already produced annual NATA-derived concentration surfaces for each pollutant of interest and used them to generate geographically weighted exposure estimates, the next question was whether the CARB benzene data along with the NATA benzene data could produce improved surfaces over time.

A number of different approaches of varying difficulty and generality have been proposed to accomplish this kind of task. One specific approach to spatiotemporal integration of simulation and measurement data that has recently been posted to CRAN (the Comprehensive R Archive Network) is the **SpatioTemporal** R package by members of the Multi-Ethnic Study of Atherosclerosis and Air Pollution (MESA Air). (See https://CRAN.R-project.org/package=SpatioTemporal.) In our context, this package models the value of a log concentration at location s and time t, $y(s, t)$, as

$$y(s,t) = aM(s,t) + b_1(s)f_1(t) + b_2(s)f_2(t) + \ldots + b_m(s)f_m(t) + n(s,t)$$

where $M(s, t)$ is the NATA estimate of log concentration at (s, t); $f_1(t), f_2(t), \ldots, f_m(t)$ are m predefined smooth temporal basis functions; $b_1(s), b_2(s), \ldots, b_m(s)$ are m coefficients to the temporal basis functions, defined as spatial fields with a universal kriging structure; and $n(s, t)$ is a structured error term. In essence, the SpatioTemporal package estimation function *estimate()*, given observations y, spatiotemporal data M, location information about measurement devices X, and predefined spatial functions *f()*, solves the above equation, while the prediction function *predict()* allows for prediction, even at locations and times other than where there is observed data.

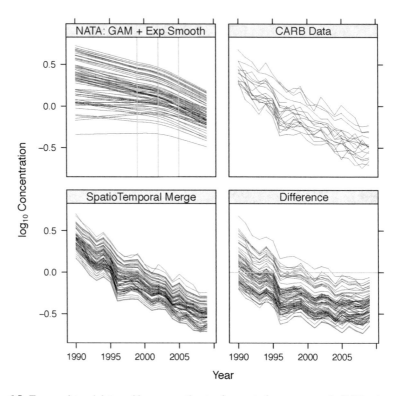

Fig. 6.5 Temporal trend data and benzene estimates for a set of census tracts in California

Functions in the **SpatioTemporal** package were used to merge the NATA-derived benzene surfaces from step 2 for 1990 through 2009 (i.e., "prior" spatiotemporal knowledge) with the CARB data ("measurement data") to produce smoothed "posterior" estimates for each census tract and year combination, where each census tract was represented by its centroid. A number of dimensions m were explored. However, all dimensions m greater than one resulted in singularities during the attempted fit. Hence, $m = 1$ was used. Finally, these merged annual data for 1990 through 2009 were extrapolated back to 1978 using the same methods as above to produce merged annual surfaces for 1978 through 2009.

The four panels in Fig. 6.5 show the dramatic effect that including actual measurement data had on the trend lines for census tracts. The upper left panel (*NATA: GAM + Exponential Smoothing*) shows the smoothed temporal trend lines for 123 California census tracts, including those where CARB data were available. The three vertical lines show the years where actual NATA simulation data were available: 1999, 2002, and 2005. Note that the trend lines are linear (on a log scale) for years before 1999 and after 2005, reflecting the assumption of constant slope outside of the region where NATA data exists. The upper right panel (*CARB Data*) shows the actual CARB data for the 23 census tracts where there were a sufficient number of observations (at least five) to detect a trend. Here we see a more dramatic trend in the years before 1999 than was captured by simply extrapolating the NATA data. The bottom left panel (*SpatioTemporal Merge*) shows the result of applying the functions in the SpatioTemporal package with one trend term to the combined NATA and CARB data to obtain predicted values. In this case the structure of the trend in the merged data closely captures the trend observed in the CARB data but not so much in the NATA data. Finally, the bottom right panel (*Difference*) shows the difference in census tract log concentrations between the merged data (lower left) and the NATA data (upper left). The NATA predictions for a census tract largely exceed the merged data predictions for that census tract, except for some tracts in the earlier years. In all likelihood, the dramatic differences in the temporal concentration between NATA simulations and CARB measurements means that any risk estimates derived therefrom will also change noticeably when one moves from risk estimates based on NATA simulation data only to risk estimates based on a more complete exposure picture that (a) incorporates measurement data, and (b) incorporates data over a longer period of time without having to resort to extrapolation.

In addition to the estimated census-tract specific predicted log concentrations, confidence intervals for those predictions were also calculated. These confidence intervals differed dramatically in size, depending on whether or not there was an actual sensor in the census tract. As might be expected, the confidence intervals were much broader for census tracts without sensors.

The above analysis demonstrates that the values we could obtain for estimated census tract log concentrations over time depended rather dramatically on the model assumptions used. While the NATA approach provides complete coverage over the time and space of interest, it is based on interpolating and extrapolating data present for only three distinct years (1999, 2002, and 2005). On the other hand, exploiting sensor measurement provides actual data over a longer period of time, but only for a limited number of census tracts. And, as Fig. 6.5 shows, necessary assumptions about the temporal evolution of average tract concentrations can drive the eventual temporal structure of the entire data set, as well as providing results with reduced confidence where no actual data was ever measured. This highlights the limitations inherent in attempting to model exposure estimates in the absence of real data.

The example for benzene, one of the contaminants for which measured data are more widely available and which represents a well-established carcinogen, illustrates the potential for uncertainty that exists for estimating individual exposure based on modeled, monitored, or even combined data. There is, unfortunately, no gold standard for specific exposures, during specific time periods at a specific geographic scale that can encompass the broad view for a project like this. While actual measurement data is appealing, in reality it is only available for a restricted few areas of the state, and even in that case, measurement at the monitor may not represent exposures over a broader area such as census tract. In the case we explored, exposure attributes would be highly dependent on the year of the difference between NATA estimates and the combined NATA+CARB estimates (Fig. 6.5). Although it is difficult to specify how risk estimate might be affected, in general, measurement error reduces risk ratio estimates. But that's true only if the measurement error is random. In this case, there's a temporal trend for measurement error, so bias may depend on which (temporal) exposure is being evaluated. While ultimately these efforts serve as an example of a feasible approach that can be used to combine measured and modeled air pollutant data, they also underscore the importance of fully evaluating the spatiotemporal patterns and gaps in the data prior to implementing these approaches.

6.4   Section IV: Integration of Residential Histories with Environmental Exposures

Exposure estimates for each residential address for each participant-year combination was estimated in three steps: (1) determining the (x, y) locations for all the residential addresses for that participant in that year; (2) calculating an annual exposure estimate for each (x, y) location using one of the methods described above; and (3) combining the exposure estimates according to the length of time spent at each location.

Step 1: Calculating Residential Locations. The first step involved obtaining the geographic locations for a resident for a given year from a set of text addresses for that year. This task was handled by modern address standardization software (ZP4), coupled with geospatial techniques that are well-developed in ArcGIS. Hence, available text-based residential addresses were translated to an (x,y) location, which was then associated with the appropriate year 2000 census tract.

Step 2: Estimating an Exposure from Concentration Surfaces. Given a set of locations and a set of concentration surfaces, we estimated average annual exposures using the simple weighted average method described above in addition to the more complex model-based methods outlined in the **SpatioTemporal** package.

Step 3: Combining Estimates. Finally, CTS participants moved from place to place over time. Hence, cumulative estimates needed to take into account this residential mobility by taking weighted averages. If multiple addresses in different locations were reported for the same year, time-weighted averaging of the exposure estimates were used for each location to produce one exposure value. Women were excluded from any analysis if they had one or more addresses that could not be geocoded or whose location did not have a matching year 2000 census tract, and hence could not be assigned an exposure value for at least 1 year. Cumulative exposures over several years for women with complete address information, was calculated using a weighted average based on the proportion of years living at each residence. Note that while the majority of the participants stayed at the same address (63%) during the follow-up period, there were also a substantial number of participants who moved and for whom a single address might misrepresent exposures of interest.

The integration of the exposure surfaces with residential histories is comparatively one of the most straightforward steps in our overall approach to assigning individual-level exposures to ambient air pollutants. It can be readily achieved through the calculation of simple weighted averages or via the **SpatioTemporal** package which allows for incorporation of more complex model assumptions. The choice of the optimal approach for integrating residential history data with exposure data needs, however, to take into account the specific data that is being integrated and to respect any spatiotemporal limitations to those data.

6.5   Section V: Conclusions/Summary

While there exist rich data resources for assessing residential history profiles for large studies where direct data collection for individuals may not be practical, none are without limitations and caveats, both for constructing residential histories and for estimating exposures to environmental agents of concern. In the example provided here there were a number of lessons learned, as well as insights for future directions.

As enumerated above, lessons learned underscore the challenges in dealing with data gaps for each step in the process: gaps in personal address information, gaps in data from vital records, and gaps in the temporal and spatial availability of environmental exposure information. As the availability and quality of electronically available data is expected to grow as we move into the future, these approaches are likely to become more fruitful. However, the overarching lessons learned for each step in our approach was that (a) there is no equal for careful data review, quality assurance, and sensitivity analysis to assess the viability and appropriateness of using data developed through these approaches for specific studies for health risks, and (b) the environmental exposure estimates may still depend critically on the methods used and completeness of the data.

With the expanding availability of electronic sources of information, it may be possible for future cohorts to characterize lifetime patterns of residential history, hence ameliorating many of the data gaps otherwise inherent in approaches relying on the use of external files. Likewise, as environmental attribute data become more available for time periods of relevance the general approach here may become more useful for large-scale studies encompassing long time periods, broad geographic areas, and large numbers of participants. It is also worth noting that residential locations do not necessarily account for where people spend extended periods during the day, so future strategies to assess workplace history locations, or other important daily activities may be important for assessing estimates of exposure over time.

Increasing interest in geographic information system (GIS) tools and improvements in exposure assessment offer many research opportunities for large-scale studies, such as the CTS. Notably, the growing ability to integrate attribute data from GIS analyses with personal self-reported information and with biomarkers of exposure and/or effect lay the groundwork for better understanding the influence of our physical environment on health and well-being in the future.

Acknowledgements *This work was funded in part from NCI grants R01CA170394 (Reynolds) and R01CA77398 (Bernstein).*

References

1. Doll R. Urban and rural factors in the aetiology of cancer. Int J Cancer. 1991;47(6):803–10.
2. Laden F, Spiegelman D, Neas LM, Colditz GA, Hankinson SE, Manson JE, Byrne C, Rosner BA, Speizer FE, Hunter DJ. Geographic variation in breast cancer incidence rates in a cohort of U.S. women. J Natl Cancer Inst. 1997;89(18):1373–8.
3. Nasca PC, Burnett WS, Greenwald P, Brennan K, Wolfgang P, Carlton K. Population density as an indicator of urban-rural differences in cancer incidence, upstate New York, 1968-1972. Am J Epidemiol. 1980;112(3):362–75.
4. Parkin DM, Bray F, Ferlay J, Pisani P. Global cancer statistics, 2002. CA Cancer J Clin. 2005;55(2):74–108.
5. Pisani P. Breast cancer: geographic variation and risk factors. J Environ Pathol Toxicol Oncol. 1992;11(5–6):313–6.
6. Reynolds P, Hurley S, Goldberg DE, Anton-Culver H, Bernstein L, Deapen D, Horn-Ross PL, Peel D, Pinder R, Ross RK, et al. Regional variations in breast cancer among California teachers. Epidemiology. 2004;15(6):746–54.
7. Reynolds P, Hurley SE, Quach AT, Rosen H, Von Behren J, Hertz A, Smith D. Regional variations in breast cancer incidence among California women, 1988-1997. Cancer Causes Control. 2005;16(2):139–50.
8. Shottenfeld D, Fraumeni J. Cancer epidemiology and prevention. 3rd ed. New York: Oxford University Press; 2006.
9. Robbins AS, Brescianini S, Kelsey JL. Regional differences in known risk factors and the higher incidence of breast cancer in San Francisco. J Natl Cancer Inst. 1997;89(13):960–5.
10. Brody JG, Rudel RA. Environmental pollutants and breast cancer. Environ Health Perspect. 2003;111(8):1007–19.
11. Fernandez SV, Russo J. Estrogen and xenoestrogens in breast cancer. Toxicol Pathol. 2010;38(1):110–22.
12. Wolff MS, Weston A. Breast cancer risk and environmental exposures. Environ Health Perspect. 1997;105(Suppl 4):891–6.
13. Hurley S, Hertz A, Nelson DO, Layefsky M, Von Behren J, Bernstein L, Deapen D, Reynolds P. Tracing a path to the past: exploring the use of commercial credit reporting data to construct residential histories for epidemiologic studies of environmental exposures. Am J Epidemiol. 2017;185(3):238–46.
14. Jacquez GM, Slotnick MJ, Meliker JR, AvRuskin G, Copeland G, Nriagu J. Accuracy of commercially available residential histories for epidemiologic studies. Am J Epidemiol. 2011;173(2):236–43.
15. Wheeler DC, Wang A. Assessment of residential history generation using a public-record database. Int J Environ Res Public Health. 2015;12(9):11670–82.
16. Cohn BA. Developmental and environmental origins of breast cancer: DDT as a case study. Reprod Toxicol. 2011;31(3):302–11.
17. Cohn BA, Wolff MS, Cirillo PM, Sholtz RI. DDT and breast cancer in young women: new data on the significance of age at exposure. Environ Health Perspect. 2007;115(10):1406–14.
18. Colditz GA, Bohlke K, Berkey CS. Breast cancer risk accumulation starts early: prevention must also. Breast Cancer Res Treat. 2014;145(3):567–79.
19. Gray JM, Rasanayagam S, Engel C, Rizzo J. State of the evidence 2017: an update on the connection between breast cancer and the environment. Environ Health. 2017;16(1):94.
20. Institute of Medicine of the National Academies. Breast Cancer and the environment: a life course approach. Washington, D.C.: National Academy of Sciences; 2014.

21. Bernstein L, Allen M, Anton-Culver H, Deapen D, Horn-Ross PL, Peel D, Pinder R, Reynolds P, Sullivan-Halley J, West D, et al. High breast cancer incidence rates among California teachers: results from the California teachers study (United States). Cancer Causes Control. 2002;13(7):625–35.
22. Dallal CM, Sullivan-Halley J, Ross RK, Wang Y, Deapen D, Horn-Ross PL, Reynolds P, Stram DO, Clarke CA, Anton-Culver H, et al. Long-term recreational physical activity and risk of invasive and in situ breast cancer: the California teachers study. Arch Intern Med. 2007;167(4):408–15.
23. Horn-Ross PL, Canchola AJ, West DW, Stewart SL, Bernstein L, Deapen D, Pinder R, Ross RK, Anton-Culver H, Peel D, et al. Patterns of alcohol consumption and breast cancer risk in the California teachers study cohort. Cancer Epidemiol Biomark Prev. 2004;13(3):405–11.
24. Horn-Ross PL, Hoggatt KJ, West DW, Krone MR, Stewart SL, Anton H, Bernstei CL, Deapen D, Peel D, Pinder R, et al. Recent diet and breast cancer risk: the California teachers study (USA). Cancer Causes Control. 2002;13(5):407–15.
25. Keegan TH, Hurley S, Goldberg D, Nelson DO, Reynolds P, Bernstein L, Horn-Ross PL, Gomez SL. The association between neighborhood characteristics and body size and physical activity in the California teachers study cohort. Am J Public Health. 2012;102(4):689–97.
26. Lee E, Schumacher F, Lewinger JP, Neuhausen SL, Anton-Culver H, Horn-Ross PL, Henderson KD, Ziogas A, Van Den Berg D, Bernstein L, et al. The association of polymorphisms in hormone metabolism pathway genes, menopausal hormone therapy, and breast cancer risk: a nested case-control study in the California teachers study cohort. Breast Cancer Res. 2011;13(2):R37.
27. Ma H, Henderson KD, Sullivan-Halley J, Duan L, Marshall SF, Ursin G, Horn-Ross PL, Largent J, Deapen DM, Lacey JV Jr, et al. Pregnancy-related factors and the risk of breast carcinoma in situ and invasive breast cancer among postmenopausal women in the California teachers study cohort. Breast Cancer Res. 2010;12(3):R35.
28. Marshall SF, Clarke CA, Deapen D, Henderson K, Largent J, Neuhausen SL, Reynolds P, Ursin G, Horn-Ross PL, Stram DO, et al. Recent breast cancer incidence trends according to hormone therapy use: the California teachers study cohort. Breast Cancer Res. 2010;12(1):R4.
29. Reynolds P, Goldberg D, Hurley S, Nelson DO, Largent J, Henderson KD, Bernstein L. Passive smoking and risk of breast cancer in the California teachers study. Cancer Epidemiol Biomark Prev. 2009;18(12):3389–98.
30. Reynolds P, Hurley S, Goldberg DE, Anton-Culver H, Bernstein L, Deapen D, Horn-Ross PL, Peel D, Pinder R, Ross RK, et al. Active smoking, household passive smoking, and breast cancer: evidence from the California teachers study. J Natl Cancer Inst. 2004;96(1):29–37.
31. Saxena T, Lee E, Henderson KD, Clarke CA, West D, Marshall SF, Deapen D, Bernstein L, Ursin G. Menopausal hormone therapy and subsequent risk of specific invasive breast cancer subtypes in the California teachers study. Cancer Epidemiol Biomark Prev. 2010;19(9):2366–78.
32. West-Wright CN, Henderson KD, Sullivan-Halley J, Ursin G, Deapen D, Neuhausen S, Reynolds P, Chang E, Ma H, Bernstein L. Long-term and recent recreational physical activity and survival after breast cancer: the California teachers study. Cancer Epidemiol Biomark Prev. 2009;18(11):2851–9.
33. Garcia E, Hurley S, Nelson DO, Gunier R, Hertz A, Reynolds P. Evaluation of Hazardous Air Pollutants Data for an Epidemiologic Study of Breast Cancer Risk. In: Poster at the ISES 2011 Conference, Baltimore MD; 2011.
34. Hurley S, Goldberg D, Nelson D, Hertz A, Horn-Ross PL, Bernstein L, Reynolds P. Light at night and breast cancer risk among California teachers. Epidemiology. 2014;25(5):697–706.
35. Lipsett MJ, Ostro BD, Reynolds P, Goldberg D, Hertz A, Jerrett M, Smith DF, Garcia C, Chang ET, Bernstein L. Long-term exposure to air pollution and cardiorespiratory disease in the California teachers study cohort. Am J Respir Crit Care Med. 2011;184(7):828–35.
36. Liu R, Nelson DO, Hurley S, Hertz A, Reynolds P. Residential exposure to estrogen disrupting hazardous air pollutants and breast cancer risk: the California teachers study. Epidemiology. 2015;26(3):365–73.

37. Ostro B, Hu J, Goldberg D, Reynolds P, Hertz A, Bernstein L, Kleeman MJ. Associations of mortality with long-term exposures to fine and ultrafine particles, species and sources: results from the California teachers study cohort. Environ Health Perspect. 2015;123(6):549–56.
38. Ostro B, Lipsett M, Reynolds P, Goldberg D, Hertz A, Garcia C, Henderson KD, Bernstein L. Long-term exposure to constituents of fine particulate air pollution and mortality: results from the California teachers study. Environ Health Perspect. 2010;118(3):363–9.
39. Reynolds P, Hurley SE, Goldberg DE, Yerabati S, Gunier RB, Hertz A, Anton-Culver H, Bernstein L, Deapen D, Horn-Ross PL, et al. Residential proximity to agricultural pesticide use and incidence of breast cancer in the California teachers study cohort. Environ Res. 2004;96(2):206–18.
40. List of consumer reporting companies. https://files.consumerfinance.gov/f/201604_cfpb_list-of-consumer-reporting-companies.pdf.
41. https://www.lexisnexis.com/en-us/products/public-records.page.
42. Garcia E, Hurley S, Nelson DO, Gunier RB, Hertz A, Reynolds P. Evaluation of the agreement between modeled and monitored ambient hazardous air pollutants in California. Int J Environ Health Res. 2014;24(4):363–77.
43. Garcia E, Hurley S, Nelson DO, Hertz A, Reynolds P. Hazardous air pollutants and breast cancer risk in California teachers: a cohort study. Environ Health. 2015;14:14.
44. National Air Toxics Assessment. http://www.epa.gov/ttn/atw/natamain/.
45. Air Quality Section Planning and Technical Support Division: State and Local Air Monitoring Network Plan. In. Sacramento: California Environmental Protection Agency; 2009.

Chapter 7
Systematic Review of Geospatial Approaches to Breast Cancer Epidemiology

Caroline A. Thompson, Sindana Ilango, Joseph Gibbons, Atsushi Nara, and Ming-Hsiang Tsou

Abstract In recent years, the application of spatial analysis in the context of epidemiologic surveillance and research has increased exponentially. Today, the use of spatial statistics extend beyond descriptive mapping to analyze and visualize the underlying spatial patterns of human dynamics; offering epidemiologists and public health researchers new and richer ways to visualize illness, and understand of the underlying spatial dynamics of cancer. For cancer prevention and control, such methods facilitate visualization of high risk areas and identification of spatially heterogeneous risk factors, both of which aid in prioritizing regions that would benefit from additional health resources, such as screening programs and treatment services. Although these sophisticated spatial methodologies are widely available, they have been slow to adoption in the field of cancer epidemiology, and conventional "nonspatial" statistical methods are still most commonly used to describe and understand the burden of breast cancer, and the relative contribution of social and geographic disparities. In this chapter, we seek to better understand how geospatial methods are being applied to understand the epidemiology of breast cancer. We conducted a systematic literature review to describe the contexts in which geospatial

C. A. Thompson (✉) · S. Ilango
School of Public Health, San Diego State University, San Diego, CA, USA

Department of Family Medicine and Public Health, University of California San Diego, San Diego, CA, USA
e-mail: caroline.thompson@sdsu.edu

J. Gibbons
Department of Sociology, San Diego State University, San Diego, CA, USA

Center for Human Dynamics in the Mobile Age, San Diego State University, San Diego, CA, USA

A. Nara · M.-H. Tsou
Center for Human Dynamics in the Mobile Age, San Diego State University, San Diego, CA, USA

Department of Geography, San Diego State University, San Diego, CA, USA

© Springer Nature Switzerland AG 2019
D. Berrigan, N. A. Berger (eds.), *Geospatial Approaches to Energy Balance and Breast Cancer*, Energy Balance and Cancer 15, https://doi.org/10.1007/978-3-030-18408-7_7

methods have been employed, including the types of research questions, populations studied, sophistication of the techniques employed, and disciplinary composition of the author groups. We assess the strengths and limitations of these approaches
and offer guidance on future directions with spatial breast cancer epidemiology.

Keywords Geospatial epidemiology · Cancer epidemiology · Systematic review ·
Cancer disparities · Spatial statistics · Spatial regression

7.1 Introduction

The use of geographic information in health surveillance and research dates back to
the first epidemiologists. In recent decades, the innovation of digital geographic
information systems (GIS) technology has allowed for the visualization, integration, manipulation, and analysis of spatial information at an unprecedented scale.
Over the last 20 years, the application of spatial analysis in the context of epidemiologic surveillance and research has increased exponentially [1]. Today, the use of
spatial statistics extend beyond descriptive mapping to analyze and visualize the
underlying spatial patterns of human dynamics; offering epidemiologists and public
health researchers new and richer ways to visualize illness, and understand of the
underlying spatial structures that contribute to patterns of exposures and disease
occurrence within and between localities that cannot be easily ascertained with the
multi-level strategies typically used in health research [2].

GIS is frequently used in the study of infectious rather than chronic disease [3].
One reason for this is person-to-person contagion and the shorter time period
between exposure to causal agent and disease onset. We also see GIS and spatial
statistics applied frequently in environmental exposures, such as pesticide spraying,
and residential power lines or industrial plants. Leveraging spatial methods for
studying such exposures seem intuitive, because the most important moderator of
the magnitude of risk is proximity to regions of concentrated exposures. In contrast,
many chronic diseases (including cancer) have complex causal pathways and long
induction periods which result in substantial challenges to using GIS effectively.
Thus, while sophistication of spatial techniques is evolving rapidly, outside of environmental exposures these methods are more rarely leveraged for studies of cancer
epidemiology, or their value may be under-realized in this research area.

Malignancies are now the first or second leading cause of death for most
Americans [4]. In 2018, it is estimated that 266,120 women will be diagnosed with
and 40,920 will die from breast cancer [4]. Routine screening can help detect breast
cancers at an early stage, when treatment is more likely to be successful. Despite
this, attendance to screening is less likely in minorities, immigrants, and persons of
lower socioeconomic status, contributing to potentially preventable mortality in
these populations. Many of the factors that account for social disparities in incidence and mortality from breast cancer are inextricably linked to geography. Areas
with mostly nonwhite populations, the result of racial segregation or ethnic enclaves,

are defined by both their members and the environment in which they live. Even in predominantly non-Hispanic White areas, neighborhoods or regional boundaries separate people along socio-economic lines. Attendance at regular screenings has also been linked to healthcare access [5]. Underutilization of screening has been found to be associated with socio-economic barriers, factors of racial segregation, as well as more social and cultural factors, for which their full effects are mostly felt at a local level [6]. Mapping allows a visualization of high risk areas that face these disparities to help prioritize regions that would benefit from additional health resources, such as cancer control programs and interventions [7]. Conventional "nonspatial" statistical methods widely used to describe and understand the burden of breast cancer, and the contribution of social and geographic disparities are criticized for their inability to estimate the influence of neighborhood effects on outcomes [8]. Although more sophisticated methodologies exist, they have been slow to adoption in the field of cancer epidemiology or application to the study of breast cancer incidence and mortality.

In this chapter, we seek to better understand how geospatial methods are being applied to understand the epidemiology of breast cancer. We conducted a systematic literature review to describe the contexts in which geospatial methods have been employed, including the types of research questions, populations studied, sophistication of the techniques employed, and disciplinary composition of the author groups. We assess the strengths and limitations of these approaches, and offer guidance on future directions with spatial breast cancer epidemiology. Specifically, we considered five questions to address with review of the selected literature, and the following sections are structured accordingly. These questions were: (1) Who is utilizing geospatial methods to conduct research on the epidemiology of breast cancer? (2) What journals are publishing the work? (3) What sources of data and cancer outcomes are being analyzed with spatial methods? (4) What types of spatial analytical methods are being implemented to describe and understand the role of geography in the burden of cancer? And, finally, (5) What is the research finding?

7.2   Methods for Article Search and Review

The search team was comprised of four members. We identified literature by searching through three library databases: MEDLINE, PubMed, and Web of Science. To capture research articles published after GIS was more accessible to researchers, the search was limited to peer-reviewed journal articles published between January 1994 through December 2017 written in English, and conducted in U.S. populations. We searched titles and abstracts using keywords that combined "breast cancer" with one or more geospatial terms, specifically we used the following query:

(("breast cancer" [Title/Abstract] AND ("geographic information" [Title/Abstract] OR "GIS" [Title/Abstract] OR "geographic disparity" [Title/Abstract] OR "geographic analysis" [Title/Abstract] OR "space-time" [Title/Abstract] OR "spatial analysis" [Title/Abstract] OR "spatial epidemiology" [Title/Abstract] OR "spatial mismatch" [Title/Abstract] OR "spatio-temporal analysis" [Title/Abstract])) AND ("1994/01/01" [PDAT] : "2017/12/31" [PDAT])

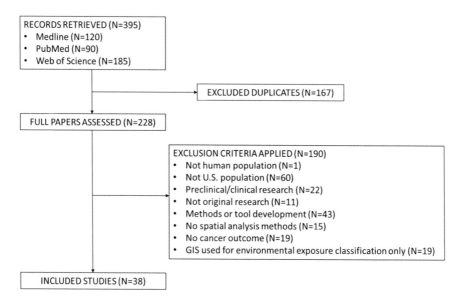

Fig. 7.1 Flow diagram of literature review

Since our focus was to understand how research groups are applying spatial methods to understand the epidemiology of breast cancer, we selected articles that described observational research which was population-based, in humans, and which incorporated a spatial analytic technique, to evaluate the occurrence of, treatment of, or mortality from, breast cancer as the outcome. Studies conducted outside the U.S, studies conducted on non-human populations, meta-research, commentaries, technical papers that described a new methodology, prevention trials (i.e., studies of interventions not specifically linked to breast cancer outcomes), and studies that used GIS only as a means to create maps (with no additional spatial analysis) or to classify the environmental exposures (e.g., pesticides, radiation) were excluded from the review (Fig. 7.1). All retrieved articles' titles and abstracts were independently reviewed to determine if the study met our inclusion criteria. Duplicates across the two databases were removed. Selected articles were read to classify information about journal type, author group composition, cancer outcome, outcome data sources, geographical coverage, types of geospatial analyses performed, key findings, and described limitations.

Listed authors and department affiliations in each journal article were examined to determine the disciplinary nature of the writing group. If multiple affiliations were listed for an author, the first was used for tabulations. If no affiliation was listed, the author's current department was obtained via an internet search. Author writing groups were classified as all-university affiliated, non-university affiliated, or affiliated with both, again using the first affiliation for each author. We classified journal subject area and category according to SCImago Journal & Country Rank, which is a publicly available portal that includes the journals and country scientific indicators developed from the information contained in the Scopus® database. For each reviewed article, we extracted the following details: data source and type of cancer outcome measure(s) (e.g., incidence, prevalence, mortality, risk, survival, etc. from breast cancer), study location and geographic unit of analysis, motivation for use of spatial techniques, types of spatial analytic methods used, and noted limitations. Classifications were not mutually exclusive; studies were grouped into all relevant categories as indicated by our review. Key thematic elements and limitations of the research were then identified based on our review of the research findings.

7.3   Results of Article Search and Review

The initial literature search yielded 228 unique research articles before the exclusion criteria were applied. Application of inclusion and exclusion criteria resulted in 38 final articles for review (Fig. 7.1; Table 7.1).

7.3.1   Who is Performing and Publishing the Research?

Examining author affiliations revealed a variety of disciplines represented. Eighty-nine percent of articles included authors in health-related fields. This includes affiliations with medicine, public health, cancer registries, and hospitals. The second most represented discipline was geography (34%). The remaining authors represented fields in the areas of physical sciences, statistics/math, social sciences, and biological sciences. About half of the studies were written by authors from only one discipline, 42% of studies were written by members from two disciplines, and 11% involved members from three or more disciplines. Tian et al. [9] included authors from health, geography, and physical sciences; Williams et al. [10] and Sheehan et al. [11] had authors from health, social sciences, and statistics departments; Mandal et al. [12] included authors from health, biological sciences, and mathematics. The two most common multidisciplinary authorship teams integrated experts from health and geography (24%) and health and other fields (26%). Author groups with members in multiple disciplines and author groups that include departments of geography appear to be increasing over time (Fig. 7.2). As depicted in Table 7.2, 63% of the studies we reviewed included authors from only academic institutions. The remaining author groups included authors from non-academic settings, including national public health organizations [13], county or statewide public health departments [11, 14–18], hospitals [19–23], and private technology companies [9, 24].

Sixteen studies (42%) were published in journals that are categorized as being medical in nature, with sub-categories such as oncology, public health, and health services. One article each was published in a predominantly social science or geo-

Table 7.1 Articles reviewed (N = 38 articles)

First author, year	Article title	Journal
Anderson, 2014 [30]	Breast cancer screening, area deprivation, and later-stage breast cancer in Appalachia: Does geography matter?	Health Services Research
Bambhroliya, 2012 [41]	Spatial analysis of county-level breast cancer mortality in Texas	Journal of Environmental and Public Health
Beyer, 2016 [28]	New spatially continuous indices of redlining and racial bias in mortgage lending: links to survival after breast cancer diagnosis and implications for health disparities research	Health & Place
Chien, 2013 [38]	Efficient mapping and geographic disparities in breast cancer mortality at the county-level by race and age in the U.S.	Spatial and Spatiotemporal Epidemiology
Crabbe 2015 [36]	Secular trends, race, and geographic disparity of early-stage breast cancer incidence: 25 years of surveillance in Connecticut	American Journal of Public Health
Dai 2010 [42]	Black residential segregation, disparities in spatial access to health care facilities, and late-stage breast cancer diagnosis in metropolitan Detroit	Health & Place
DeGuzman, 2017 [45]	Impact of urban neighborhood disadvantage on late stage breast cancer diagnosis in Virginia	Journal of Urban Health
Gregorio, 2017 [34]	Geography of breast cancer incidence according to age & birth cohorts	Spatial and Spatiotemporal Epidemiology
Han, 2004 [20]	Geographic clustering of residence in early life and subsequent risk of breast cancer (United States)	Cancer Causes and Control
Han, 2005 [25]	Assessing spatio-temporal variability of risk surfaces using residential history data in a case control study of breast cancer	International Journal of Health Geographics
Highfield, 2013 [22]	Spatial patterns of breast cancer incidence and uninsured women of mammography screening age	Breast Journal
Hsu 2004 [39]	Evaluating the disparity of female breast cancer mortality among racial groups – a spatiotemporal analysis	International Journal of Health Geographics
Huang 2009 [16]	Does distance matter? Distance to mammography facilities and stage at diagnosis of breast cancer in Kentucky	Journal of Rural Health
Jacquez 2013 [24]	Residential mobility and breast cancer in Marin County, California, USA	International Journal of Environmental Research and Public Health
Kulldorff 1997 [13]	Breast cancer clusters in the northeast United States: a geographic analysis	American Journal of Epidemiology
Lin, 2017 [48]	Geographic variations of colorectal and breast cancer late-stage diagnosis and the effects of neighborhood-level factors	Journal of Rural Health

(continued)

Table 7.1   (continued)

First author, year	Article title	Journal
Liu, 2016 [43]	Risks of developing breast and colorectal cancer in association with incomes and geographic locations in Texas: a retrospective cohort study	BMC Cancer
MacKinnon, 2007 [17]	Detecting an association between socioeconomic status and late stage breast cancer using spatial analysis and area-based measures	Cancer Epidemiology, Biomarkers and Prevention
Mandal, 2009 [12]	Spatial trends of breast and prostate cancers in the United States between 2000 and 2005	International Journal of Health Geographics
Nichols, 2014 [49]	The geographic distribution of mammography resources in Mississippi	Online Journal of Public Health Informatics
Onitilo, 2014 [23]	Geographical and seasonal barriers to mammography services and breast cancer stage at diagnosis	Rural and Remote Health
Roche, 2002 [14]	Use of a geographic information system to identify and characterize areas with high proportions of distant stage breast cancer	Journal of Public Health Management and Practice
Roche, 2017 [15]	Disparities in female breast cancer stage at diagnosis in New Jersey: a spatial-temporal analysis	Journal of Public Health Management and Practice
Schootman, 2009 [44]	The role of poverty rate and racial distribution in the geographic clustering of breast cancer survival among older women: a geographic and multilevel analysis	American Journal of Epidemiology
Schootman, 2010 [19]	Temporal trends in geographic disparities in small-area breast cancer incidence and mortality, 1988–2005	Cancer Epidemiology, Biomarkers and Prevention
Scott, 2017 [35]	Geospatial analysis of inflammatory breast cancer and associated community characteristics in the United States	International Journal of Environmental Research and Public Health
Sheehan, 2000 [11]	Geographic assessment of breast cancer screening by towns, zip codes, and census tracts	Journal of Public Health Management and Practice
Sheehan, 2004 [18]	The geographic distribution of breast cancer incidence in Massachusetts 1988–1997, adjusted for covariates	International Journal of Health Geographics
Sheehan, 2005 [37]	A space-time analysis of the proportion of late stage breast cancer in Massachusetts, 1988–1997	International Journal of Health Geographics
Tarlov, 2009 [21]	Characteristics of mammography facility locations and stage of breast cancer at diagnosis in Chicago	Journal of Urban Health
Tian, 2010 [40]	Female breast cancer mortality clusters within racial groups in the United States	Health & Place
Tian, 2012 [9]	Identifying risk factors for disparities in breast cancer mortality among African-American and Hispanic women	Women's Health Issues

(continued)

Table 7.1 (continued)

First author, year	Article title	Journal
Vieira, 2005 [26]	Spatial analysis of lung, colorectal, and breast cancer on Cape Cod: an application of generalized additive models to case-control data	Environmental Health
Vieira, 2008 [27]	Spatial-temporal analysis of breast cancer in upper Cape Cod, Massachusetts	International Journal of Health Geographics
Wang, 2008 [47]	Late-stage breast cancer diagnosis and health care access in illinois	Professional Geographer
Wang, 2010 [62]	Healthcare access, socioeconomic factors and late-stage cancer diagnosis: an exploratory spatial analysis and public policy implication	International Journal of Public Policy
Williams, 2015 [10]	Rural-urban difference in female breast cancer diagnosis in Missouri	Rural and Remote Health
Yao, 2013 [29]	Radiation therapy resources and guideline-concordant radiotherapy for early-stage breast cancer patients in an underserved region	Health Services Research

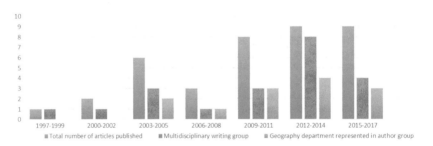

Fig. 7.2 Articles published by year and type of authorship group (N = 38 articles)

spatial journal, and the rest were published in journals with two or more categories: medicine and social sciences (21%), medicine and information sciences (16%), and medicine and environmental sciences (16%). About 25% of articles published in medical journals included authors with affiliations in departments of geography (data not shown).

7.3.2 Source and Type of Cancer Outcome Data

Statewide cancer registry data was by far the most common source of outcome data (58%). Cancer registries typically provide details about patient-level cancer diagnosis, treatment and vital status, but not consistently for all U.S. states. Mechanisms of reporting varied by state. Data was additionally retrieved from national and statewide sources of vital statistics, the Surveillance, Epidemiology and End Results

Table 7.2 Characteristics of reviewed articles: authorship groups, cancer outcomes, data source and region (N = 38 articles reviewed)

Article characteristics	N (%)	Article characteristics, (contd)	N (%)
Journal category		Outcome data source[a]	
Medicine only	16 (42.1)	Statewide cancer registry	22 (57.9)
Medicine & Social Sciences	8 (21.0)	SEER cancer registry[c]	3 (7.9)
Medicine & Informatics	6 (15.8)	Other national cancer registry[d]	4 (10.5)
Medicine & Environmental Science	6 (15.8)	Hospital cancer registry	1 (2.6)
Earth & Planetary Science	1 (2.6)	Case-control study	5 (13.2)
Social Sciences	1 (2.6)	Vital statistics registry	4 (10.5)
Author disciplines represented[a]		Geographic unit of analysis	
Public Health/Medicine	34 (89.5)	Exact Address	8 (21.0)
Geography	13 (34.2)	Census block group	3 (7.9)
Physical Sciences	3 (7.9)	Census tract	12 (31.6)
Statistics/Math	4 (10.5)	Zip code	3 (7.9)
Social Sciences	7 (18.4)	County	12 (31.6)
Biological Sciences	1 (2.6)	Geographic study coverage	
No. disciplines in author group		Single City	3 (7.9)
One	18 (47.3)	Multiple cities in one state	2 (5.3)
Two	16 (42.1)	Sub-county region	2 (5.3)
Three or more	4 (10.5)	Single county	1 (2.6)
Composition of author groups		Multiple county region in one state	4 (10.5)
Health only	15 (39.5)	Single state	18 (47.3)
Geography only	3 (7.9)	Multiple state contiguous region	2 (5.3)
Health and geography	9 (23.7)	SEER[c] program regions	2 (5.3)
Health and other	10 (26.3)	Nationwide	4 (10.5)
Geography and other	1 (2.6)	State-specific study locations (n = 30)[a,e]	
Author Institutional Affiliation		Connecticut	2 (6.7)
University only	24 (63.2)	Illinois	3 (10.0)
Government only	2 (5.3)	Kentucky	3 (10.0)
Hospital only	1 (2.6)	Massachusetts	5 (16.7)
University + other[b]	11 (28.9)	New Jersey	2 (6.7)
Cancer outcome type[a]		New York	2 (6.7)

(continued)

Table 7.2 (continued)

Article characteristics	N (%)	Article characteristics, (contd)	N (%)
Overall incidence	8 (21.0)	Texas	4 (13.3)
Stage-specific incidence	17 (44.7)	Wisconsin	2 (6.7)
Odds of breast cancer	5 (13.2)	Other[f]	7 (23.3)
Cancer-specific mortality	9 (23.7)	Urbanicity of target population	
Survival time	1 (2.6)	Urban	8 (21.0)
Treatment receipt	1 (2.6)	Rural	6 (15.8)
		Mixed	24 (63.2)

[a]These categories are not mutually exclusive
[b]Other includes government, industry, hospital, or research foundation
[c]Surveillance Epidemiology and End Results Program
[d]Including National Program of Cancer Registries (NPCR), and United States Cancer Statistics (USCS)
[e]Excluding studies that were regional or nationwide
[f]The following states had one study each: California, Florida, Michigan, Mississippi, Missouri, South Dakota, Virginia

(SEER) program (8%) and other sources of national cancer statistics such as the National Program of Cancer Registries (NPCR), and United States Cancer Statistics (USCS) (11%). Three different population-based case-control studies of breast cancer which collected lifetime residential history were described in five papers [20, 24–27] (Table 7.2).

With regard to type of cancer outcome, most studies fell into three categories: studies of the overall incidence of breast cancer (21%), stage-specific incidence of breast cancer (45%), breast cancer mortality (24%). For the case-control studies, the outcome was odds of breast cancer (13%). One article each studied survival time after breast cancer diagnosis [28] and receipt of radiation therapy for treatment-eligible breast cancer patients [29].

7.3.3   Study Regions and Geographic Unit of Analysis

Articles reviewed covered a wide range of geographical coverage areas and target populations. Most conducted their study across a single state (47%). Others studied a single city or greater metropolitan area (8%), multiple neighboring cities (5%), a sub-county region (5%), across multiple neighboring counties that are, for example, served by the same healthcare system (11%), across multiple neighboring states in a specific region of the country (5%), and nationwide (11%). Two studies focused a set of contiguous counties across multiple states in the rural Appalachian region [29, 30] in the eastern part of the U.S. Research groups that used SEER for cancer outcome data (5%) were able to examine the association of interest in SEER participating states and regions. SEER states are CA, CT, IA, KY, LA, NJ, NM, and

UT. Regions that are also part of the SEER program are in MI GA, and WA. It became apparent that there are regions in the U.S. that published studies fitting our selection criteria more frequently than other regions. More than half of the studies reviewed were conducted in New England and the East North Central regions of the country. There were comparatively fewer studies conducted in the Mountain and Pacific regions (Table 7.2).

The geographic unit of analysis reflected the granularity available through the data sources, with a strong emphasis on ensuring protection of private health information for administrative data sources. Units ranged from individual address-level (most granular), to county-level (least granular). Individual-level addresses were available in the case-control studies, a hospital records-based study [23], and two of the statewide cancer registry studies [16, 21]. The most common units were census tracts (32%) and counties (32%). These units were used more frequently than using zip codes or zip code areas, which together, comprised 8% of the studies.

7.3.4   Spatial Methods

We classified the authors' motivation for use of spatial analytic techniques broadly in to four categories: (1) to model spatial variation in an outcome variable, including the need to "fill in" sparse data; (2) to identify spatial clusters of an outcome variable; (3) to measure proximity and travel distance to health care services for use as an exposure variable; and (4) to identify factors associated with the spatial and temporal distribution of disease. Accordingly, spatial techniques were grouped into the following categories: (1) spatial interpolation methods, which leverage the underlying spatial distribution to estimate risk across space, and address sparse data issues by accounting for uncertainty in local measurement and spatial dependence between neighboring measurements; (2) global and local spatial statistics, which are a broad class of methods that analyze and test how traits, events, or relationships are distributed over space; (3) proximity analysis to classify healthcare accessibility based on spatial and non-spatial factors such as distance, cost, and quality of services; and (4) spatiotemporal analysis, which describe the stability and change of values across space over time. As depicted in Table 7.3, these geospatial analytic methods were further divided into more specific methodologies, distinguished by the level of detail described in the literature.

The most prevalent type of spatial analysis was the spatial cluster analysis, which is used to identify a geographic area with significantly elevated risk of the outcome of interest. Generally, a cluster of disease is a region with higher than expected levels of the outcome variable. More rigorously, a cluster should reflect a higher than expected likelihood of disease that persists after accounting for other known influences [31]. Cluster statistics can be implemented with point location or aggregated data, and they can detect regions with higher than expected levels of cancer both globally and locally. Global cluster methods (e.g., Moran's I) test for global autocorrelation of an outcome variable, but do not identify specific clusters.

Table 7.3 Geospatial analytic methods used in reviewed literature (N = 38)

Geospatial analytic method[a, b]	N (%)
Spatial Smoothing and Interpolation	5 (13.2)
Kernel density estimation (n = 3)	
Empirical Bayes smoothing (n = 2)	
Proximity Analysis	11 (28.9)
Euclidian distance (n = 1)	
Network distance and travel time (n = 7)	
Two-step floating catchment area (n = 4)	
Adaptive spatial filtering (n = 1)	
Spatial Cluster Analysis	25 (65.8)
Global Spatial cluster statistics (N = 24)	
Moran's I (n = 5)	
Oden's Ipop (n = 2)	
k-function (n = 1)	
Local Spatial cluster statistics	
The Getis-Ord Gi (n = 2)	
Q statistics (n = 1)	
Local indicators of spatial association (LISA) (n = 4)	
Spatial Regression Models (n = 6)	
Spatial scan statistic (n = 12)	
Structured additive regression models (n = 1)	
Local generalized additive regression models (n = 2)	
Spatial lag regression models (n = 2)	
Geographic weighted regression (n = 2)	
Spatiotemporal Statistics	5 (13.2)
Space and Time Scan Statistic (n = 5)	
Space-time k function (n = 1)	

[a]These categories are not mutually exclusive
[b]Spatial analytic methods were classified using techniques described in publication method sections. Specificity of methods descriptions varied across articles and journals

Local methods (e.g., Getis-Ord Gi∗) can define the locations and extent of the clusters in a region. The spatial scan statistic uses a circular or elliptical scanning window to identify cluster patterns, and employs Bernoulli and Poisson model structures to compare observed and expected outcome counts while adjusting for additional explanatory variables [32]. The spatial scan statistic was used in 14 (32%) of the studies we reviewed. Indeed, this method has been widely applied in health-related research thanks in part to SaTScan, a freely available software for implementation of the method that is user-friendly to a non-specialized audience.

Five studies implemented spatiotemporal cluster analysis to understand how spatial patterns of cancer outcomes varied over space and time.

Studies which leveraged modeling to identify factors associated with the spatial distribution of a cancer outcome did so with a variety of methodological approaches. We observed both frequentist and Bayesian regression modeling that accounted for spatial covariance structures, such as simultaneous autoregressive and moving average models. We also frequently observed non-spatial models that were implemented after a spatial analysis, for example by treating the output of a cluster analysis as an outcome variable and then using logistic regression models to identify factors associated with a specific region being labeled as a hotspot in the cluster analysis. The latter has the advantage of being approachable to a wider audience but may disregard potential important spatial variations in relationships. Geographic weighted regression (GWR) models, which were used in two of the papers we reviewed, are a relatively new class of models used for exploratory spatial analysis. GWRs incorporate spatial structures of data into statistical models to generate localized regression coefficients that elucidate geographic variation in the relationships between dependent variables and covariates predictors [33].

Another common use of spatial methods was to quantify accessibility to access to health care and mammogram screening facilities through proximity analysis, including network analysis, two-step floating catchment area, and adaptive spatial filtering methods. For many of these studies, geocoded locations of cancer patients and available regional services were used to calculate drive-times and correlate them with stage of cancer diagnosis and cancer survival.

7.3.5   Key Themes in the Research Findings

7.3.5.1   Spatial and Space-Time Cluster Studies

Geospatial approaches were used to identify areas with higher or lower than expected incidence of overall or invasive breast cancer [12, 17, 18, 22, 34], incidence of inflammatory breast cancer [35], proportion of breast cancers diagnosed at an early or late stage [11, 14, 36, 37], and breast cancer mortality [13, 38–40]. Some of these investigators also examined temporal patterns to identify whether spatial clustering was also relevant to specific time periods [15, 18, 37, 40]. In an effort to elucidate possible sources of environmental exposures or exposure latency periods, the studies utilizing case-control data from Massachusetts, Western New York and California were concerned with the spatial clustering of lifetime residential history and its relationship with case/control status [20, 24–27]. Gregorio et al. examined geographic variation in breast cancer incidence in Connecticut according to age and birth cohort and found the global distribution of incidence rates across places to be more heterogeneous for younger women and later birth cohorts [34]. Many of these studies also elucidated racial/ethnic and socioeconomic disparities as explanatory factors for identified clusters, as described below.

7.3.5.2 Racial and Ethnic Disparities and Segregation

Many studies examined how the distribution of cancer outcomes across a region differ by race/ethnicity. In a study of Texas breast cancer mortality, regions with higher mortality rates had higher proportion of non-Hispanic blacks in urban areas and Hispanic blacks in border regions in Texas [41]. In Michigan, spatial analysis identified areas of greater black segregation significantly increases the risk of later stage of diagnosis [42]. In New Jersey, regions with higher than expected rates of later stage at diagnosis were found to have higher proportions of Hispanic populations and linguistically isolated households [14]. Beyer et al. used novel methods for classifying racial bias in mortgage lending and investigated association between these new measures and breast cancer survival among Black/African American women in the Milwaukee, Wisconsin metropolitan area [28]. Schootman et al., used the SEER program data to calculate measures of absolute and relative disparities their spatiotemporal analysis identified patterns of decreasing disparities over time for all breast cancer indicators except for in situ breast cancer [19].

7.3.5.3 Socioeconomic Status

Breast cancer outcomes were found to be both positively and negatively associated with geographic distribution of income across study regions. Incidence of breast cancer and proportion of cancers diagnosed at an early stage were found to be more common in regions with higher household income and insurance levels in Texas [22, 43]. These findings could be explained by availability of screening and poor spatial access to health care. In an analysis of breast cancer survival across nine SEER regions, stage at diagnosis and census-tract poverty (and patient's race in Atlanta) explained geographic variation in breast cancer survival [44]. In Florida, neighborhoods of severe and near poverty were found to be associated with higher-than-expected incidence of late stage breast cancer [17]. Inner-city poverty in urban Virginia impacts risk of late stage breast cancer diagnosis [45]. Anderson et al. used GWR techniques to identify relationships with late stage breast cancer and area deprivation in Appalachia, finding that most deprived counties had a 3.31 times greater rate of late stage cancers compared to the least deprived [30]. Because of the known high correlations between breast cancer and income level as well as between neighborhood and socioeconomic status, spatial variation in breast cancer outcomes was frequently explained by SES and was not surprisingly a very common theme in the literature reviewed.

7.3.5.4 Spatial Access to Health Care Services

Spatial network analytic methods are typically used to understand accessibility to health care through examining the flow characteristics of transportation networks [46]. Eleven studies utilized road network analyses methods to examine the role of health care distance on cancer outcomes; we did not review any studies that analyzed public transportation networks. The majority of these studies focused on rural populations, and evaluated average distance to mammography clinics, primary care providers, federally qualified health care centers and treatment facilities. In Illinois, poor geographical access to primary health care significantly increases the risk of late diagnosis among rural residents [47], and Tarlov et al. identified a positive association between number of homicides near mammography facilities and later stage at diagnosis in urban Chicago [21]. In Wisconsin, travel time to nearest mammogram center was found to be inversely related to breast cancer stage at diagnosis [10, 23]. In Kentucky, advanced diagnoses had longer than average travel distances than early stage diagnoses [16], and the limited availability of radiation therapy resources in the Appalachian region was found to be associated with disparities in receipt of guideline-concordant radiotherapy [29]. Spatial accessibility and travel time to health care facilities did not explain variation in breast cancer outcomes in studies in South Dakota, Texas and Mississippi [9, 48, 49]. Use of GIS to classify accessibility to cancer health services seems to be a growing area of research with increasingly sophisticated methodology. However, point-based (as opposed to area-based) approaches are likely more valid for making inference in individual-level data.

7.3.6   Limitations of Spatial Approaches

Reviewed articles described similar limitations in spatial approaches in their discussion sections. Most articles commented on their limited accuracy, resulting from imprecise geocoding and data restricted to aggregation at specific geographical unit of analysis. Aggregation to different units of analysis, or areal units, leads to a number of considerations. First is the concern of 'ecological fallacy', the issue of misattributing relations identified at a population level, in this case the areal unit, to the individual level [50–52]. The second concern is the similar Modifiable Areal Unit Problem (MAUP), the arbitrary creation of aerial units, such as assigning neighborhood boundaries that local residents would not recognize, or misusing areal units made for one purpose for another, such as using zip code data meant for the postal service for health service assessment [53, 54]. These two concepts describe the same problem and are often interchangeably used by different disciplines. The arbitrary selection of boundary may influence generated estimates [55]. The second most common limitation described was missing or unavailable data, followed by not accounting for spatiotemporal variation in analyses. Inadequate power, lack of generalizability outside study population and region, and measurement error were also commonly described limitations.

7.4   Discussion

The use of geospatial methods can provide powerful insight into the relationship between spatial characteristics and cancer outcomes. We have conducted a systematic literature review to describe the recent use of geospatial techniques in understanding the epidemiology of breast cancer. Boulos et al. [56] conducted a systematic literature review examining the use of GIS in oncological research. Their findings are similar to ours; while the use of geospatial methods in cancer research is increasing, it is underutilized, and findings are often inconsistent and may be due to differences in employed methodologies, geographical region, and units of analyses. Gomez et al. [57] had similar findings in their review of neighborhood and built environmental factors and cancer outcomes.

The studies we reviewed varied substantially in the questions addressed and regions studied. Our review was restricted to studies conducted within the US for more comparability across data sources and screening policies. We were not surprised to find that a majority of the studies reviewed addressed issues of race/ethnicity, SES, or spatial access to health care as those factors are attributed to disparities in the cancers of interest, and also frequently co-vary with geolocation. We were also not surprised to find that the majority of studies used cancer registry data (or SEER) as their primary source of outcome data. We were more surprised to find, however, that some parts of the country were significantly overrepresented, while other regions were absent. The SEER registries include 18 geographic regions and cover only 28% of the U.S. population. Advantages to using SEER are the relative ease in access to data, and data harmonization across regions. The National Program of Cancer Registries (NPCR), established in 1992 by Congress via the Cancer Registries Amendment Act requires that all U.S. states have cancer registration systems. Complexity of the process to access these data for research varies from state-to-state [58]. Excluding three nationwide analyses, the studies we reviewed accessed data in a total of 23 U.S. states (or regions within those states), leaving the other 27 not represented at all.

The analytic methods and software used in the literature varied substantially in terms of its sophistication and application. Geospatial approaches surveyed ranged from visualization of cancer instances with GIS to advanced spatiotemporal statistics. The more sophisticated methods have demonstrated the ability to identify clusters of cancer outcomes as well as to model the local association of outcomes on possible predictors, while accounting for the spatial autocorrelation in both the predictors and the outcome. In spite of this promise, comparatively few of the existing studies draw on these more advanced methods. One reason for this lack of systematized agreement in geospatial techniques is the relative newness of geospatial methods in cancer epidemiology. Institutions like the NCI have taken strides to address this inconsistency by introducing easy to use mapping software (e.g., SaTScan, which was heavily represented in the literature we reviewed). However, differences in the knowledge base of researchers may be important. One way to deal with this issue is more emphasis on multidisciplinary collaborative teams, pairing cancer epidemiologists and oncologists with geoscientists and other spatial scientists to pool skills, maximizing the potential of the geospatial cancer studies. Indeed, our findings may suggest that multidisciplinary author groups, or author groups that include members of geography department facilitate the use of more sophisticated advanced spatial methods.

Cancer is a life-threatening disease and particularly sensitive public health concern. The kind of data needed to conduct studies of incidence and mortality at a local area level, such as street addresses, census blocks or even zip codes are considered protected health identifiers (PHI) because of their potential to reveal patient identity. It is generally difficult to gain access to these data at the smallest unit of geographic analysis, and when obtained, data use agreements often prevent mapping them in areas with small case numbers or sparse populations. Advances in geospatial sciences have yielded methods to mask the privacy of data, such as merging similar areas of small populations, or to otherwise obtain regions of comparable populations that do not necessarily reflect boundaries provided on maps and maintain geoprivacy [59, 60]. These have been incorporated into social science and public health research with modest success [61]. However, one can argue that the rarity, severity, and sensitivity of this disease add up to an imperative to incorporate such methods in cancer epidemiology. Despite this, we saw limited use of them in our review.

Our literature review is subject to limitations. Our inclusion and exclusion criteria limit the generalizability of our findings, for example, we excluded studies conducted outside of the U.S. Further, we may not have described all the ways that cancer researchers are using geography. Spatial methods are important in exposure studies, which we did not include. Many studies were excluded for their use of mapping only. For our tabulations, there remains a possibility of misclassifying authors by using their first listed affiliation. We assumed this department and/or affiliation reflected the field of expertise of the author in order to classify authorship groups. In particular, public health and medical departments frequently employ spatial scientists, so our metric of Geography department authorship should not be considered a proxy for the representation of spatial expertise. Misclassification may have also occurred when categorizing spatial methods. Spatial methods of the reviewed literature were described and subsequently classified using text descriptions from the methods sections of the journal articles. The level of detail describing the analyses varied greatly across journals. For example, articles published in journals geared toward geography/spatial science audiences did not detail out basic methods to the extent an article published in a health science journal would. The lack of consistency might result in misclassification of methods implemented.

We evaluated the existing usage of geospatial methods for breast cancer epidemiology to guide future uses of this approach. Our summarization of this literature suggests that the adoption of geospatial methods in cancer epidemiology has been slow going and that spatial methods are not uniformly being used to their full potential. A key limitation of this slow adoption seems to be a lack of awareness of the full scope of methods available. This could be improved by increased accessibility to cancer outcomes data, strategic use of methods to maintain health privacy, and pooling research specialties through more inter-disciplinary collaborations. Understanding spatial dynamics of cancer outcomes and their relationship with other spatially varying characteristics, such as race, income, and availability of services, is important to inform policy and prevention efforts.

References

1. Korycinski RW, Tennant BL, Cawley MA, Bloodgood B, Oh AY, Berrigan D. Geospatial approaches to cancer control and population sciences at the United States cancer centers. Cancer Causes Control. 2018;29(3):371–7.
2. Yang TC, Matthews SA. Understanding the non-stationary associations between distrust of the health care system, health conditions, and self-rated health in the elderly: a geographically weighted regression approach. Health Place. 2012;18(3):576–85.
3. Miranda ML, Casper M, Tootoo J, Schieb L. Putting chronic disease on the map: building GIS capacity in state and local health departments. Prev Chronic Dis. 2013;10:E100.
4. Society AC. Cancer facts & figures 2016. In: Society AC, ed. Atlanta 2016.
5. Alford-Teaster J, Lange JM, Hubbard RA, et al. Is the closest facility the one actually used? An assessment of travel time estimation based on mammography facilities. Int J Health Geogr. 2016;15(1):8.
6. Dean L. The role of social capital in African-American women's use of mammography. Soc Sci Med. 2014;104:148–56.
7. Musa GJ, Chiang PH, Sylk T, et al. Use of GIS mapping as a public health tool-from Cholera to Cancer. Health Serv Insights. 2013;6:111–6.
8. Fotheringham S, Brunsdon C, Charlton M. Geographically weighted regression: the analysis of spatially varying relationships. New York: Wiley; 2003.
9. Tian N, Goovaerts P, Zhan FB, Chow TE, Wilson JG. Identifying risk factors for disparities in breast cancer mortality among African-American and Hispanic women. Women's Health Issues Publ Jacobs Inst Women's Health. 2012;22:e267–76.
10. Williams F, Jeanetta S, O'Brien DJ, Fresen JL. Rural-urban difference in female breast cancer diagnosis in Missouri. Rural Remote Health. 2015;15:3063.
11. Sheehan TJ, Gershman ST, MacDougall LA, et al. Geographic assessment of breast cancer screening by towns, zip codes, and census tracts. J Public Health Manag Pract. 2000;6:48–57.
12. Mandal R, St-Hilaire S, Kie JG, Derryberry D. Spatial trends of breast and prostate cancers in the United States between 2000 and 2005. Int J Health Geogr. 2009;8:53.
13. Kulldorff M, Feuer EJ, Ba M, Freedman LS. Breast cancer clusters in the northeast United States: a geographic analysis. Am J Epidemiol. 1997;146:161–70.
14. Roche LM, Skinner R, Weinstein RB. Use of a geographic information system to identify and characterize areas with high proportions of distant stage Breast Cancer. J Public Health Manag Pract. 2002;8:26–32.
15. Roche LM, Niu X, Stroup AM, Henry KA. Disparities in female Breast Cancer stage at diagnosis in New Jersey: a spatial-temporal analysis. J Public Health Manag Pract. 2017;23(5):477–86.
16. Huang B, Dignan M, Han D, Johnson O. Does distance matter? Distance to mammography facilities and stage at diagnosis of breast cancer in kentucky. J Rural Health. 2009;25:366–71.
17. MacKinnon JA, Duncan RC, Huang Y, et al. Detecting an association between socioeconomic status and late stage breast cancer using spatial analysis and area-based measures. Cancer Epidemiol Biomark Prev Publ Am Assoc Cancer Res Am Soc Prev Oncol. 2007;16:756–62.
18. Joseph Sheehan T, DeChello LM, Kulldorff M, Gregorio DI, Gershman S, Mroszczyk M. The geographic distribution of breast cancer incidence in Massachusetts 1988 to 1997, adjusted for covariates. Int J Health Geogr. 2004;3:17.

19. Schootman M, Lian M, Deshpande AD, et al. Temporal trends in geographic disparities in small-area breast cancer incidence and mortality, 1988 to 2005. Cancer Epidemiol Biomark Prev Publ Am Assoc Cancer Res Am Soc Prev Oncol. 2010;19:1122–31.

20. Han D, Rogerson PA, Nie J, et al. Geographic clustering of residence in early life and subsequent risk of Breast Cancer (United States). Cancer Causes Control. 2004;15:921–9.

21. Tarlov E, Zenk SN, Campbell RT, Warnecke RB, Block R. Characteristics of mammography facility locations and stage of breast cancer at diagnosis in Chicago. J Urban Health. 2009;86:196–213.

22. Highfield L. Spatial patterns of breast cancer incidence and uninsured women of mammography screening age. Breast J. 2013;19(3):293–301.

23. Onitilo AA, Liang H, Stankowski RV, et al. Geographical and seasonal barriers to mammography services and breast cancer stage at diagnosis. Rural Remote Health. 2014;14(3):2738.

24. Jacquez GM, Barlow J, Rommel R, et al. Residential mobility and breast cancer in Marin County, California, USA. Int J Environ Res Public Health. 2013;11:271–95.

25. Han D, Rogerson PA, Bonner MR, et al. Assessing spatio-temporal variability of risk surfaces using residential history data in a case control study of breast cancer. Int J Health Geogr. 2005;4:9.

26. Vieira V, Webster T, Weinberg J, Aschengrau A, Ozonoff D. Spatial analysis of lung, colorectal, and Breast Cancer on Cape Cod: an application of generalized additive models to case-control data. Environ Health Glob Access Sci Source. 2005;4:11.

27. Vieira VM, Webster TF, Weinberg JM, Aschengrau A. Spatial-temporal analysis of breast cancer in upper Cape Cod, Massachusetts. Int J Health Geogr. 2008;7:46.

28. Beyer KM, Zhou Y, Matthews K, Bemanian A, Laud PW, Nattinger AB. New spatially continuous indices of redlining and racial bias in mortgage lending: links to survival after breast cancer diagnosis and implications for health disparities research. Health Place. 2016;40:34–43.

29. Yao N, Matthews SA, Hillemeier MM, Anderson RT. Radiation therapy resources and guideline-concordant radiotherapy for early-stage breast cancer patients in an underserved region. Health Serv Res. 2013;48(4):1433–49.

30. Anderson RT, Yang TC, Matthews SA, et al. Breast cancer screening, area deprivation, and later-stage breast cancer in appalachia: does geography matter? Health Serv Res. 2014;49:546–67.

31. Wakefield JC, Kelsall JE, Morris SE. Clustering, cluster detection and spatial variation in risk. In: Elliott P, Wakefield JC, Best NG, Briggs DJ, editors. Spaital epidemiology- methods and applications. Oxford: Oxford University Press; 2000. p. 128–52.

32. Kulldorff M, Nagarwalla N. Spatial disease clusters: detection and inference. Stat Med. 1995;14(8):799–810.

33. Nakaya T, Fotheringham AS, Brunsdon C, Charlton M. Geographically weighted poisson regression for disease association mapping. Stat Med. 2005;24(17):2695–717.

34. Gregorio DI, Ford C, Samociuk H. Geography of breast cancer incidence according to age & birth cohorts. Spat Spatiotemporal Epidemiol. 2017;21:47–55.

35. Scott L, Mobley LR, Il'yasova D. Geospatial analysis of inflammatory Breast Cancer and associated community characteristics in the United States. Int J Environ Res Public Health. 2017;14(4)

36. Crabbe JCF, Gregorio DI, Samociuk H, Swede H. Secular trends, race, and geographic disparity of early-stage breast cancer incidence: 25 years of surveillance in Connecticut. Am J Public Health. 2015;105:e64–70.

37. Sheehan TJ, DeChello LM. A space-time analysis of the proportion of late stage breast cancer in Massachusetts, 1988 to 1997. Int J Health Geogr. 2005;4:15.

38. Chien LC, Yu HL, Schootman M. Efficient mapping and geographic disparities in breast cancer mortality at the county-level by race and age in the U.S. Spat Spatiotemporal Epidemiol. 2013;5:27–37.

39. Ed Hsu C, Jacobson H, Soto Mas F. Evaluating the disparity of female breast cancer mortality among racial groups – a spatiotemporal analysis. Int J Health Geogr. 2004;3:4.

40. Tian N, Gaines Wilson J, Benjamin Zhan F. Female breast cancer mortality clusters within racial groups in the United States. Health Place. 2010;16:209–18.
41. Bambhroliya AB, Burau KD, Sexton K. Spatial analysis of county-level breast cancer mortality in Texas. J Environ Public Health. 2012;2012:959343.
42. Dai D. Black residential segregation, disparities in spatial access to health care facilities, and late-stage breast cancer diagnosis in metropolitan Detroit. Health Place. 2010;16:1038–52.
43. Liu Z, Zhang K, Du XL. Risks of developing breast and colorectal cancer in association with incomes and geographic locations in Texas: a retrospective cohort study. BMC Cancer. 2016;16:294.
44. Schootman M, Jeffe DB, Lian M, Gillanders WE, Aft R. The role of poverty rate and racial distribution in the geographic clustering of breast cancer survival among older women: a geographic and multilevel analysis. Am J Epidemiol. 2009;169:554–61.
45. DeGuzman PB, Cohn WF, Camacho F, Edwards BL, Sturz VN, Schroen AT. Impact of urban neighborhood disadvantage on late stage Breast Cancer diagnosis in Virginia. J Urban Health. 2017;94(2):199–210.
46. Hensher DA. Handbook of transport geography and spatial systems. Oxford: Elsevier; 2004.
47. Wang F, McLafferty S, Escamilla V, Luo L. Late-stage Breast Cancer diagnosis and health care access in illinois. Prof Geogr J Assoc Am Geogr. 2008;60:54–69.
48. Lin Y, Wimberly MC. Geographic variations of colorectal and Breast Cancer late-stage diagnosis and the effects of neighborhood-level factors. J Rural Health. 2017;33(2):146–57.
49. Nichols EN, Bradley DL, Zhang X, Faruque F, Duhé RJ. The geographic distribution of mammography resources in Mississippi. Online J Public Health Informatics. 2014;5:226.
50. Robinson WS. Ecological correlations and the behavior of individuals. Am Sociol Rev. 1950;15(3):351–7.
51. Subramanian SV, Jones K, Kaddour A, Krieger N. Revisiting Robinson: the perils of individualistic and ecologic fallacy. Int J Epidemiol. 2009;38(2):342–60; author reply 370-343
52. Commentary FG. Is the social world flat? W.S. Robinson and the ecologic fallacy. Int J Epidemiol. 2009;38(2):368–70.. author reply 370-363
53. Flowerdew R, Manley DJ, Sabel CE. Neighbourhood effects on health: does it matter where you draw the boundaries? Soc Sci Med. 2008;66(6):1241–55.
54. Haynes R, Daras K, Reading R, Jones A. Modifiable neighbourhood units, zone design and residents' perceptions. Health Place. 2007;13(4):812–25.
55. Gehlke CE, Biehl K. Certain effects of grouping upon the size of the correlation coefficient in census tract material. J Am Stat Assoc. 1934;29(185):169–70.
56. Boulos DNK, Ghali RR, Ibrahim EM, Boulos MNK, AbdelMalik P. An eight-year snapshot of geospatial cancer research (2002-2009): clinico-epidemiological and methodological findings and trends. Med Oncol. 2011;28:1145–62.
57. Gomez SL, Shariff-Marco S, DeRouen M, et al. The impact of neighborhood social and built environment factors across the cancer continuum: current research, methodological considerations, and future directions. Cancer. 2015;121(14):2314–30.
58. Cancer Registry Research Approval Process: Classification of States by Level of Approval Required. In: 2016.
59. Rushton G, Armstrong MP, Gittler J, et al. Geocoding in cancer research: a review. Am J Prev Med. 2006;30(2 Suppl):S16–24.
60. Mu L, Wang F, Chen VW, Wu XC. A place-oriented, mixed-level regionalization method for constructing geographic areas in health data dissemination and analysis. Ann Assoc Am Geogr. 2014;105(1):48–66.
61. Kounadi O, Leitner M. Why does geoprivacy matter? The scientific publication of confidential data presented on maps. J Empir Res Hum Res Ethics. 2014;9(4):34–45.
62. Wang F, Luo L, McLafferty S. Healthcare access, socioeconomic factors and late-stage cancer diagnosis: an exploratory spatial analysis and public policy implication. Int J Public Policy. 2010;5:237–58.

Part II
Environment and Context

Chapter 8
Studying the Influence of the Neighborhood Obesogenic Environment on Breast Cancer in Epidemiological Cohorts: The Multiethnic Cohort

Shannon M. Conroy, Salma Shariff-Marco, Yurii B. Shvetsov, Jennifer Jain, Loïc Le Marchand, Lynne R. Wilkens, Scarlett Lin Gomez, and Iona Cheng

Abstract The obesogenic environment, defined as neighborhood social and built environment attributes that promote a positive energy balance and obesity, has only recently been considered for its role in shaping racial/ethnic disparities in obesity-related cancer outcomes. Applying a multilevel framework, the influence of the neighborhood obesogenic environment on breast cancer incidence was examined in the Multiethnic Cohort Study (MEC), with attention to differential associations in four major racial/ethnic groups—African American, Japanese American, Latino, and white. This chapter describes the approaches used to characterize the neighborhood obesogenic environment in the MEC, provides an overview of key findings in relation to post-menopausal breast cancer incidence, and discusses challenges and opportunities in neighborhood contextual studies of breast cancer. Findings to date suggest that a composite metric of neighborhood socioeconomic status is an independent risk factor for breast cancer across diverse populations, and that attributes of the built environment (e.g., mixed-land use and unhealthy food environments) have varying effects on breast cancer incidence by race/ethnicity. Future neighborhood stud-

S. M. Conroy · S. Shariff-Marco · S. L. Gomez · I. Cheng (✉)
Department of Epidemiology and Biostatistics, University of California, San Francisco, San Francisco, CA, USA

Helen Diller Family Comprehensive Cancer Center, University of California, San Francisco, CA, USA
e-mail: iona.cheng@ucsf.edu

Y. B. Shvetsov · L. Le Marchand · L. R. Wilkens
Population Sciences in the Pacific Program, University of Hawaii Cancer Center, Honolulu, HI, USA

J. Jain
Department of Epidemiology and Biostatistics, University of California, San Francisco, San Francisco, CA, USA

© Springer Nature Switzerland AG 2019
D. Berrigan, N. A. Berger (eds.), *Geospatial Approaches to Energy Balance and Breast Cancer*, Energy Balance and Cancer 15, https://doi.org/10.1007/978-3-030-18408-7_8

ies in the MEC will capitalize on novel longitudinal geospatial methods, expand to additional neighborhood measures, and integrate genetic and biomarker data. Robust epidemiologic cohorts integrating geospatial- and individual-level data are imperative to delineate and understand the key neighborhood attributes that impact breast cancer development, with the potential to ultimately impact public policies.

Keywords Breast neoplasms · Neighborhood environment · Obesity · Race/ethnicity · Socioeconomic status · Cohort studies

8.1 Introduction

Breast cancer is the most common cancer among women of all major U.S. racial/ethnic groups [1, 2]. In 2012–2016, age-adjusted incidence rates of breast cancer were highest among non-Hispanic whites (NHWs) at 136.6 per 100,000, followed by African Americans (124.0), Asian Americans/Pacific Islanders (AAPIs; 100.1), and Hispanics (97.2) [1]. Incidence rates increased between 2007 and 2016 among minorities, particularly in AAPIs (0.9% per year), while rates among NHWs remained stable [1]. Minorities relative to NHWs are more likely to be diagnosed with more clinically aggressive tumor subtypes based on joint expression of tumor markers for estrogen receptor (ER), progesterone receptor (PR), and human epidermal growth factor 2 (HER2) such as the higher prevalence of triple-negative subtypes (ER-, PR-, HER2-) in African Americans and Latinos [3]. AAPIs represents a heterogeneous group with substantial variability in migration patterns, acculturation, English language proficiency, socioeconomic status (SES), health behaviors, lifestyles, and culture [4–6], and differences in breast cancer incidence have been observed in AAPI sub-populations with incidence rates in Japanese Americans and Native Hawaiians approaching or surpassing that of NHWs [7, 8].

Racial/ethnic differences in breast cancer risk are partially explained by racial/ethnic-specific differences in the distribution of established risk factors for breast cancer, including reproductive (e.g., ages at first menarche, first birth, and menopause, parity, hormone therapy use) and behavioral factors (e.g., diet, physical activity, alcohol intake) [9–11]. These factors reflect the fact that research has largely focused on individual-level exposures, while the influence of the contextual environments in which these risk factors operate remain poorly understood. Neighborhood attributes of the social and built environments are recognized as an important context that can independently or synergistically impact health outcomes [12–15].

Neighborhood social and built environments are hypothesized to influence breast cancer development [16]. Empirical evidence of the role of residential neighborhoods in breast cancer incidence are largely from cancer registry studies using individual-level data on demographics, tumor characteristics, and area-level census data describing neighborhood contextual features for the residence at diagnosis [16, 17]. Neighborhood socioeconomic status (nSES), encompassing area-based attributes of education, income, poverty, occupation, or multidimensional composite measures have been associated with breast cancer incidence in population-based registry studies [17]. More pronounced magnitude of effects of nSES and breast cancer incidence have been seen in Latinos and AAPIs in comparison to NHWs (e.g., age-adjusted incidence rate ratios comparing living in the highest versus lowest nSES areas: 1.8 in Latino, 1.7 in AAPI, and 1.3 in NHW) [18]. Population-based case-control studies [19–21] additionally support nSES as an independent risk factor for breast cancer while accounting for individual-level risk factors, including education, established reproductive, hormonal, and behavioral risk factors for breast cancer, and built environment attributes. In the Black Women's Health Study, a prospective study of African American women aged 21–69 years from 17 states across the United States, higher nSES was associated with increased ER+ breast cancer risk, but associations were attenuated after adjustment for individual-level risk factors [22]. Another social environment factor, ethnic enclaves, reflecting areas with high ethnic concentrations of residents that maintain cultural identities and behaviors that differ from surrounding areas, has been associated with lower breast cancer risk among Hispanic women independent of nSES [23, 24] and individual-level immigration and established risk factors [24]. The few studies of built environments and breast cancer risk have focused on urbanization and support associations of increased risk [17]. Expanding on the few studies examining the independent and joint associations of contextual- and individual-level risk factors are important for further delineating the impact of specific aspects of neighborhoods on breast cancer risk.

The multifactorial etiology of breast cancer reflects an interplay of biologic, social, behavioral, and environmental factors, requiring a multi-level conceptual approach [12], such as the ecosocial theory [25] or the cells-to-society framework [12, 26]. While multiple pathways have been hypothesized by which neighborhood attributes can influence health and cancer outcomes [16], this chapter focuses on understanding the contribution of the neighborhood obesogenic environment in relation to breast cancer development. Neighborhood environments have been established as determinants of obesity and obesity-related disparities [14, 27–30]. It is increasingly recognized that interventions targeting obesity must account for social and neighborhood context to be successful and sustainable. With this recognition, there has been a shift in obesity prevention strategies to look beyond individual factors with consideration of the role of the obesogenic environment [31–33], encompassing neighborhood attributes of an individual's geospatial surroundings relevant to promoting weight gain and obesity [34]. The neighborhood obesogenic environment may be particularly relevant for postmenopausal women as excess adiposity is among the few modifiable risk factors for breast cancer [35] and obesity influences breast cancer risk differentially across race/ethnicity [36]. Moreover, disparities in the neighborhood obesogenic environment may contribute to the unequal burden of breast cancer across racial/ethnic groups.

Studies of neighborhoods and obesity have focused on nSES and built environments [37–40]. Lower nSES has consistently been positively associated with obesity [38]. and, furthermore, negatively impacts social and built environments [41, 42]. In a landmark randomized study, Moving to Opportunity, low-income families living in high-poverty neighborhoods received housing vouchers to move to healthier,

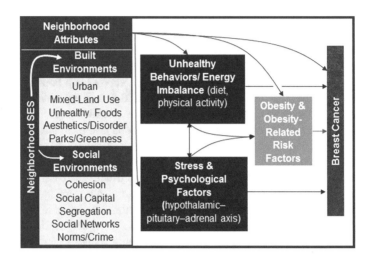

Fig. 8.1 Neighborhood socioeconomic status (SES), built environments, and social environments are hypothesized to influence breast cancer through obesogenic pathways that include health behaviors resulting in energy imbalance, stress, and psychological factors negatively influencing the hypothalamic–pituitary–adrenal axis. Obesity-related risk factors for breast cancer include inflammation, adipokines, insulin resistance, and lipid profiles

low-poverty neighborhoods, and showed modest but potentially important reductions in the prevalence of extreme obesity, demonstrating the potential health benefits of healthy residential neighborhoods [43]. Specific neighborhood attributes associated with obesity and/or higher body mass index (BMI; kg/m^2) include higher density of unhealthy food outlets/restaurants,[44–46], lower walkability (e.g., street connectivity, density of walkable destinations) [47–49], higher traffic density [50, 51], lower proximity to parks [48, 52], and lower residential greenness [53]. Building from conceptual models of neighborhood attributes relevant for unhealthy behaviors/energy balance, obesity, and breast cancer [16, 41, 42, 54, 55], Fig. 8.1 shows a framework for examining the role of neighborhood environments on breast cancer risk. In addition to operating through energy balance, some neighborhood attributes (e.g., nSES, social disorder, crime) may also promote a chronic stress response [56–59] that, in turn, contributes to response of the neuroendocrine-autonomic nervous system leading to the accumulation of excess body fat [60] and can influence breast cancer development [61]. Evidence is also accumulating that neighborhood obesogenic environments adversely impact obesity-related biological profiles (e.g., systemic inflammation and insulin resistance [62–64]) that have been linked with increased breast cancer risk [65, 66].

   In this chapter, we describe our characterization of the neighborhood obesogenic environment within the MEC with a focus on key findings of these factors and breast cancer risk in four major U.S racial/ethnic groups—African Americans, Japanese Americans, Latinos, and whites. The MEC is a large population-based prospective study established in 1993–1996 to investigate risk factors for cancer, largely focusing on diet, health-related behaviors, and genetic factors in a diverse sample of racial/ethnic minorities [67, 68]. We describe here our multi-level contextual studies leveraging the wealth of questionnaire data in the MEC that we have spatially linked via residential geocodes to the CA Neighborhoods Data System (CNDS) [69], an integrated system of small area-level measures of the social and built environments for CA, that have been leveraged for epidemiologic investigations of neighborhood attributes and health outcomes [21, 70–77]. In addition to demonstrating the utility of multi-level neighborhood studies within prospective cohorts of cancer, we discuss caveats and highlight directions and opportunities for future studies.

8.2   MEC Infrastructure

The MEC enrolled 96,810 men and 118,441 women aged 45–75 years at recruitment, primarily from five main racial/ethnic groups: African Americans and Latinos largely recruited from CA (predominantly LA County) and Japanese Americans, Native Hawaiians, and whites largely recruited from HI [67]. Participants entered the cohort by voluntarily completing a baseline 26-page, self-administered mailed questionnaire from 1993 through 1996, collecting information on demographics, anthropometry, smoking history, medical and reproductive histories, family history of cancer, diet, and physical activity. The population-based sampling frames included drivers' license records in both states, supplemented with voter registration lists in HI and Health Care Financing Administration (Medicare) files in CA.

MEC prospectively collected risk factor information and health outcomes. A 4-page follow-up questionnaire was sent in 1998–2002, 2008–2012 and 2012–2016 and currently in 2018–2022 [78]. A repeat of the 26-page baseline questionnaire was sent in 2003–2008. Incident breast cancers are identified through routine linkage with the state-mandated CA Cancer Registry and the HI Tumor Registry; both registries participate in the National Cancer Institute's Surveillance, Epidemiology, and End Results (SEER) program. Breast tumor characteristics available from the cancer registries include hormone receptor status, stage, and tumor size. Deaths are identified by linkage to the CA and HI state death-certificate files and to the National Death Index for deaths occurring in other states. Administrative data on chronic diseases, such as diabetes, is captured through linkage with administrative sources, including Medicare claims [79], health plans in HI [80], and hospital discharge data in CA [81].

8.3   MEC Residential Histories

The MEC has maintained up-to-date addresses on participants since enrollment with the collection of baseline residential addresses. Address updates are obtained prospectively at various time points as part of routine follow-up activities, including annual newsletters, follow-up questionnaires (every 5 years), and through linkages to administrative data sources, such as the USPS change of address database and Medicare. Since baseline (1993–1996), addresses are updated annually and have been used to create a residential history for each MEC participant. Addresses have been geocoded to latitude and longitude coordinates using parcel data as available or street centerline. Geocodes from 1993–1996 (baseline), 1997–2006, and 2007–2013 have been spatially linked to 1990, 2000, and 2010 U.S. Census block groups, respectively. Census block groups, the smallest geographic census unit for which Census Bureau tabulates data, represent an average of 1500 residents in CA and HI and serve as the primary neighborhood unit for contextual studies of cancer within the MEC. Comparison of prior studies of various census geography measures (block group, census tract, zip code) have shown meaningful associations of census block group measures and health outcomes, demonstrating their utility for defining neighborhoods for health studies [82].

8.4 Neighborhood Obesogenic Environment

Geospatial data from the CNDS were operationalized for characterizing the neighborhood obesogenic environment in the CA MEC as described previously [70]. While current efforts are underway to define some of these measures for HI participants in the MEC, here we focus on the CA MEC. Neighborhood attributes were selected *a priori* based on available literature supporting higher levels of obesity or BMI associated with neighborhood attributes [37–40]; specifically, lower nSES, lower population density, higher proportion of residents commuting by car/motorcycle, more unhealthy food outlets, fewer neighborhood amenities measured by number of businesses, recreational facilitates, and parks, lower street connectivity as a measure of walkability, and higher traffic density. These neighborhood attributes were defined using Census, American Community Survey (ACS), business listings derived from Walls & Associates' National Establishment Time-Series Database from 1990–2008 [83], farmers' markets listings from the CA Department of Food and Agriculture [84], parks and street networks from Navteq's NavStreets database [85], and traffic data from the CA Department of Transportation (2000) [86] curated in the CNDS.

Census block group-level data were appended to MEC participants' residential histories. Composite nSES measures were derived from principal components analysis of Census (1990, 2000) and ACS (2007–2011) data on income, housing, occupation, and education [18, 87]. Other census-based measures included population density (1990, 2000, 2010 Census) and percent of residents who commute to work by car/motorcycle per block group (1990, 2000 Census; 2007–2011 ACS).

Neighborhood amenities, food environment, street connectivity, and traffic density were measured using a geographic information system (GIS) [88]. For analyses based on participants' baseline residential addresses, we quantified number of businesses, farmers' markets, and parks within a one-mile pedestrian network distance, street connectivity within a 1600 meter buffer, and traffic density within 500 meter buffer. For longitudinal analyses based on participants' residential histories, these neighborhood measures were quantified based on census block group. The number of businesses was based on annual average count across three-year activity windows (1990–1992, 1999–2001, 2006–2008), offering more stability in estimates due to business turnover compared to 1 year windows. Unhealthy food environments were conceptualized by the restaurant environment index (REI), the ratio of unhealthy to healthy restaurants, and the retail food environment index (RFEI), the ratio of unhealthy to healthy food outlets [89]. Walkability was quantified by the gamma index measure of street connectivity [90], defined as the ratio of actual number of street segments to maximum possible number of intersections within a 1600 meter buffer. Traffic density was estimated from vehicle miles within a 500 meter buffer of a participant's geocoded residence [91]. To more fully characterize a neighborhood's obesogenic environment, we derived factors from principal components factor analysis of nine built environment attributes at the block-group level [71]. Specifically, we identified four neighborhood factors: an "urban environment" factor characterized by high population density, high street connectivity, low percent commute by car/motorcycle, and high traffic density; a "mixed-land development" factor characterized by high recreational facilities per population, and high businesses per population; an "unhealthy food outlets" factor characterized by high ratio of unhealthy to healthy restaurants and a high ratio of unhealthy to healthy retail establishments; and a "parks" factor characterized by high number of parks per population.

8.5   Geographic Distribution of Neighborhood Obesogenic Factors

As CA MEC participants resided primarily in LA County (95% at baseline), their residential neighborhoods represent diverse geographic areas with heterogeneous distributions in neighborhood obesogenic factors across race/ethnicity. Figure 8.2 shows the geospatial distribution of residential baseline addresses for CA MEC participants residing in LA County for African American, Japanese American, Latino, and white women (Fig. 8.2a) and composite nSES for 1990 census block groups in CA with quintiles based on the distribution for block groups in LA County (Fig. 8.2b). At baseline, most African American (67%) and Latino women (58%) lived in low-SES (quintiles 1–2) neighborhoods while the majority of Japanese American (58%) and white women (54%) lived in high-SES (quintiles 4–5) neighborhoods (Fig. 8.2) [70]. A higher proportion of African American women lived in more urban environments (quintile 4–5; 53%) than Latino (38%), white (24%) and Japanese American (22%) women. Most African American (63%) and Latino women (55%) lived in neighborhoods characterized by low mixed-land use (quintile 1–2) while about one-third of white (38%) and Japanese American (36%) women lived in this type of neighborhood. The proportion of women living in

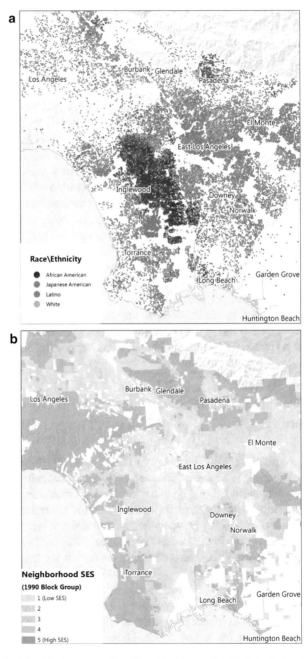

Fig. 8.2 (**a**) Residential addresses at baseline (1993–1996), Multiethnic Cohort female participants, Los Angeles County; (**b**) neighborhood socioeconomic status (SES) composite index for 1990 U.S. Census block groups, quintiles based on distribution for block groups in Los Angeles County

neighborhoods characterized by more unhealthy food outlets was similar across racial/ethnic groups (~28%).The geospatial distribution for mixed-land use and unhealthy food outlets in LA County is shown in Fig. 8.3.

8.6   Obesity, Energy-Balance, and Neighborhood Obesogenic Factors

Body fat, physical activity, and dietary intake vary by race/ethnicity in postmenopausal MEC women. In an analysis of the 23,006 (39%) Latino, 20,266 (35%) African American, 9115 (16%) white, and 6296 (11%) Japanese American postmenopausal MEC women living in CA at baseline, a substantially higher proportion of African Americans (38%) were obese ($\geq$ 30 kg/m^2) compared to Latinos (29%), whites (21%), and Japanese Americans (5%) [70]. Compared to other racial/ethnic groups, African Americans had a higher consumption of processed red meat and lower consumption of vegetables, Latinos were less educated (i.e., $\leq$ high school graduate), more likely to have no moderate/vigorous recreational activity, higher consumption of red meats and daily caloric intake, and whites had higher daily moderate/vigorous activity, lower consumption of red meats (including processed red meats), and higher consumption of dairy products [70]. The substantial variation in the distribution in lifestyle factors captured via extensive questionnaires provide a broad representation of individual-level risk factors to be considered in analyses of neighborhood environments and health outcomes.

Living in lower SES neighborhoods was consistently associated with obesity across all racial/ethnic groups with evidence of a dose response relationship across quintiles, except among Japanese Americans (Fig. 8.4) [70]. These associations with obesity were independent of individual modifiable (i.e., smoking, alcohol intake, hours of moderate and vigorous activity per day, dietary intake of red meat, vegetables, fruits, and total calories), obesity-related factors (i.e., age, marital status, education, BMI at age 21, reproductive history, menopausal status, hormone replacement therapy), and built environment attributes. A greater magnitude of effects of two-fold higher odds of obesity compared to normal BMI (18.5–24.9 kg/m^2) was observed for living in the lowest versus highest nSES quintile in African American women (adjusted odds ratio = 2.07, 95% confidence interval (CI) = 1.62–2.65) and white women (2.50, 1.73–3.61) compared to 45% higher odds in Latino (1.45, 1.17–1.79) women. Racial/ethnic differences with a larger magnitude of effect for the nSES–obesity association in whites compared with African American women has also been suggested in other studies [27].

Modifiable health behaviors (i.e., smoking, alcohol intake, physical activity, dietary intake) explained, in part, the nSES and obesity associations. In African American, Latino, and white women, the addition of modifiable health behaviors attenuated odd ratios 19–26% when added to models adjusted for age, marital status, BMI at age 21, education and reproductive factors [70]. The nSES-obesity associations remained significant with further adjustment for built environment attributes

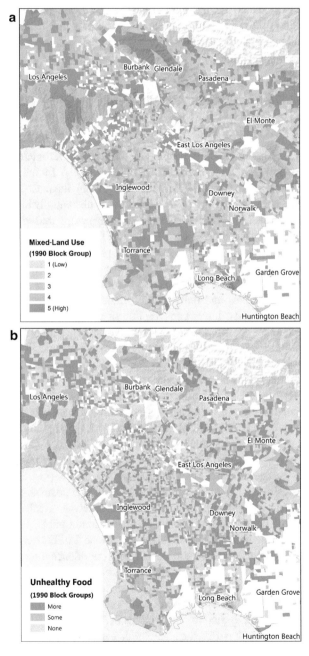

Fig. 8.3 Composite neighborhood obesogenic factors for 1990 U.S. Census block groups, Los Angeles County; (**a**) mixed-land use defined as more businesses and more recreational facilities per population, quintiles based on distribution of block groups in Los Angeles County; (**b**) unhealthy food environment defined as higher ratio of unhealthy restaurants and retail food outlets

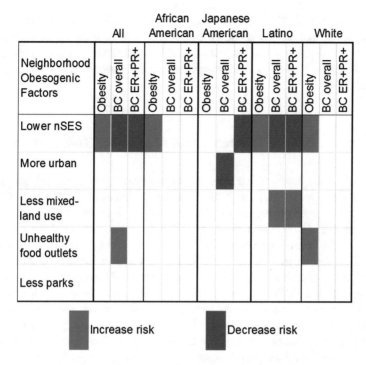

Fig. 8.4 The neighborhood obesogenic factors and risk of obesity and breast cancer risk, Multiethnic Cohort, 1993–2010. Increase and decrease risk estimates from multinomial logistic regression models for odds of obesity (≥ 30 kg/m^2) compared to normal (<18.5–24.9 kg/m^2) weight, and Cox proportional hazards models for invasive breast cancer (BC) or hormone receptor-positive tumors [estrogen receptor or progesterone receptor (BC ER + PR+)]. All models adjusted for adjusted age, race/ethnicity for all women, individual-level risk factors, clustering effect of block groups, and all neighborhood obesogenic factors

(5–11% attenuation). The attenuation in the racial/ethnic-specific associations between nSES and obesity demonstrate the complex underlying relationships contributing to health disparities.

Associations between obesogenic built environment attributes and likelihood of being obese at cohort entry varied by race/ethnicity while accounting for individual factors and nSES. Living in neighborhoods with a higher proportion of residents commuting by car or motorcycle was associated with higher odds of being obese in white women only, while an opposite pattern of association was seen for Latino women with lower odds of being obese [70]. However, individual-level commuting patterns were not collected in the MEC and may account for the observed differential association in white and Latino women. Living in neighborhoods with lower density of businesses was associated with being obese among African American and white women and more unhealthy food outlets was associated with obesity only among white women [92]. There was no evidence of associations of obesity with urbanicity, mixed-land use, nor parks (Fig. 8.4). Other measures of parks, such as park characteristics [93], perceived park quality [94], size of parks [52], access to walking trails, and neighborhood greenness [53] may be more important determinants for obesity and should be considered in future studies. Future longitudinal studies in the MEC will examine neighborhood environments and change in BMI over follow-up.

8.7 Breast Cancer Incidence and Modifiable Risk Factors

In the MEC, the age-adjusted incidences rate of breast cancer display striking racial/ethnic disparities [11, 68]. In 2007–2011, Native Hawaiian (572.1 per 100,000) women experienced the highest incidence rate of breast cancer followed by African American (427.6), Japanese American (326.7), white (322.4), US-born Latino (310.7), and foreign-born Latino (240.7) women. Notably, the incidence rates in Japanese American women were comparable to white women in the MEC. While Latino women experienced the lowest incidence rates of breast cancer in the cohort; incidence rates in US-born Latino women approached those of white women. Leveraging the wealth of individual-level data, the MEC has shown that racial/ethnic variation in established risk factors for breast cancer—reproductive history, weight, hormone replacement therapy use, and alcohol consumption— accounted for differences in risk among African Americans, Japanese Americans, and US-born and foreign-born Latinos in comparison to whites, but not among Native Hawaiians [11].

Various measures of body size have been associated with breast cancer risk within the MEC. There was a 38% significantly increased risk of breast cancer in obese compared to normal weight (20.0–24.9 kg/m^2) postmenopausal women [95]. The magnitude of the obesity effect was significantly different across racial/ethnic groups, highest at 82% increased risk in Native Hawaiians and 59% in Japanese Americans and no significant association in Latinos. Obesity and breast cancer risk associations were also more pronounced for more advanced (82%) than for localized (22%) tumors. Both BMI at baseline and weight gain since age 21 were associated with breast cancer risk [95]. Each 5 kg of adult weight gain conferred a 7% increased risk of breast cancer in postmenopausal MEC women, ranging from 3% in Latinos to 16% in Japanese Americans. When BMI and adult weight gain were modeled simultaneously, adult weight gain was a more important predictor than baseline BMI, demonstrating the importance of maintaining a healthy weight through adulthood for the prevention of postmenopausal breast cancer.

8.8 Neighborhood Obesogenic Factors and Breast Cancer

We conducted a prospective investigation of neighborhood obesogenic factors and breast cancer risk among 48,247 postmenopausal MEC women in CA with 2341 breast cancer cases identified after a median of 17 years of follow-up. This study

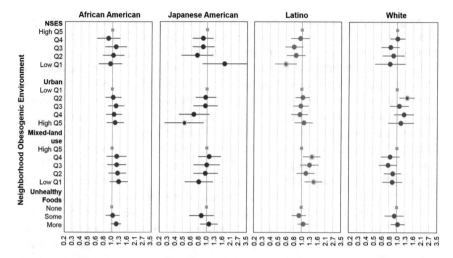

Fig. 8.5 Neighborhood obesogenic environments and breast cancer risk, Multiethnic Cohort, 1993–2010. Hazards ratios (HR) and 95% confidence intervals for invasive breast cancer adjusting for age, individual-level risk factors, clustering effect of block group, and all neighborhood obesogenic factors. Quintiles (Q) based on distribution for block groups in Los Angeles County. Yellow boarder around HR represent statistically significant associations (*P* < 0.05)

identified differential associations of neighborhood obesogenic factors and breast cancer risk by race/ethnicity (Fig. 8.4). NSES was the strongest obesogenic factor associated with breast cancer risk independent of adult BMI, adult weight gain since age 21 years, education, established reproductive and hormonal risk factors, behavioral risk factors (alcohol intake, vigorous-moderate activity, dietary intake), and mammography use. Living in the lowest- versus highest-SES neighborhoods (quintile 1 vs. 5) was associated with 21% decreased risk (adjusted hazard ratio, 95% confidence interval) for invasive breast cancer risk in all women (0.79, 0.66–0.95) and a more pronounced, 40% decreased risk in Latinos (0.60, 0.43–0.85; Fig. 8.5). The nSES–breast cancer associations appeared somewhat stronger for hormone receptor–positive tumors compared with all tumors in white and Latino women, with a suggestive association in Japanese Americans (quintile 2-low vs. 5-high: 0.44, 0.23–0.86; P_{trend} = 0.20; Fig. 8.4). Results were also similar with and without adjustment for behavioral risk factors, BMI at baseline, and adult weight gain since age 21 years. Furthermore, the associations were unlikely to be related to access to mammographic screening, as analyses were adjusted for ever having had a mammogram, and analyses specific for early- or late- stage breast cancer yielded similar results. These results contribute to the growing body of epidemiologic evidence documenting positive nSES associations with breast cancer risk independent of individual-level SES (mostly measured as education) and established reproductive, hormonal, and behavioral risk factors for breast cancer [19–22, 96, 97]. Moreover, these findings in the MEC speak to the role of nSES and breast cancer risk in minority populations.

Neighborhood obesogenic built environment factors were associated with breast cancer risk independent of individual risk factors and nSES. Having more compared to no unhealthy food outlets was associated with 10% higher risk overall (1.10, 1.00–1.21). Differential association across racial/ethnic groups were evident for urban environments and mixed land use (Fig. 8.5). Living in the highest versus lowest quintile of urban neighborhoods was associated with a 51% lower risk among Japanese Americans (0.49, 0.26–0.90), and highest versus lowest quintile of mixed-land use was associated with a 32% (0.68, 0.52–0.91) lower risk of breast cancer in Latinos. In general, established breast cancer risk factors account for a small proportion of breast cancer risk in Latinos [98] and Japanese Americans [11], suggesting neighborhood factors may account for the unexplained variability in breast cancer risk among these groups. The heterogeneous associations in Latinos and Japanese Americans may reflect early-life exposures unique to Latinos living in lower-SES or more mixed-land use neighborhoods or to Japanese Americans living in urban environments such as exposures related to hygiene and infectious diseases [99]. Studies support heterogeneity in nSES-breast cancer risk associations by neighborhood racial/ethnic composition or ethnic enclaves [24, 100]. The development and maintenance of closer ethnic ties, stronger cultural mores and ethnically distinct resources for Japanese Americans and Latinos likely have beneficial effects on breast cancer risk. Residing in ethnic enclaves may offer these benefits and subsequently protect against breast cancer independent of nSES [23, 24, 101]. Further studies are needed to understand the racial/ethnic-specific contextual role of the neighborhood on breast cancer risk [16].

8.9 Neighborhood Exposure Change, Residential Mobility, and Breast Cancer Risk

Neighborhood social and built environments are dynamic, changing over time [102–104]. Favorable changes in neighborhood attributes have been associated with improved health outcomes such as healthier food/physical activity environments and reductions in BMI [105] and improved nSES and lower mortality rates [106]. Unfavorable changes have been associated with worsening health outcomes [106–108]. In addition, neighborhood exposure over time may have cumulative impact on health outcomes. Thus, accounting for changes in neighborhood attributes would help to more accurately assess neighborhood-health associations.

Measurement and quantification of neighborhood change involves a number of methodological challenges. First, it requires neighborhood data from several time points or census periods with consistent geospatial areas across time points. Conversion of data between different areal units (e.g., between block groups and census tracts) may introduce additional measurement error. Second, the neighborhood unit boundaries often do not exactly match across the time periods, making it difficult to measure temporal change on the scale of neighborhood units. Few studies have examined neighborhood change in its relation to health [106, 109, 110] and in particular its effect on cancer incidence and mortality [107, 111, 112].

Due to the above considerations, we have focused on study participants and their neighborhood exposure, rather than characterizing neighborhood attributes and using them as spatial variables in the analysis. For every participant, change in the exposure to each of the neighborhood obesogenic factor was defined as a shift up or down by at least one category level (e.g., a change from quintile 3 to 4) between the participant's baseline and any subsequent address or between census periods. Relative risk of breast cancer was estimated for upward and downward direction of change, using 'no change' (same distribution quintile) as the reference category.

A special focus in our analysis was disentangling the two types of change in the neighborhood exposure: that due to an individual's change of physical residence, or move, and that due to changes in the neighborhood, such as redevelopment or deterioration. We accounted for this difference through participants' moving status. Study participants were classified as movers if they had more than one residential address during follow-up or non-movers if they had only one residential address. For example, in the MEC from 1993–2010, the majority (58%) of women did not physically change residence and a small proportion (7%) of women had more than two moves. Movers resided at the same address for on average 6.5 years. Moving to a more favorable neighborhood environment has been shown to improve health outcomes [43, 113].

In the MEC, we examined change in neighborhood obesogenic factors and breast cancer risk, accounting for baseline level of the respective obesogenic factor. Over a median of 17 years of follow-up in the MEC, we observed significant associations (hazard ratio, 95% CI) between change to less mixed-land use neighborhoods (across quintiles) relative to no-change (same quintile strata) and increased risk of breast cancer among nonmovers (1.20, 1.02–1.41), but no associations in movers (0.94, 0.75–1.18). This association in nonmovers is consistent with the observed association of lower mixed-land use reported at baseline (1993–1996) and increased breast cancer risk in Latino women (Fig. 8.5). It is possible that the neighborhood contextual effect of mixed-land use on breast cancer risk becomes diffused/attenuated among movers. Associations with change in other neighborhood obesogenic factors (i.e., nSES, urbanicity, unhealthy food environments, parks) did not reach statistical significance. Our results suggest that mixed-land use is important to consider in longitudinal studies of cancer and energy balance [102, 109].

8.10   Opportunities for Long-Term Neighborhood Exposure

The wealth of address information within the MEC offers the opportunity to examine long-term neighborhood exposures and breast cancer outcomes while applying a life-course perspective. The residential history information within the MEC are being augmented and enhanced via linkage to commercial databases [114], and may provide the opportunity to obtain addresses prior to cohort entry and/or missing address information. With such data, we will enhance our understanding of neighborhoods and breast cancer risk over an extended period in an individual's adult life.

Life-course approaches represent dynamic spatial-temporal frameworks of cumulative exposure over an individual's life and the sequence of exposure over a residential trajectory in relation to breast cancer risk [115]. Life-course approaches are especially relevant for breast cancer given the increasing recognition that risk is likely influenced by early-life exposures and relevant windows over a woman's life. Epidemiological studies have examined cumulative effects as weighted sums of neighborhood exposures over a specific period for each participant [116, 117]. For example, a weighted sum is computed over all residential addresses and/or census periods throughout the study period and weighted by the length of residence at each address. To properly implement this approach, one needs to ensure that the neighborhood attributes are measured using the same geographic scale and point of reference across all time points or census periods. Some neighborhood attributes, especially composite measures such as nSES, are dependent on census data at a single time point of reference that may not be equivalent across time periods (e.g. 1990 and 2000 US Census). To address this issue, time-invariant measures of census data have been developed to make unbiased inferences about neighborhood change [118]. Constructing residential trajectories is another approach in measuring residential change [119, 120]. In our longitudinal analysis, we compared the baseline address and subsequent address at time of event, without accounting for what happened in between. However, a monotonic positive shift in the level of a neighborhood attribute may have a different impact on an individual compared to a negative shift followed by a positive shift of greater magnitude. Thus, one could compare stable to more variable trajectories, such as a trajectory reflecting steady positive (or negative) shift to that where both positive and negative shifts occurred over time. Heinonen and colleagues used a similar construct in their analysis of residential trajectories of obesogenic neighborhood environments in relation to marriage and parenthood [120]. Employing life-course methods in future studies, coupled with the wealth of residential history data in the MEC, will make a significant contribution to our understanding of relevant long-term neighborhood exposures and breast cancer risk.

8.11 Strengths and Limitations

The MEC provides a diverse study population that allows for well-powered, longitudinal studies of neighborhood impact on cancer outcomes among diverse racial/ethnic groups. The extensive questionnaire data and substantial variation in the distribution of dietary intake and lifestyle factors provide a broad representation of individual-level risk factors. CA MEC participants resided primarily in LA County and their residential neighborhoods represent diverse geographic areas, providing a wide spectrum of variation in nSES and built environment attributes that characterize the obesogenic environment. We examined associations between the neighborhood obesogenic environment at baseline as well as change over time for these attributes and breast cancer. Several limitations should be considered. While there is efficiency in leveraging secondary geospatial data, depending on administrative boundaries for defining neighborhoods may introduce bias or lack of participants' perceptive neighborhood environment [121]. Focusing on place of residence does not capture participants' activity space of the entire obesogenic experience, such as workplace that may also reflect their access to recreational facilities and their food environment. Additionally, we did not have self-reported data on how participants' perceive or interact with their environment nor information on participants' space–time trajectories [121]. Our residential history data enabled us to identify movers and non-movers over the follow-up and change in neighborhood environments; however we are unable to account for selective mobility bias [121]. Our multilevel regression analyses have accounted for the nested nature of individuals within block groups and we have applied different approaches to consider temporal changes in neighborhood environments over time. However, we have not yet accounted for spatial considerations in modeling neighborhood exposures with breast cancer risk; such methods have recently become available and will be applied in future analyses that will account for space and time in neighborhood impacts on breast cancer risk.

8.12   Future Directions

The current findings in the MEC underscore how different attributes of the neighborhood obesogenic environment differentially influence breast cancer risk among African American, Japanese American, Latino, and white women. In the field of cancer epidemiology, there is increasing recognition and calls for similar well-designed prospective studies that can integrate detailed individual- with small area neighborhood-level data to identify the full spectrum of multilevel factors that contribute to breast cancer risk, particularly in regards to racial/ethnic disparities. Furthermore, prospective studies of neighborhood factors on breast cancer risk are needed to determine the causal relationships between the neighborhood environment and health outcomes. This is central to the establishment of a foundation for the next set of translational research studies that will test multilevel interventions that address modifiable neighborhood factors in experimental and quasi-experimental designs [42].

Future directions for contextual studies of breast cancer in the MEC are centered on several research areas. First, as nSES, a composite measure of multiple social and economic domains, has been shown to have strong effects on obesity and breast cancer within the MEC, it is essential to try and delineate the relevant pathways that shape health behaviors and influence breast cancer development. Thus, future MEC studies aim to investigate specific components of nSES such as percent poverty, unemployment, housing availability as well as neighborhood measures of social stress (Fig. 8.1), such as racial residential segregation, racial/ethnic composition, and ethnic enclaves for their role in breast cancer disparities with the goal of achieving health equity for all vulnerable populations [16, 101] as further described in Chap. 15. Second, in addition to secondary geospatial data that characterizes availability of resources and/or presence of attributes, studies capturing information on perceived neighborhood resources and experience/use are important and likely relate more to health behaviors and outcomes of individuals. Third, neighborhood audits via new technologies such as Google Street View, social media, mobile devices, and apps may enhance the collection of neighborhood attributes for future studies of breast cancer survival in contemporary periods. With the absence of historical audit or social media data since enrollment of this cohort, we are unable to use such data for etiologic studies of breast cancer risk. Lastly, with adopting a "cells-to-society" framework, we will extend our future neighborhood studies to incorporate both downstream and upstream factors. For downstream factors, we plan to incorporate data on biological factors such as obesity-related biomarkers, methylation data, and genetic susceptibility markers for breast cancer. Initial findings among women in the MEC have shown that residence in neighborhoods of lower nSES or population density was strongly associated with higher circulating levels of C-reactive protein, a systemic marker of inflammation, independent of BMI, modifiable risk factors (smoking, physical activity, diet), menopausal status and hormone therapy use, comorbidities, and nonsteroidal anti-inflammatory drug use. These findings suggest inflammation as a possible biological mechanism by which the neighborhood environment may operate (Fig. 8.1) [122]. For upstream factors, we plan to integrate data on city, county, and state policies that may impact social determinants of health such as governmental regulations related to housing and racial segregation or health care policies that influence health care insurance or mammography screening. With a more integrated approach of extending contextual studies of breast cancer in the MEC, we aim to gain a better understanding of the complex interactions and joint associations driving breast cancer risk and racial/ethnic disparities.

8.13   Conclusions

The MEC is uniquely positioned to contribute to neighborhood health research in examining differential associations of neighborhood attributes and health outcomes across racial/ethnic minorities (African Americans, Japanese Americans, Latinos, and Native Hawaiians). The MEC has shown the important role of nSES as a risk factor for obesity and breast cancer risk independent of individual demographics, diet, lifestyle factors, and health behaviors. Furthermore, certain neighborhood obesogenic attributes demonstrated racial/ethnic-specific associations with breast cancer. These findings in the MEC set the foundation for further research in evaluating the underlying contextual determinants and biological mechanisms by which the neighborhood obesogenic environment influences breast cancer risk. Moreover, additional prospective studies of breast cancer with appropriate analytic methods are needed to examine the spatial and temporal variation in contextual factors in a multiethnic setting of diverse populations that also capture time-varying changes in individual-level behaviors. Ultimately, this geospatial research has translational potential in improving health in neighborhoods through urban planning, policy intervention, and community building, in particular among vulnerable populations that experience an unequal burden of breast cancer.

References

1. Howlader N, Noone AM, Krapcho M, Miller D, Brest A, Yu M, Ruhl J, Tatalovich Z, Mariotto A, Lewis DR, Chen HS, Feuer EJ, Cronin KA (eds). SEER Cancer Statistics Review, 1975–2016, National Cancer Institute. Bethesda, MD, https://seer.cancer.gov/csr/1975_2016/, based on November 2018 SEER data submission, posted to the SEER web site, April 2019.
2. DeSantis CE, Fedewa SA, Goding Sauer A, Kramer JL, Smith RA, Jemal A. Breast cancer statistics, 2015: convergence of incidence rates between black and white women. CA Cancer J Clin. 2016;66(1):31–42.
3. Howlader N, Altekruse SF, Li CI, et al. US incidence of breast cancer subtypes defined by joint hormone receptor and HER2 status. J Natl Cancer Inst 2014; 106(5). PMC4580552.
4. Asian & Pacific Islander American Health Forum. Snapshot: Asian American, Native Hawaiian, and Pacific Islander Health. 2017. www.APIAHF.org. Accessed Sept 2018.
5. Tseng W, McDonnell DD, Takahashi L, Ho W, Lee C, Wong S. Ethnic health assessment for Asian Americans, Native Hawaiians and Pacific Islanders in California. San Francisco: Asian & Pacific Islander American Health Forum. 2010. www.APIAHF.org. Accessed Sept 2018.
6. Asian Pacific American Legal Center and Asian American Justice Center. A Community of Contrasts – Asian Americans in the United States: 2011. Washington, DC: Asian American Center for Advancing Justice. 2013. www.aajc.advancingjustice.org. Accessed Sept 2018.
7. Torre LA, Sauer AM, Chen MS Jr, Kagawa-Singer M, Jemal A, Siegel RL. Cancer statistics for Asian Americans, Native Hawaiians, and Pacific Islanders, 2016: converging incidence in males and females. CA Cancer J Clin. 2016;66(3):182–202. PMC5325676
8. Gomez SL, Von Behren J, McKinley M, et al. Breast cancer in Asian Americans in California, 1988–2013: increasing incidence trends and recent data on breast cancer subtypes. Breast Cancer Res Treat. 2017;164:139–47.
9. Chlebowski RT, Chen Z, Anderson GL, et al. Ethnicity and breast cancer: factors influencing differences in incidence and outcome. J Natl Cancer Inst. 2005;97(6):439–48.
10. Gathani T, Ali R, Balkwill A, et al. Ethnic differences in breast cancer incidence in England are due to differences in known risk factors for the disease: prospective study. Br J Cancer. 2014;110(1):224–9. PMC3887283
11. Pike MC, Kolonel LN, Henderson BE, et al. Breast cancer in a multiethnic cohort in Hawaii and Los Angeles: risk factor-adjusted incidence in Japanese equals and in Hawaiians exceeds that in whites. Cancer Epidemiol Biomark Prev. 2002;11(9):795–800.
12. Warnecke RB, Oh A, Breen N, et al. Approaching health disparities from a population perspective: the National Institutes of Health Centers for Population Health and Health Disparities. Am J Public Health. 2008;98(9):1608–15. PMC2509592
13. Bell CN, Thorpe RJ Jr, LaVeist TA. The role of social context in racial disparities in self-rated health. J Urban Health. 2018;95(1):13–20. PMC5862697
14. Bleich SN, Thorpe RJ Jr, Sharif-Harris H, Fesahazion R, Laveist TA. Social context explains race disparities in obesity among women. J Epidemiol Community Health. 2010;64(5):465–9. PMC3099623

15. LaVeist T, Pollack K, Thorpe R Jr, Fesahazion R, Gaskin D. Place, not race: disparities dissipate in Southwest Baltimore when blacks and whites live under similar conditions. Health Aff. 2011;30(10):1880–7.
16. Gomez SL, Shariff-Marco S, DeRouen M, et al. The impact of neighborhood social and built environment factors across the cancer continuum: current research, methodological considerations, and future directions. Cancer. 2015;121(14):2314–30. 4490083
17. Akinyemiju TF, Genkinger JM, Farhat M, Wilson A, Gary-Webb TL, Tehranifar P. Residential environment and breast cancer incidence and mortality: a systematic review and meta-analysis. BMC Cancer. 2015;15:191. 4396806
18. Yost K, Perkins C, Cohen R, Morris C, Wright W. Socioeconomic status and breast cancer incidence in California for different race/ethnic groups. Cancer Causes Control. 2001;12(8):703–11.
19. Robert SA, Strombom I, Trentham-Dietz A, et al. Socioeconomic risk factors for breast cancer: distinguishing individual- and community-level effects. Epidemiology. 2004;15(4):442–50.
20. Webster TF, Hoffman K, Weinberg J, Vieira V, Aschengrau A. Community- and individual-level socioeconomic status and breast cancer risk: multilevel modeling on Cape Cod, Massachusetts. Environ Health Perspect. 2008;116(8):1125–9. PMC2516595
21. Conroy SM, Shariff-Marco S, Koo J, et al. Racial/ethnic differences in the impact of neighborhood social and built environment on breast cancer risk: the Neighborhoods and Breast Cancer Study. Cancer Epidemiol Biomark Prev. 2017;26:541–52.
22. Palmer JR, Boggs DA, Wise LA, Adams-Campbell LL, Rosenberg L. Individual and neighborhood socioeconomic status in relation to breast cancer incidence in African-American women. Am J Epidemiol. 2012;176(12):1141–6. PMC3571232
23. Keegan TH, John EM, Fish KM, Alfaro-Velcamp T, Clarke CA, Gomez SL. Breast cancer incidence patterns among California Hispanic women: differences by nativity and residence in an enclave. Cancer Epidemiol Biomark Prev. 2010;19(5):1208–1218.2895619.
24. Gomez SL, Shariff-Macro S, Yang J, et al. Abstract nr B26: Individual- and neighborhood-level immigration factors and breast cancer risk among Latinas in the San Francisco Bay Area: the Neighborhoods and Breast Cancer (NABC) Study. Proceedings of the Sixth AACR Conference: The Science of Cancer Health Disparities; Dec 6–9, 2013; Atlanta, GA. Philadelphia (PA): AACR; Cancer Epidemiol Biomarkers Prev 2014; 23 (11 Suppl). https://doi.org/10.1158/1538-7755.DISP13-B26; 2014.
25. Krieger N. Theories for social epidemiology in the 21st century: an ecosocial perspective. Int J Epidemiol. 2001;30(4):668–77.
26. Gehlert S, Rebbeck T, Lurie N, Warnecke R, Paskett E, Goodwin JS. Cells to society: overcoming health disparities. Washington, DC; 2007.
27. Do DP, Dubowitz T, Bird CE, Lurie N, Escarce JJ, Finch BK. Neighborhood context and ethnicity differences in body mass index: a multilevel analysis using the NHANES III survey (1988–1994). Econ Hum Biol. 2007;5(2):179–203. 2587036
28. Robert SA, Reither EN. A multilevel analysis of race, community disadvantage, and body mass index among adults in the US. Soc Sci Med. 2004;59(12):2421–34.
29. Kirby JB, Liang L, Chen HJ, Wang Y. Race, place, and obesity: the complex relationships among community racial/ethnic composition, individual race/ethnicity, and obesity in the United States. Am J Public Health. 2012;102(8):1572–8. PMC3464818
30. Dubowitz T, Heron M, Bird CE, et al. Neighborhood socioeconomic status and fruit and vegetable intake among whites, blacks, and Mexican Americans in the United States. Am J Clin Nutr. 2008;87(6):1883–91. PMC3829689
31. Khan LK, Sobush K, Keener D, et al. Recommended community strategies and measurements to prevent obesity in the United States. MMWR Recomm Rep. 2009;58(RR-7):1–26.
32. Park BZ, Cantrell L, Hunt H, Farris RP, Schumacher P, Bauer UE. State public health actions to prevent and control diabetes, heart disease, obesity and associated risk factors, and promote school health. Prev Chronic Dis. 2017;14:E127. PMC5724997
33. Rutledge GE, Lane K, Merlo C, Elmi J. Coordinated approaches to strengthen state and local public health actions to prevent obesity, diabetes, and heart disease and stroke. Prev Chronic Dis. 2018;15:E14. PMC5798214

34. Swinburn B, Egger G, Raza F. Dissecting obesogenic environments: the development and application of a framework for identifying and prioritizing environmental interventions for obesity. Prev Med. 1999;29(6. Pt 1):563–70.
35. World Cancer Research Fund/American Institute for Cancer Research. Continuous update project expert report 2018. Diet, nutrition, physical activity and breast cancer. Available at dietandcancerreport.org.
36. Bandera EV, Maskarinec G, Romieu I, John EM. Racial and ethnic disparities in the impact of obesity on breast cancer risk and survival: a global perspective. Adv Nutr. 2015;6(6):803–19. PMC4642425
37. Mackenbach JD, Rutter H, Compernolle S, et al. Obesogenic environments: a systematic review of the association between the physical environment and adult weight status, the SPOTLIGHT project. BMC Public Health. 2014;14:233. PMC4015813
38. Leal C, Chaix B. The influence of geographic life environments on cardiometabolic risk factors: a systematic review, a methodological assessment and a research agenda. Obes Rev. 2011;12(3):217–30.
39. Feng J, Glass TA, Curriero FC, Stewart WF, Schwartz BS. The built environment and obesity: a systematic review of the epidemiologic evidence. Health Place. 2010;16(2):175–90.
40. Papas MA, Alberg AJ, Ewing R, Helzlsouer KJ, Gary TL, Klassen AC. The built environment and obesity. Epidemiol Rev. 2007;29:129–43.
41. Suglia SF, Shelton RC, Hsiao A, Wang YC, Rundle A, Link BG. Why the neighborhood social environment is critical in obesity prevention. J Urban Health. 2016;93(1):206–12. PMC4794461
42. Diez Roux AV, Mair C. Neighborhoods and health. Ann NY Acad Sci. 2010;1186:125–45.
43. Ludwig J, Sanbonmatsu L, Gennetian L, et al. Neighborhoods, obesity, and diabetes—a randomized social experiment. N Engl J Med. 2011;365(16):1509–19. PMC3410541
44. Li F, Harmer P, Cardinal BJ, Bosworth M, Johnson-Shelton D. Obesity and the built environment: does the density of neighborhood fast-food outlets matter? Am J Health Promot. 2009;23(3):203–209. 2730045.
45. Pruchno R, Wilson-Genderson M, Gupta AK. Neighborhood food environment and obesity in community-dwelling older adults: individual and neighborhood effects. Am J Public Health. 2014;104(5):924–9. PMC3987600
46. Xu Y, Wang F. Built environment and obesity by urbanicity in the U.S. Health Place. 2015:34, 19–29. PMC4497827
47. Muller-Riemenschneider F, Pereira G, Villanueva K, et al. Neighborhood walkability and cardiometabolic risk factors in Australian adults: an observational study. BMC Public Health. 2013;13:755. PMC3844350
48. Wen M, Kowaleski-Jones L. The built environment and risk of obesity in the United States: racial-ethnic disparities. Health Place. 2012;18(6):1314–22. 3501580
49. Creatore MI, Glazier RH, Moineddin R, et al. Association of neighborhood walkability with change in overweight, obesity, and diabetes. JAMA. 2016;315(20):2211–20.
50. Boehmer TK, Lovegreen SL, Haire-Joshu D, Brownson RC. What constitutes an obesogenic environment in rural communities? Am J Health Promot. 2006;20(6):411–21.
51. Powell-Wiley TM, Ayers CR, de Lemos JA, et al. Relationship between perceptions about neighborhood environment and prevalent obesity: data from the Dallas heart study. Obesity (Silver Spring). 2013;21(1):E14–21. PMC3602329
52. Rundle A, Quinn J, Lovasi G, et al. Associations between body mass index and park proximity, size, cleanliness, and recreational facilities. Am J Health Promot. 2013;27(4):262–9. PMC3696994
53. Villeneuve PJ, Jerrett M, Su JG, Weichenthal S, Sandler DP. Association of residential greenness with obesity and physical activity in a US cohort of women. Environ Res. 2018;160:372–84. PMC5872815
54. Diez Roux AV, Mujahid MS, Hirsch JA, Moore K, Moore LV. The impact of neighborhoods on CV risk. Glob Heart. 2016;11(3):353–63. PMC5098701
55. Glass TA, McAtee MJ. Behavioral science at the crossroads in public health: extending horizons, envisioning the future. Soc Sci Med. 2006;62(7):1650–71.

56. Burdette AM, Hill TD. An examination of processes linking perceived neighborhood disorder and obesity. Soc Sci Med. 2008;67(1):38–46.
57. Matthews SA, Yang TC. Exploring the role of the built and social neighborhood environment in moderating stress and health. Ann Behav Med. 2010;39(2):170–83. 4017772
58. Glass TA, Rasmussen MD, Schwartz BS. Neighborhoods and obesity in older adults: the Baltimore memory study. Am J Prev Med. 2006;31(6):455–63. 1851911
59. Taylor SE, Repetti RL, Seeman T. Health psychology: what is an unhealthy environment and how does it get under the skin? Annu Rev Psychol. 1997;48:411–47.
60. Kyrou I, Chrousos GP, Tsigos C. Stress, visceral obesity, and metabolic complications. Ann N Y Acad Sci. 2006;1083:77–110.
61. Antonova L, Aronson K, Mueller CR. Stress and breast cancer: from epidemiology to molecular biology. Breast Cancer Res. 2011;13(2):208. PMC3219182
62. Keita AD, Judd SE, Howard VJ, Carson AP, Ard JD, Fernandez JR. Associations of neighborhood area level deprivation with the metabolic syndrome and inflammation among middle- and older- age adults. BMC Public Health. 2014;14:1319. PMC4364504
63. King KE, Morenoff JD, House JS. Neighborhood context and social disparities in cumulative biological risk factors. Psychosom Med. 2011;73(7):572–9. PMC3216672
64. Merkin SS, Basurto-Davila R, Karlamangla A, et al. Neighborhoods and cumulative biological risk profiles by race/ethnicity in a national sample of U.S. adults: NHANES III. Ann Epidemiol. 2009;19(3):194–201. PMC3428227
65. Nimptsch K, Pischon T. Obesity biomarkers, metabolism and risk of cancer: an epidemiological perspective. Recent Results Cancer Res. 2016;208:199–217.
66. Rose DP, Vona-Davis L. Biochemical and molecular mechanisms for the association between obesity, chronic inflammation, and breast cancer. Biofactors. 2014;40(1):1–12.
67. Kolonel LN, Henderson BE, Hankin JH, et al. A multiethnic cohort in Hawaii and Los Angeles: baseline characteristics. Am J Epidemiol. 2000;151(4):346–57. 4482109
68. Kolonel LN, Altshuler D, Henderson BE. The multiethnic cohort study: exploring genes, lifestyle and cancer risk. Nat Rev Cancer. 2004;4(7):519–27.
69. Gomez SL, Glaser SL, McClure LA, et al. The California Neighborhoods Data System: a new resource for examining the impact of neighborhood characteristics on cancer incidence and outcomes in populations. Cancer Causes Control. 2011;22(4):631–47. 3102646
70. Conroy SM, Shariff-Marco S, Yang J, et al. Characterizing the neighborhood obesogenic environment in the multiethnic cohort: a multi-level infrastructure for cancer health disparities research. Cancer Causes Control. 2018;29(1):167–83. PMC5806518
71. Conroy SM, Clarke C, Yang J, et al. Contextual impact of neighborhood obesogenic factors on postmenopausal breast cancer: the Multiethnic Cohort. Cancer Epidemiol Biomark Prev. 2017;26:480–9.
72. Shariff-Marco S, Von Behren J, Reynolds P, et al. Impact of social and built environment factors on body size among breast cancer survivors: the Pathways Study. Cancer Epidemiol Biomark Prev. 2017;26:505–15.
73. Sposto R, Keegan TH, Vigen C, et al. The effect of patient and contextual characteristics on racial/ethnic disparity in breast cancer mortality. Cancer Epidemiol Biomark Prev. 2016;25(7):1064–72. PMC4930680
74. Cheng I, Shariff-Marco S, Koo J, et al. Contribution of the neighborhood environment and obesity to breast cancer survival: the California Breast Cancer Survivorship Consortium. Cancer Epidemiol Biomark Prev. 2015;24(8):1282–90. PMC4687960
75. Shariff-Marco S, Yang J, John EM, et al. Intersection of race/ethnicity and socioeconomic status in mortality after breast Cancer. J Community Health. 2015;40(6):1287–99. PMC4628564
76. Keegan TH, Shariff-Marco S, Sangaramoorthy M, et al. Neighborhood influences on recreational physical activity and survival after breast cancer. Cancer Causes Control. 2014;25(10):1295–308. 4194215
77. Shariff-Marco S, Yang J, John EM, et al. Impact of neighborhood and individual socioeconomic status on survival after breast cancer varies by race/ethnicity: the Neighborhood and Breast Cancer Study. Cancer Epidemiol Biomark Prev. 2014;23(5):793–811. 4018239

78. University of Hawaii Cancer Center. The Multiethnic Cohort Study Participant Questionnaires https://www.uhcancercenter.org/for-researchers/mec-questionnaires. Accessed 29 Nov 2018.
79. Setiawan VW, Virnig BA, Porcel J, et al. Linking data from the Multiethnic Cohort Study to medicare data: linkage results and application to chronic disease research. Am J Epidemiol. 2015;181(11):917–9. PMC4445395
80. Maskarinec G, Erber E, Grandinetti A, et al. Diabetes incidence based on linkages with health plans: the Multiethnic Cohort. Diabetes. 2009;58(8):1732–8. PMC2712787
81. State of California Office of Statewide Health Planning and Development. Data and Reports https://oshpd.ca.gov/data-and-reports/. Accessed Aug 2018.
82. Krieger N, Chen JT, Waterman PD, Soobader MJ, Subramanian SV, Carson R. Geocoding and monitoring of US socioeconomic inequalities in mortality and cancer incidence: does the choice of area-based measure and geographic level matter?: the Public Health Disparities Geocoding Project. Am J Epidemiol. 2002;156(5):471–82.
83. Walls & Associates. National Establishment Time-Series (NETS) Database, 2009 Oakland, 2008.
84. California Department of Food and Agriculture. California certified farmers' market Database. Sacramento. 2010.
85. NavTeq. NAVSTREETS street data reference manual v3.7. Chicago: NavTeq. 2010.
86. California Department of Transportation. Highway performance and monitoring system. Sacramento, CA. 2004.
87. Yang J, Schupp CW, Harrati A, Clarke C, Keegan THM, Gomez SL. Developing an area-based socioeconomic measure from American Community Survexy data. Fremont: Cancer Prevention Institute of California; 2014.
88. ArcGIS. Environmental Systems Research Institute, Inc., 2011.
89. Babey SH, Diamant AL, Hastert TA, et al. Designed for disease: the link between local food environments and obesity and diabetes. Los Angeles: California Center for Public Health Advocacy, Policy-Link, and the UCLA Center for Health Policy Research; 2008.
90. Berrigan D, Pickle LW, Dill J. Associations between street connectivity and active transportation. Int J Health Geogr. 2010;9:20. 2876088
91. Gunier RB, Hertz A, Von Behren J, Reynolds P. Traffic density in California: socioeconomic and ethnic differences among potentially exposed children. J Expo Anal Environ Epidemiol. 2003;13(3):240–6.
92. Shariff-Macro S, Tao L, Yang J, et al. Development of neighborhood "obesogenic factors" and its applicability to obesity and cancer studies in diverse populations: the Multiethnic Cohort Study. Ninth American Association for Cancer Research Conference on the Science of Cancer Health Disparities in Racial/Ethnic Minorities and the Medically Underserve; September 25–28, 2016; Fort Lauderdale
93. Stark JH, Neckerman K, Lovasi GS, et al. The impact of neighborhood park access and quality on body mass index among adults in New York City. Prev Med. 2014;64:63–8. 4314092
94. Bai H, Wilhelm Stanis SA, Kaczynski AT, Besenyi GM. Perceptions of neighborhood park quality: associations with physical activity and body mass index. Ann Behav Med. 2013;45(Suppl 1):S39–48.
95. White KK, Park SY, Kolonel LN, Henderson BE, Wilkens LR. Body size and breast cancer risk: the Multiethnic Cohort. Int J Cancer. 2012;131(5):E705–16. PMC4484854
96. Hastert TA, Beresford SA, Sheppard L, White E. Disparities in cancer incidence and mortality by area-level socioeconomic status: a multilevel analysis. J Epidemiol Community Health. 2015;69(2):168–76.
97. Torio CM, Klassen AC, Curriero FC, Caballero B, Helzlsouer K. The modifying effect of social class on the relationship between body mass index and breast cancer incidence. Am J Public Health. 2010;100(1):146–51. PMC2791249
98. Hines LM, Risendal B, Slattery ML, et al. Comparative analysis of breast cancer risk factors among Hispanic and non-Hispanic white women. Cancer. 2010;116(13):3215–23. PMC2922031
99. Dowd JB, Zajacova A, Aiello A. Early origins of health disparities: burden of infection, health, and socioeconomic status in U.S. children. Soc Sci Med. 2009;68(4):699–707. PMC2670067

100. Eschbach K, Mahnken JD, Goodwin JS. Neighborhood composition and incidence of cancer among Hispanics in the United States. Cancer. 2005;103(5):1036–44. PMC1853250

101. Fang CY, Tseng M. Ethnic density and cancer: a review of the evidence. Cancer. 2018;124(9):1877–903. PMC5920546

102. Hirsch JA, Grengs J, Schulz A, et al. How much are built environments changing, and where?: Patterns of change by neighborhood sociodemographic characteristics across seven U.S. metropolitan areas. Soc Sci Med. 2016;169:97–105. PMC5075249

103. Hirsch JA, Green GF, Peterson M, Rodriguez DA, Gordon-Larsen P. Neighborhood sociodemographics and change in built infrastructure. J Urban. 2017;10(2):181–97. PMC5353850

104. Versey HS. A tale of two Harlems: gentrification, social capital, and implications for aging in place. Soc Sci Med. 2018;214:1–11.

105. Barrientos-Gutierrez T, Moore KAB, Auchincloss AH, et al. Neighborhood physical environment and changes in body mass index: results from the Multi-Ethnic Study of Atherosclerosis. Am J Epidemiol. 2017;186(11):1237–45. PMC5860514

106. Xiao Q, Berrigan D, Powell-Wiley TM, Matthews CE. Ten-year change in neighborhood socioeconomic deprivation and rates of total, cardiovascular disease, and cancer mortality in older US adults. Am J Epidemiol. 2018;187(12):2642–50. PMC6269245

107. Zhang D, Matthews CE, Powell-Wiley TM, Xiao Q. Ten-year change in neighborhood socioeconomic status and colorectal cancer. Cancer. 2019;125(4):610–617. https://doi.org/10.1002/cncr.31832

108. Powell-Wiley TM, Cooper-McCann R, Ayers C, et al. Change in neighborhood socioeconomic status and weight gain: Dallas Heart Study. Am J Prev Med. 2015;49(1):72–9. PMC4476924

109. Hirsch JA, Moore KA, Barrientos-Gutierrez T, et al. Built environment change and change in BMI and waist circumference: Multi-Ethnic Study of Atherosclerosis. Obesity (Silver Spring). 2014;22(11):2450–7. PMC4224985

110. Wing JJ, August E, Adar SD, et al. Change in neighborhood characteristics and change in coronary artery calcium: a longitudinal investigation in the MESA (Multi-Ethnic Study of Atherosclerosis) cohort. Circulation. 2016;134(7):504–13. PMC4991627

111. Barrett RE, Cho YI, Weaver KE, et al. Neighborhood change and distant metastasis at diagnosis of breast cancer. Ann Epidemiol. 2008;18(1):43–7.

112. Cho YI, Johnson TP, Barrett RE, Campbell RT, Dolecek TA, Warnecke RB. Neighborhood changes in concentrated immigration and late stage breast cancer diagnosis. J Immigr Minor Health. 2011;13(1):9–14.

113. Chiu M, Rezai MR, Maclagan LC, et al. Moving to a highly walkable neighborhood and incidence of hypertension: a propensity-score matched cohort study. Environ Health Perspect. 2016;124(6):754–60. PMC4892930

114. Stinchcomb DG, Roeser A. NCI/SEER residential history project technical report. Rockville, MD2016.

115. Morenoff JD, Lynch JW. What makes a place healthy? Neighborhood influences on racial/ethnic disparities in health over the life course. In: Anderson NB, Bulatao RA, Cohen B, National research council (U.S.). panel on race ethnicity and health in later life., eds. Critical perspectives on racial and ethnic differences in health in late life. Washington, D.C.: National Academies Press; 2004: 406 p.

116. Carson AP, Rose KM, Catellier DJ, et al. Cumulative socioeconomic status across the life course and subclinical atherosclerosis. Ann Epidemiol. 2007;17(4):296–303.

117. Lemelin ET, Diez Roux AV, Franklin TG, et al. Life-course socioeconomic positions and subclinical atherosclerosis in the Multi-Ethnic Study of Atherosclerosis. Soc Sci Med. 2009;68(3):444–51. PMC5444463

118. Miles JN, Weden MM, Lavery D, Escarce JJ, Cagney KA, Shih RA. Constructing a time-invariant measure of the socio-economic status of U.S. census tracts. J Urban Health. 2016;93(1):213–32. PMC4794463

119. Murray ET, Diez Roux AV, Carnethon M, Lutsey PL, Ni H, O'Meara ES. Trajectories of neighborhood poverty and associations with subclinical atherosclerosis and associated risk

factors: the Multi-Ethnic Study of Atherosclerosis. Am J Epidemiol. 2010;171(10):1099–108. PMC2877469

120. Boone-Heinonen J, Howard AG, Meyer K, et al. Marriage and parenthood in relation to obesogenic neighborhood trajectories: the CARDIA study. Health Place. 2015;34:229–40. PMC4496281

121. Kwan M. The limits of the neighborhood effect: contextual uncertainties in geographic, environmental health, and social science research. Ann Am Assoc Geogr. 2018;108(6):1482–90.

122. Conroy SM, Canchola AJ, Shariff-Marco S, et al. Neighborhood obesogenic environment and obesity-related biomarkers in the Multiethnic Cohort: potential underlying mechanisms for obesity-related cancers. NCI Conference on Geospatial Approaches to Cancer Control and Population Sciences; September 12–14, 2016; NIH Campus, Bethesda.

Chapter 9
Spatial Analyses of Environmental Exposures and Breast Cancer: Natural Vegetation, Ambient Air Pollution and Outdoor Light at Night as Examples

Natalie DuPré, Jaime E. Hart, and Peter James

Abstract In this chapter, several environmental exposures are highlighted that are relevant to breast cancer epidemiology such as natural vegetation/greenness, air pollutants, and outdoor light at night exposures. Each section gives an overview of the rationale and potential mechanisms behind these exposures, followed by a description of the available epidemiologic literature with respect to breast cancer incidence and survival, and then a summary of the challenges and next steps for this area of research. Throughout the chapter, epidemiologic concepts such as exposure measurement, confounding, effect modification and mediation are discussed in context with the environmental exposure. Environmental exposures may play an important role in breast cancer prevention and survival after a diagnosis of breast cancer through a direct influence on biologic pathways and/or via their influence on vital behaviors of energy balance relevant to breast cancer epidemiology (e.g. physical activity and circadian patterns). As one may expect with diseases of long latency such as breast cancer and for studies of environmental exposures, there are chal-

N. DuPré (✉)
Brigham and Women's Hospital, Channing Division of Network Medicine,
Boston, MA, USA

Department of Epidemiology and Population Health, University of Louisville, School of
Public Health and Information Sciences, Louisville, KY, USA
e-mail: natalie.dupre@louisville.edu

J. E. Hart
Channing Division of Network Medicine, Department of Medicine,
Brigham and Women's Hospital and Harvard Medical School, Boston, MA, USA

Department of Environmental Health, Harvard T.H. Chan School of Public Health,
Boston, MA, USA

P. James
Division of Chronic Disease Research Across the Lifecourse (CoRAL), Department of
Population Medicine, Harvard Medical School and Harvard Pilgrim Health Care Institute,
Boston, MA, USA

© Springer Nature Switzerland AG 2019   189
D. Berrigan, N. A. Berger (eds.), *Geospatial Approaches to Energy Balance and Breast
Cancer*, Energy Balance and Cancer 15, https://doi.org/10.1007/978-3-030-18408-7_9

lenges to these spatial analyses of breast cancer environmental determinants, particularly with regards to obtaining personal-level measurements of environmental exposures at the appropriate time window within the life course. Understanding the multi-level context of breast cancer incidence and survival after a diagnosis of breast cancer is needed and has potential to explain the geographic variation of breast cancer risk and mortality.

Keywords Environmental exposure · Breast cancer epidemiology · Greenness · Vegetation · Air pollution · Outdoor light at night

9.1   Introduction

Historical migration studies highlighted the importance of environmental and lifestyle factors in breast cancer etiology. Specifically, these studies consistently observed that immigrants to the US and their children experienced an upward shift of breast cancer rates approaching the breast cancer rates of women in the US compared to lower rates of their native counterparts [1–3]; this rapid upward shift cannot be explained by germline genetics. In addition, geographic variation in breast cancer incidence and mortality rates across countries, as well as within countries, highlight the possibility that differing distributions of breast cancer risk factors, including environmental exposures, may play an important role in driving these patterns [4–6].

Modifiable lifestyle factors such as weight gain, physical activity, alcohol consumption, breastfeeding, and menopausal hormone therapy use have been well-established for their associations with breast cancer incidence and account for approximately one-third of post-menopausal breast cancers in the US [7]. Ecosocial theory explains that while health behaviors are the function of individual choices, these choices are made within the context of community-level factors [8]. These community-level factors, which often have a geospatial or environmental component, can create opportunities or barriers to partake in healthier behaviors, or may directly influence health outcomes. Researchers are now working to identify multilevel interventions (e.g. modifiable community-level factors and individual-level interventions) to promote cancer prevention behaviors. As part of the effort to identify additional risk factors that explain the remainder of breast cancer risk, novel spatial and contextual environmental factors have been gaining attention in the US through research initiatives from the Interagency Breast Cancer & Environment Research Coordinating Committee and the Institute of Medicine [9, 10]. Consideration of spatial and contextual features that influence survival after a breast cancer diagnosis is also warranted, as over three million women in the US are living with a breast cancer diagnosis [11]. Expanding the framework of cancer research from single factors to incorporate multifactorial causes is needed to understand the complex relationships between social, behavioral, molecular, environmental, and historical factors that influence cancer incidence and progression [12–14]. In this chapter, we highlight environmental factors that may influence behavior and biology germane to breast tumor development and/or progression. We focus on studies exploring the impacts of natural vegetation, air pollutants, and outdoor light at night on breast cancer incidence, variation in intermediate markers of breast cancer risk, and disease survival. Throughout the chapter, we will highlight epidemiologic concepts that include, but are not limited to, exposure measurement, confounding, effect modification and mediation as they relate to the geospatial exposures discussed in this chapter: natural vegetation/greenness, air pollutants, and outdoor light at night.

9.2 Natural Vegetation and Breast Cancer

9.2.1 Rationale and Mechanisms

Natural vegetation, or greenness, as well as green spaces, such as parks, gardens, and forests, have been evaluated in relation to a variety of healthy behaviors—most notably physical activity—and health outcomes (e.g., obesity, mental health, birth and developmental outcomes, allergies, cardiovascular disease, and mortality) [15–18]. The health benefits of exposure to natural vegetation have been conceptualized in a biopsychosocial framework that encompasses several domains [19]. That is, exposure to natural vegetation may build capacities (e.g., promote physical activity and social cohesion), restore capacities (e.g., mental restoration, physiological stress recovery, and immune functioning), and reduce harm (e.g., from ambient pollutants, noise, and temperature extremes) [19, 20]. Elements of this framework, such as physical activity, social engagement, and ambient pollutants (discussed later in this chapter), have been associated independently with breast cancer incidence and/or breast cancer specific mortality, but few studies have directly examined the relation between greenness and incidence of breast cancer or breast cancer-specific mortality. Furthermore, breast cancer patients experience a variety of quality of life issues, particularly regarding mental health, social cohesion, and stress, and therefore may be an important population to benefit from green space exposures or interventions. Here, we evaluate elements of the biopsychosocial domains of greenness, modified from Markevych et al. [19], that influence factors that are particularly relevant to breast cancer outcomes (Table 9.1).

9.2.1.1 Physical Activity

Physical inactivity is one of the few well-established and modifiable breast cancer risk factors [21] and is associated with higher rates of breast cancer-specific mortality and cancer-related symptoms for breast cancer patients [22, 23]. In the US, the majority of women with breast cancer do not meet physical activity guidelines of ≥ 150 min per week of moderate activity or ≥ 75 min per week of vigorous activity [24]. While physical activity duration and intensity have been

Table 9.1 Domains and selected factors, modified from Markevych et al. through which natural vegetation/greenness exposure may influence breast cancer incidence and survival

Greenness domains	Selected factors associated with higher greenness exposure	Relevance of factors with regards to breast cancer epidemiology	Key conclusions for future breast cancer work
Build capacities	Physical activity promotion	Physical inactivity is a modifiable risk factor for breast cancer incidence and breast cancer specific mortality	Optimal environments to promote physical activity and identification of the barriers to their utilization, particularly for communities with high breast cancer risk, may provide valuable insight on strategies to reduce breast cancer risk and improve survival
	Encourages social cohesion	Social support has benefits for breast cancer specific survival, and other important quality of life components after a diagnosis of breast cancer	The benefits of greenness exposure via encouraging social cohesion may be particularly relevant among breast cancer patient populations, and remains to be addressed.
Restore capacities	Mental health benefits and stress reduction	A breast cancer diagnosis is a psychological stressor that impacts mental health in cancer patients and chemotherapy treatment is anecdotally a concern among breast cancer patients who believe it affects their cognitive abilities.	More research is needed to determine whether cancer patient populations may benefit from greater exposure to nature both in their communities and in hospital care settings.
Reduce harm	Reduces exposure to air pollutants	Air pollution exposure in adulthood has generally not been strongly associated with breast cancer incidence; however, post-diagnosis $PM_{2.5}$ exposure has been consistently associated with higher breast cancer specific-mortality.	The interplay between greenness and air pollution on the development of breast cancer has not been explicitly explored.

studied extensively in relation to breast cancer incidence and survival, details on the environments in which the activities take place and their accessibility may provide valuable insight on strategies to reduce breast cancer risk and improve survival. Within a large cohort of women (The Sister Study Cohort, comprised of women who have a sister diagnosed with breast cancer), those who resided in areas with the highest tertile of green cover (i.e., forests, shrub lands, or herbaceous land covers) and open green spaces had higher physical activity levels compared to those in the lowest tertile of green space, and this relationship was seen in all types of areas (urban/suburban or rural/small towns) [25]. Moreover, those with higher green space exposure were less likely to be obese, and the reported associations were more strongly protective among those with low incomes [25]. Several studies have suggested that physical activity has larger benefits in terms of short-term physiological and psychological outcomes when performed in greener areas [17]. Thus, for breast cancer prevention and survival, as well as for other health outcomes, it is vital to study optimal environments to promote physical activity and identify the barriers that exist preventing their utilization [26]. This may be particularly true for populations that largely do not meet physical activity recommendations, such as women with a breast cancer diagnosis [24] and communities at high risk of aggressive breast cancer, e.g., women with a family history of breast cancer and African-American women [13, 27–29].

9.2.1.2 Social Cohesion

In addition to greenness building capacities such as physical activity, greenness may promote social cohesion [15, 17–19]. Social isolation has shown profound effects on promoting breast tumors in rats [30]. In humans, social engagement metrics have been linked with health-promoting behaviors such as usage of screening mammography [31, 32], though the role of social engagement on breast cancer incidence is limited [33]. Among women diagnosed with breast cancer, social support has benefits for breast cancer specific survival, from quality of life metrics, psychological distress, to breast cancer-specific mortality, and all-cause mortality [34–41].

9.2.1.3 Mental Health

The demonstrated social cohesion, mental health benefits, and stress reducing properties of greenness [19] may be particularly useful among women diagnosed with breast cancer. Being diagnosed with breast cancer increased risk of suicide within 1 year of diagnosis [42]. Also, patients report experiences of short-term loss of mental acuity after treatment with chemotherapy, often called "chemo brain"— though this condition is not well understood [43]. Extending the work on the restorative properties of green space to improve mental health and cognition [44], and reduce psychological distress and depression [16, 45–48] for cancer patients is a potential avenue for breast cancer survivorship research. Future research should focus on how exposure to nature, both in one's community and in hospitals treating cancer patients, might have mental health benefits among breast cancer patients.

9.2.1.4 Reduction of Deleterious Exposures

Greenness may be linked to health due to the fact that green environments may reduce exposure to factors such as air pollution, which is strongly related to mortality, cardiovascular diseases, and respiratory diseases such as lung cancer

[49]. Studies have demonstrated that natural vegetation is negatively correlated with air pollutants, such as $PM_{2.5}$ and NO_2, such that greener areas have lower levels of air pollutants [50]. The relevance of air pollution and breast cancer epidemiology is discussed in Sect. 3, though air pollution research has not often simultaneously considered greenness. The interplay between greenness and air pollution (e.g. whether they are mediators or effect modifiers and/or whether the association between greenness and the breast cancer is independent of air pollution levels and vice versa) on the development of breast cancer should be more explicitly explored.

9.2.2   Epidemiologic Evidence

As of 2018, three epidemiologic studies have directly assessed greenness or access to green spaces in relation to breast cancer incidence [51–53]. They have used a variety of exposure measures [17, 20] such as distance to nearest green space, type of green space within a certain area surrounding a residence that are derived from land use datasets and Geographic Information System (GIS)-based approaches, as well as measures generated from satellite-data that objectively capture fluctuations in exposure over time. Because chlorophyll in vegetation absorbs visible light for photosynthesis and reflects near-infrared light, natural vegetation levels (i.e. greenness) can be quantified from satellite sensors that measure the wavelength of light in images using a ratio of reflected near-infrared and visible light, called the Normalized Difference Vegetation Index (NDVI), which is a commonly used measure in epidemiologic literature of greenness.

The association between greenness and breast cancer incidence has been evaluated in two cohort studies and one case-control study. Within the prospective cohort study of Nurses' Health Study II with questionnaires mailed to the participants' address every 2 years, 109,643 female participants were followed from 1989–2013 of whom 3458 developed invasive breast cancer [51]. Cumulative average residential greenness was measured using NDVI measurements in July of each year (summertime greenness to maximize variability) from 1989–2013 and were updated over follow-up. Women who resided in the top quintile of greenness had a 13% lower hazard of developing breast cancer compared to those in the lowest quintile of exposure (95% CI 0.75, 1.01; p-value for trend = 0.02) after adjusting for many known and suspected breast cancer risk factors [51]. A majority of the participants in this study (approximately 84%) lived in metropolitan areas; however, there was no evidence of effect modification by urban/rural status, which suggests that the relationship between greenness and mortality was consistent across both urban and rural areas. In a large statutory health insurance cohort of 1.9 million beneficiaries in Saxony, Germany, postal-code level estimates of greenness in 2007 were weakly and inversely associated with breast cancer risk for a 10% increase in NDVI (Relative Risk [RR] = 0.96 95% CI 0.92 0.99), but analyses were only adjusted for age [52]. In a Spanish case-control study of 1129 breast cancer cases and 1619 controls matched on age and area, residential proximity to urban green spaces (e.g. gardens, zoos, and urban parks), agricultural green areas and surrounding NDVI were examined [53]. Compared to those who did not live within 300 meters to an urban green space, living within 100 meters of an urban green area was associated with 44% lower odds of breast cancer (95% CI 0.41, 0.76) and within 100–300 meters was associated with a 29% lower odds of breast cancer (95% CI 0.53, 0.96) after adjusting for age, education, socioeconomic status indices, and parity. However, protective effects were not observed with proximity to agricultural green spaces within 300 meters compared to those who did not live within 500 meters from an agricultural area (Odds Ratio [OR] = 1.25 95% CI 0.99, 1.56) or NDVI (Odds Ratio [OR] = 1.17 95% CI 1.06, 1.28) [53].

A few studies of greenness addressed total cancer mortality [18] or lung cancer mortality [45, 54], but no studies have examined breast cancer specific mortality. Among 108,630 women in the Nurses' Health Study followed from 2000 to 2008, of whom 8604 died from any cause and 3363 died from cancer, higher cumulative average NDVI was associated with lower hazard of nonaccidental all-cause mortality and with lower risk of cancer-specific mortality (Quintile 5 versus Quintile 1, Hazard Ratio [HR] = 0.87 95% CI 0.78, 0.97) in fully-adjusted models [18]. Variability in mental health and social engagement mediated this relationship between NDVI and lower cancer mortality by approximately 20% and 10%, respectively, and to a lesser extent was mediated by physical activity or air pollution. It remains uncertain whether this reduction in total cancer mortality with higher greenness exposure was driven by breast cancer mortality, though breast cancer deaths likely comprised a majority of the cancer mortality cases in women. Future studies should determine whether the observed association of greenness and lower cancer mortality are driven by lower breast cancer specific mortality and identify the extent to which other factors may mediate this association.

9.2.3 Summary: Challenges and Next Steps

In summary, the main mechanisms that greenness may operate through to influence breast cancer outcomes will likely stem from promoting physical activity, social cohesion, cancer screening, and mental health restoration. It is too soon to draw conclusions about the relationship between natural vegetation exposure and breast cancer incidence or mortality (Table 9.2); however, the potential health benefits of greenness exposure are very relevant to breast cancer prevention strategies and may improve prognostic and quality of life factors for women with breast cancer.

Existing epidemiologic studies can help to frame future research considerations, particularly in terms of exposure definition, confounding, effect modification, and mediation. In terms of exposures definition, epidemiologic studies use a variety of measures to classify greenness exposure that each have their own strengths and limitations. The NDVI measure of greenness at one's residence is frequently used in epidemiologic research as an objective measure of greenness but does not distinguish the specific uses or accessibility of specific green spaces and hence may cap-

Table 9.2 Selected epidemiologic studies of multiple exposures of natural vegetation, air pollutants, and outdoor light at night in relation to breast cancer outcomes

Exposure	Study design	First author (year)	Overall findings
Greenness, green space	Cohort	Datzmann et al. (2018)	• Suggestive inverse associations between greenness and breast cancer risk that may depend on the specific exposure proxies used
		James (2017)	
	Case-control	O'Callaghan Gordo et al. (2018)	
Ambient Particulate Matter (PM)	Cohort	Reding et al. (2015)	• PM exposures during adulthood have not been associated with incidence of breast cancer • Adult-life $PM_{2.5}$ may be associated with higher mammographic density among women without breast cancer • Higher $PM_{2.5}$ exposure after diagnosis may be associated with higher breast cancer-specific mortality rates
		Hart et al. (2016)	
		Zorana Jovanovic Andersen et al. (2017)	
		Zorana J. Andersen et al. (2017)	
		Yaghjyan et al. (2017)	
		N. C. DuPre et al. (2017)	
		Hu et al. (2013)	
		Tagliabue et al. (2016)	
		N. DuPre et al. (2017)	
Ambient NO_2 or NO_X	Cohort	Raaschou-Nielsen et al. (2011)	• Exposures during adulthood have not been consistently associated with breast cancer risk • Some studies have observed elevated risks of specific breast cancer subtypes and or among subgroups of women
		Reding et al. (2015)	
		Huynh et al. (2015)	
		Zorana Jovanovic Andersen et al. (2017)	
		Zorana J. Andersen et al. (2017)	
	Case-control	Crouse et al. (2010)	
		Hystad et al. (2015)	
		Goldberg et al. (2017)	
Proxies for traffic pollution based on roadway characterization	Cohort	Hart et al. (2016)	• Traffic proxies have not been consistently associated with breast cancer risk or mammographic density
		Zorana J. Andersen et al. (2017)	
		Shmuel, White, and Sandler (2017)	
		Raaschou-Nielsen et al. (2011)	
		N. C. DuPre et al. (2017)	
Circulating PAH-DNA adducts	Case-control	Gammon et al. (2004)	• Circulating levels of PAH-DNA adducts have been associated with elevated breast cancer risk • Risk may depend on genetic polymorphisms in specific DNA nuclear repair genes
		Crew et al. (2007)	
		Shen et al. (2008)	
		Saieva et al. (2011)	
		Shen et al. (2017)	
		Agudo et al. (2017)	
		Niehoff et al. (2017)	

(continued)

Table 9.2 (continued)

Exposure	Study design	First author (year)	Overall findings
Ambient PAH from traffic	Case-control	Nie et al. (2007)	• Little evidence of associations with breast cancer risk • Suggestions of gene-environment interactions with DNA repair genes
		Mordukhovich et al. (2016b, 2016a)	
		White et al. (2016)	
		Niehoff et al. (2017)	
Hazardous air pollutants	Cohort	Liu et al. (2015)	• Limited consistent evidence of adverse associations of airborne endocrine disrupting chemicals or mammary carcinogens on breast cancer incidence
		Garcia et al. (2015)	
		Hart et al. (2018)	
Outdoor light at night	Case-control	Bauer et al. (2013)	• Elevated risk of breast cancer with higher outdoor light at night exposure in case-control studies and cohort studies • Associations may be modified by demographic and lifestyle factors
		Keshet-Sitton et al. (2016)	
		Garcia-Saenz et al. (2018)	
	Cohort	Hurley et al. (2014)	
		James et al. (2017)	

ture distinct constructs. This was exemplified in the breast cancer case-control study in Spain that observed very different associations with breast cancer incidence depending on the exposure metric chosen [55]. A few novel methods to improve upon the greenness exposure definition may provide insight on specific greenness qualities, such as machine learning and Google Street View methods [56] as well as incorporating time-activity patterns to understand how participants interact with green spaces [57]. Future studies should assess the contributors of confounding and control for confounding particularly by socioeconomic status in analyses of breast cancer incidence and survival. The associations between greenness and breast cancer outcomes may also differ by effect modifiers such as geographic regions, built environment characteristics (e.g., neighborhood walkability) and urbanicity, which will shed light on to the true construct of what it means to live and play in green areas that may differ depending on where one lives (e.g. living in a very green area in rural areas may represent a different construct versus living in a very green area in a city). Prospective cohort studies and nested case-control studies will be optimal to disentangle the temporal factors that mediate the relationship between greenness and breast cancer incidence and breast cancer mortality, particularly by physical activity levels, mental health, social cohesion, and ambient pollution. Future research should assess both the direct impact of greenness on breast cancer outcomes that may suggest some underlying biological role of greenness on cancer development, as well as its indirect pathways through promoting capacities (i.e., physical activity and social cohesion) and restoring capacities (i.e. mental health).

Conducting research on the role of greenness in breast cancer survivorship, extending to breast cancer mortality and mental health outcomes, may also be beneficial for breast cancer research.

9.3 Ambient Air Pollutants and Breast Cancer

9.3.1 Rationale and Mechanisms

Outdoor air pollution is a ubiquitous ambient exposure that is inhaled at higher doses during physical exertion [58–61]. As such, it is important to consider air pollution within the context of geospatial factors, energy balance, and breast cancer risk. Ambient air pollution and particulate matter were classified as human carcinogens by the World Health Organization (WHO) International Agency for Research on Cancer (IARC) primarily based on the evidence available for lung cancer at the time of the panel review [62]. Prospective cohort studies have been published since the panel review on air pollution and ambient particulate matter in relation to breast carcinogenesis. We focus on the literature examining ambient particulate matter, oxides of nitrogen, as well as other more specific constituents of airborne exposures such as polycyclic aromatic hydrocarbons (PAHs), airborne mammary carcinogens, and endocrine disrupting airborne chemicals.

Ambient particulate matter (PM) is a complex mixture of solid and liquid particles often characterized by aerodynamic diameter (e.g. ultrafine particles [UFP], $PM_{2.5}$, PM_{10}). Smaller particles can penetrate more deeply into the lungs [63, 64]. There is convincing evidence that ambient particulate matter induces systemic inflammation, oxidative stress, and epigenetic changes [64–69] that are important mechanisms underlying carcinogenesis [70–73]. Inflammation has been shown to be particularly pertinent to breast cancer progression [73–82], with less of a role on breast cancer development in epidemiologic studies [83–89]. Particulate matter not only increases systemic inflammation and oxidative stress, but some of its components have also been directly characterized as endocrine disruptors [90] that alter hormonal systems and homeostatic systems.

Motor vehicle traffic is a major source of ambient gaseous oxides of nitrogen (NO_2 and NO_X) pollutant exposure. While nitrogen oxides are not thought of as carcinogens, they are often used as a proxy for other exposures such as PAHs that are also emitted from traffic [91]. PAHs are produced by the combustion of organic matter [92]. PAHs persist when bound to solid particulate matter, unlike gas-phase PAHs that have durations of less than a day [92]. PAHs and other air pollutants, such as diesel exhaust, or metals in ambient particulate matter, can be estrogenic and anti-estrogenic and can activate the aryl hydrocarbon receptor [90, 93–95] that plays a role in tumor development [96, 97].

9.3.2 Epidemiologic Evidence

9.3.2.1 Particulate Matter (PM)

At the time of the IARC panel review on ambient particulate matter, cohort and case-control studies of ambient particles and breast cancer primarily focused on larger total suspected particles (TSP) that are 50–100 microns in diameter, or proxies for air pollution exposure, such as proximity to roadways, industrial sources or traffic density [62]. Four prospective cohort studies have since examined ambient particulate matter exposure in relation to breast cancer incidence with broader geographic spread [98–101].

The Sister Study Cohort and the Nurses' Health Study II have examined the relationship between adult-life exposure to particulate matter and incidence of invasive breast cancer for women residing across the US. Women ages 35–74 enrolled in the Sister Study Cohort from 2003 to 2009 (N = 47,591) were followed until January 2013 and 1749 developed invasive breast cancer [98]. Residential air pollution concentrations were derived using a validated prediction model from 2006 for $PM_{2.5}$ and from 2000 for PM_{10}. After adjustment for several breast cancer risk factors, adult exposure to an interquartile range increase in $PM_{2.5}$ (3.6 $\mu g/m^3$) or PM_{10} (5.8 $\mu g/m^3$) was not associated with invasive breast cancer incidence ($PM_{2.5}$ HR of breast cancer = 1.03 95% CI 0.96, 1.11; PM_{10} HR = 0.99 95% CI 0.98,1.00) [98]. Similarly, there was no association between $PM_{2.5}$, $PM_{2.5–10}$, and PM_{10} exposures and incidence of breast cancer defined by tumor hormone receptor status. Among 115,921 participants in the Nurses' Health Study II who were followed every 2 years for incidence of invasive breast cancer confirmed by medical records, 3416 participants developed invasive breast cancer [99]. High-resolution estimates of residential ambient particulate matter were derived using validated prediction models updated from 1989–2007 [102]. After adjusting for many known breast cancer risk factors, a 10 $\mu g/m^3$ increase in PM size fractions was not associated with breast cancer incidence overall ($PM_{2.5}$ HR = 0.90 95% CI 0.79, 1.03; $PM_{2.5–10}$ HR = 1.06 95% CI 0.96, 1.17; PM_{10} HR = 1.00 95% CI 0.93, 1.07) or breast tumors defined by ER/PR status [99].

Two prospective cohort studies have examined adult-life particulate matter in relation to breast cancer incidence in Europe [100, 101]. Danish female nurses (n = 22,877) were followed from 1993–2013 for a breast cancer diagnosis ascertained from the Danish Cancer Register. After adjusting for many important and known breast cancer risk factors (i.e. age, smoking, alcohol consumption, physical activity, BMI, age at first birth, parity, age at menarche, hormone therapy, menopausal status, and oral contraceptive use), the authors observed no association between particulate matter and breast cancer incidence [100]. In a large meta-analysis of 68,806 postmenopausal participants, particulate matter and eight of its elemental constituents were estimated from land use regression models between 2008–2011 in 11 cohorts from nine European countries [101]. The authors examined the constituents of PM as a measure of likely sources of the exposure. Overall,

PM size fractions were not associated with postmenopausal breast cancer incidence ($PM_{2.5}$ HR = 1.08 95% CI 0.77, 1.51; $PM_{2.5-10}$ HR = 1.20 95% CI 0.96, 1.49; PM_{10} HR = 1.07 95% CI 0.89, 1.30); however, substantial heterogeneity existed across cohorts for $PM_{2.5}$ and in post hoc analyses removing a cohort with poor covariate information, a 5 µg/m³ increase in $PM_{2.5}$ was associated with higher rate of developing postmenopausal breast cancer (HR = 1.28 95% CI 0.99, 1.65). Single elemental constituents of $PM_{2.5}$ did not appear to drive this association [101]. In general, European studies of PM and breast cancer incidence reported largely null associations.

Studying intermediate markers of breast cancer, such as mammographic density—a strong and well-established breast cancer risk factor [103]— examines normal variation in breast tissue composition that captures a time window before disease development, which can aid in our understanding of earlier differences in breast tissue that may lead to cancer development. As of 2018, three epidemiologic studies have investigated particulate matter exposures and mammographic density. In the Breast Cancer Surveillance Consortium from five registries in New Hampshire, Vermont, New Mexico, San Francisco, and western Washington State, increased PM was associated with having more dense categories of percent mammographic density [104]. Within the Nurses' Health Study and Nurses' Health Study II, only $PM_{2.5}$ exposure was associated with slightly higher percent density among a subgroup of postmenopausal women in the Northeast, but not in other US regions or among premenopausal women [105]. A study of PM and mammographic density in the area of Utrecht, Netherlands reported no association between PM and mammographic density, although there was very little exposure variability [106].

Breast cancer survival after a diagnosis of breast cancer is a pressing concern, as breast cancer is the leading cause of cancer death worldwide [107] and the second leading cause of cancer death among women in the US (108). With the high uptake of mammography screening, many women are being diagnosed with low stage breast cancer [109] and approximately three million women in the US are living with a breast cancer diagnosis [11]. Among 255,128 women with breast cancer diagnosed between 1999–2009 in the California Surveillance Epidemiology and End Results (SEER) registry, a 5 µg/m³ increase in $PM_{2.5}$ levels at diagnosis was associated with higher breast cancer mortality (HR = 1.86 95% CI 1.12, 3.10), particularly among breast cancer patients with lower stage disease [110]. In a smaller study of 2021 women with breast cancer diagnosed between 2003–2009 from the Varese province in northern Italy with approximately half of the cases diagnosed with Stage I disease, a similar association between $PM_{2.5}$ and breast cancer specific mortality was reported (Quartile 4 vs Quartile 1: HR = 1.72 95% CI 1.08, 2.75) [111]. Additionally, among 8936 participants with confirmed Stage I-III breast cancer in the Nurses' Health Study and Nurses' Health Study II, a 10 µg/m³ increase in post-diagnosis PM exposure updated over follow-up was associated with modest increases in all-cause mortality [112] consistent with previous findings of PM and all-cause mortality in the full cohort [113]. Furthermore, among participants with Stage I disease, a 10 µg/m³ increase in $PM_{2.5}$ was associated with higher breast cancer specific-mortality (HR = 1.64 95% CI 1.11, 2.43), but not for $PM_{2.5-10}$ or PM_{10} or among women with Stage II or Stage II disease [112]. In summary, while PM exposures in adult-life were generally not associated with breast cancer incidence, $PM_{2.5}$ exposure has been consistently associated with higher breast-cancer specific mortality in the three studies available as of 2018 (Table 9.2).

9.3.2.2 Nitrogen Oxides (NO_2/NO_X) and Traffic Proxies

Nitrogen oxides are other air pollutants that predominately come from motor vehicle traffic emissions and have been studied in relation to breast cancer incidence. Case-control studies within Canada have reported elevated risks of breast cancer with increasing exposure to ambient NO_2 and NO_X [as summarized in [114]], though findings were not statistically significant [115–117]. Of two case-control studies of postmenopausal breast cancer in Montreal, Canada, significant elevated risk of postmenopausal breast cancer was reported with only one measure of exposure [116] and was observed for hormone receptor positive tumors among non-movers in Montreal [115]. However, in a case-control study across eight Canadian provinces, NO_2 exposure was not associated with postmenopausal breast cancer but was associated with elevated premenopausal breast cancer risk [117]. Cohort studies in the US and Europe have examined ambient exposure to NO_2 and NO_X and generally did not observe significant associations between NO_2/NO_X exposure and breast cancer incidence [98, 100, 101, 118] or with mammographic density [119]; however, there were specific subgroup findings in the Sister Study Cohort [98] and in the ESCAPE meta-analysis [101]. In the Sister Study Cohort of women with a family history of breast cancer, the relative risk of developing ER-positive breast cancer for a 5.8 ppb increase in 2006 NO_2 was 1.10 (95% CI 1.02, 1.19), but was null for ER-negative breast cancer [98]. Within the ESCAPE meta-analysis, a 20 $\mu g/m^3$ increase in 2008–2011 NO_X estimates was associated with modestly higher risk of postmenopausal breast cancer (HR = 1.04 95% CI 1.00, 1.08), but not NO_2 estimates [101]. Residential proximities to roadways and traffic characteristics of roads near participants' residences have not been associated with statistically significant elevations in breast cancer risk [99, 101, 118, 120] or mammographic density [105]. In summary, studies of nitrogen oxides and breast cancer risk have yielded inconsistent results across exposures types and subpopulations suggesting harmful associations, as well as null associations.

9.3.2.3 Polycyclic Aromatic Hydrocarbons (PAH)

Epidemiologic studies suggested that circulating levels of PAH-DNA adducts may be associated with elevated breast cancer risk in some [121–123], but not all studies [124, 125]. Studies of whether the association between circulating PAH-DNA adducts and breast cancer risk differs by genetics and lifestyle factors have also been explored [121, 125–128]. Effect modification [126] by genetic polymorphisms

[127, 128], familial breast cancer risk [121], BMI and weight gain [125] suggest that circulating PAH-DNA adducts may be associated with elevated breast cancer risk among those with genetic polymorphisms in certain DNA nuclear repair genes [127, 128] but may be chance findings due to issues of multiple testing and small sample sizes. Utilizing circulating biomarkers of PAH exposure in epidemiologic settings provides individual-level exposure to the diverse sources of PAHs, though it is unclear if they represent long-term PAH exposure specifically from traffic or from other sources such as smoking or grilled proteins. Studies have also estimated ambient exposure to PAHs modeled from vehicular and other emissions, traffic patterns, meteorological factors, and dispersion factors data. In studies from New York, the associations between modeled ambient PAH exposure and breast cancer risk were generally consistent with the null [125, 129–131]; however, there may be gene-environment interactions with DNA repair genes such as *ERCC2* [131] that need to be replicated in larger studies. For example, while estimated traffic PAH exposure in 1995 was not associated with breast cancer incidence in the Long Island Breast Cancer Study Project (OR = 1.01 95% CI 0.81, 1.26), there was an association between estimate traffic PAH exposure and breast cancer incidence among participants with a homozygous variant genotype of *ERCC2* after adjusting for age (OR = 2.09 95% CI 1.13, 3.90) [131]. More research is needed to understand the plausibility of these gene-environment interactions.

9.3.2.4   Other Ambient Pollutants

Cohort studies in the Nurses' Health Study II and the California Teachers Study assessed ambient exposures to airborne chemicals, some of which are considered mammary carcinogens and endocrine disruptors. Overall, there was limited evidence of adverse associations of the airborne chemicals examined on breast cancer incidence, and there was little agreement across studies [132–134].

Within the California Teachers Study, 112,379 participants were enrolled in 1995–1996 and followed through 2011 for a diagnosis of breast cancer. Twenty-four mammary gland carcinogens and eleven estrogen-disrupting chemicals were evaluated from the 2002 US Environmental Protection Agency National-Scale Air Toxics Assessment [132, 133]. In the California Teachers Study, acrylamide, benzidine, carbon tetrachloride, ethylidene dichloride, and vinyl chloride were associated with increased risks of estrogen and progesterone receptor-positive tumors (ER+/PR+) and benzene, cadmium and arsenic compounds were associated with elevated risk of hormone receptor-negative (ER-/PR-) tumors [132, 133]. Within the Nurses' Health Study II, there were no consistent trends of elevated risk of invasive breast cancer with exposure to the same chemicals assessed in the California Teachers Study, after adjustment for many breast cancer risk factors, though suggestions of elevated risk were observed with increasing exposure to 1,2-dibromo-3-chloropropane, diesel exhaust, 4-nitrophenol, dibutulphthalate and dimethyl formamide for overall and ER+ breast cancer, and elevated risk for ER-breast cancer with higher exposure to bis(2-ethylhexyl)phthalate (DEHP) [134].

9.3.3 Summary: Challenges and Next Steps

In summary (Table 9.2), while the associations between adult-life exposure to particulate matter and breast cancer incidence are generally null, studies of post-diagnosis exposure to $PM_{2.5}$ report consistent elevations in breast cancer-specific mortality and all-cause mortality for women diagnosed with localized breast cancer. This association may be restricted to those with localized disease because Stage II-IV breast tumors have already spread outside the breast such that air pollution has little effect on tumor progression at this point. Furthermore, studies of particulate matter and intermediate markers of breast cancer risk (i.e. mammographic density) suggest that particulate matter may influence early breast biology and it will be important to study early-life exposure to particulate matter in relation to breast tissue variation and tumor development. The biological mechanisms underlying this association will be an important next step in epidemiologic and animal research to establish whether environmental pollutants influence breast tissue and breast tumor progression. Studies of ambient NO_2/NO_X, traffic proxies, airborne PAH, and airborne chemicals are generally null or inconsistent with reported elevated breast cancer risk among specific subgroups or with specific exposure definitions. There are a number of key considerations for studies of air pollutants and breast cancer research that may contribute to the null findings and inconsistencies.

The prospective cohort studies described in the section above focused primarily on adult-life exposure to air pollutants due to the ages of participants at the time when exposure data was available. For example, Nurses' Health Study II participants were ages 25–42 in 1989 and PM exposure data became available in the mid-1980s when the participants were already past adolescence; hence, this precluded analyses of exposure to air pollutants during early-life. A more relevant time window of exposure for breast tumor development occurs during the time of puberty and a woman's first child birth [1, 135–137]. More research on early-life exposures to environmental pollutants is needed as higher exposure to total suspended particles [138] and modeled traffic emissions of benzo[a]pyrene (BaP) [139] at the time of birth, menarche, or first childbirth were associated with higher risk of breast cancer in a population-based case-control study in the Western New York Exposures and Breast Cancer study [138, 139]. Early-life exposures to ambient total suspended particles and traffic emission estimates were also associated with differential epigenetic methylation patterns for a few genes within breast tissue in the Western New York Exposures and Breast Cancer study and the Long Island Breast Cancer Study Project case-control study [140, 141].

Measurement error of air pollutants, like all environmental exposures, is a major challenge and likely contributes to null findings for many studies [142]. Exposure measurement error is common in research focusing on exposures at the participants' residences, as this is not the only location one spends time. Collecting personal exposure data via backpack monitors is not feasible on a large epidemiologic scale, but can aid in validation of air pollutant exposure models [113, 143]. Advances in tracking systems via Global Positioning System (GPS) and smartphone technologies may be an avenue for future research to validate exposure models and to better classify participants' dynamic movement across space and time [61]. It is also essential to update measures of air pollutants over follow-up in prospective cohort studies because air pollution changes over time [144]. Air pollutant exposure modeling is preferable to information from the monitor closest to each participant, especially in rural or suburban areas with less regulatory monitoring locations, as exposure modeling has been shown to be more strongly correlated with personal exposure measures [143].

In addition to exposure measurement error, there are additional considerations when it comes to the environmental exposure variation and definition. It is vital that there is sufficient exposure variability to be able to detect associations, which can be addressed with cohorts of participants residing across broad geographic areas. It is also important to consider that ambient particulate matter composition is heterogeneous across geography [145]. For example, the composition of particulate matter varies across the US with major differences in composition between the Eastern US and Western US [145]. These differences in composition may explain why the health effects of PM exposure has been more pronounced within certain geographic regions [146] and may explain some of the heterogeneity across studies from various geographic areas.

Given that $PM_{2.5}$ has been associated with breast cancer specific survival and there are subgroup findings for certain air pollutants and breast cancer incidence, understanding the biology underlying this association is vital. With the technological advances in –omics research, especially in tissue samples, future breast cancer epidemiologic research can integrate environmental and molecular epidemiology to study biological pathways in the breast perturbed by environmental exposures utilizing breast tissue gene expression data via transcriptomic platforms and tissue epigenomics [140, 141]. Furthermore, establishing the connection between ubiquitous air pollution exposures and breast biology in humans and with animal models is warranted.

9.4   Outdoor Light at Night and Breast Cancer

9.4.1   Rationale and Mechanisms

Since the expansion of electricity in the early 1900s, electric lighting provides a means for modern society to function. We now can work, eat, and be active at all times of the day and the night. While this ubiquitous lighting has a clear benefit to productivity and quality of life in many ways, exposure to light at night (LAN) may disrupt sleep, alter biological sequences maintained by endogenous circadian clocks, and influence diet and physical activity patterns; LAN has also been shown to be inversely correlated with natural vegetation [147]. Ultimately, these factors may have downstream consequences on breast cancer risk [148]. With a specific focus on ambient or outdoor LAN, this section examines mechanisms through which outdoor LAN may affect breast cancer risk, the evidence supporting associations between outdoor LAN and breast cancer risk, strengths and limitations of this research, and next steps to better understand whether outdoor LAN plays a role in driving breast cancer.

Exposure to LAN is thought to affect breast cancer risk because light exposure regulates the circadian system and suppresses the production of melatonin in the pineal gland [149–151]. The suprachiasmatic nucleus in the hypothalamus serves as a circadian pacemaker and is a core physiologic determinant of alertness and performance with an intrinsic period averaging 24 h [152]. Light is the primary stimulus for the circadian pacemaker, and there are multiple pathways linking circadian disruption to cancer risk. Circadian disruption may drive cancer through after-effects of melatonin suppression, altered sleep-wake patterns, cell cycle impairment, and altered clock gene function [153, 154]. Circadian disruption and altered sleep patterns may alter diets, increase energy imbalance, and lead to obesity [155], which may have downstream consequences for cancer. The melatonin pathway to cancer risk has also received substantial attention. Mechanistically, light falling onto specific retinal ganglion cells at night triggers the pineal gland to stop the release of melatonin [156]. Animal and epidemiologic studies suggest that exposure to LAN can modulate pineal gland function to decrease melatonin secretion [157, 158]. Experimental evidence shows that melatonin inhibits the growth of established tumors [159, 160], and melatonin may prevent cancer initiation due to anti-proliferative and anti-oxidant capacities, properties to enhance immune surveillance, and ability to modulate cellular and humoral responses and epigenetic alterations [161]. More specifically, decreased melatonin may drive breast cancer risk by increasing reproductive hormone levels, including estradiol, which could increase the proliferation of hormone sensitive cells in the breast [162]. Melatonin may also interact with nuclear receptors to directly affect hormone-dependent proliferation [163], or may increase the expression of the tumor suppressor gene p53 [164].

With these mechanisms in mind, epidemiologic literature has drawn fairly consistent associations between night shift work and invasive breast cancer [165, 166], so much so that shift work is currently classified as a 2A "probable human carcinogen" by the IARC [167]. The proposed mechanism through which shift work influences breast cancer risk is through increased exposure to LAN [165].

More recently, studies have demonstrated associations between outdoor LAN and breast cancer risk. Outdoor LAN is thought of as a surrogate for greater total evening and nighttime circadian-effective light exposure, as individuals living in communities with higher outdoor LAN likely drive on roads that are lit by street lighting, experience higher levels of light exposure during evening outdoor activities, and may have more outdoor light intrusion into their bedroom in the evening [168].

9.4.2 Epidemiologic Evidence

Epidemiologic studies have assessed links between outdoor LAN and breast cancer in ecological analyses [169–176], three case-control studies [177–179], and two prospective cohorts: one in California [180] and one nationwide across the US [181].

9.4.2.1 Ecological Studies

The following ecologic studies observed intriguing results between outdoor LAN and breast cancer rates, but should be interpreted cautiously due to confounding and ecologic fallacy that are inherent in most ecologic studies. Kloog et al. merged nighttime satellite images of LAN with cancer rate data from 147 localities in Israel [172]. They found that higher levels of satellite-based estimates of LAN were associated with higher breast cancer rates after adjustment for per capita income, minority ethnic composition, population density, and birth rate. In a later global analysis, the same research group observed that country-level LAN was associated with higher incidence rates of breast cancer [173]. Similar ecological studies showed positive associations between LAN and breast cancer in Korea [171], in Israel [170], in the US [174], and globally [169, 175]. A recent ecological study in Israel specifically utilized satellite data on short wavelength, or "blue" light, which is thought to have the greatest effect on melatonin suppression [176]. Consistent with this theory, blue light held a strong positive association with breast cancer incidence.

9.4.2.2 Case-Control Studies

An early case-control study examined data from the Georgia Comprehensive Cancer Registry comparing exposure to light at night for 34,053 breast cancer cases to 14,458 lung cancer controls [177]. The authors estimated that those living in high LAN exposure areas had higher odds of being a breast cancer case (OR = 1.12, 95% CI 1.04, 1.20). In analyses stratified by race, this elevated odds ratio was only observed among white participants. In an Israeli case-control study, 93 breast cancer cases were enrolled from cancer centers and matched with 185 controls recruited from friends of breast cancer patients [178]. Cases and controls were matched by age and residential area and were asked about exposure to outdoor lighting in the sleeping habitat, as well as living near strong LAN sources on questionnaires. Women who lived near strong LAN sources had higher odds of breast cancer (OR = 1.52, 95% CI 1.10, 2.12), but no elevated odds were observed for light penetrating into the bedroom. A recent case-control study in Spain examined the impact of specific spectral bands in LAN independently, including the blue spectral band that is thought to be most influential for melatonin suppression [179]. In addition to satellite-based measures, the authors also asked participants to report levels of light in the bedroom during sleeping time. In this multi-center case-control study, including 1219 breast cancer cases recruited from 23 hospitals across Spain and 1385 hospital catchment area controls, there was no difference in the odds of breast cancer for those reporting more light in the bedroom, nor for satellite-based outdoor LAN. However, when considering the blue light spectrum of outdoor LAN specifically, there was a 47% higher odds of breast cancer in the highest tertile of blue light exposure compared to the lowest tertile (OR = 1.47, 95%CI 1.00, 2.17) [179].

9.4.2.3   Prospective Studies

Two prospective cohorts have explored the relationship between outdoor LAN exposure and incident breast cancer risk. Using data from 106,731 women in the California Teachers Study, Hurley et al. linked LAN exposure data throughout follow-up to each participant's baseline (1995–1996) address [180]. The authors also asked participants to indicate the use of bright lights within the bedroom on questionnaires. Over 5000 breast cancer cases occurred over follow-up (1995–2011), demonstrating a modest association between outdoor LAN exposure and breast cancer risk (HR = 1.12, 95% CI 1.00, 1.26 for highest quintile of light exposure compared to lowest). In stratified analyses, positive associations between LAN and breast cancer were confined to women who were premenopausal at baseline, and this association among premenopausal women was only observed in women with BMI <25 kg/m². Positive associations were observed when stratifying by urban or suburban areas, as well as among different levels of neighborhood socioeconomic status. No increased breast cancer risk was observed among those who reported higher light use in the bedroom. Another prospective analysis utilized data from the nationwide Nurses' Health Study II to examine outdoor LAN and breast cancer incidence [181]. For this analysis, the authors linked outdoor LAN to each participant's residential address history throughout follow-up. Over two million person-years of follow-up, 3549 cases of breast cancer occurred, and an interquartile range increase in LAN was associated with a 5% increase in breast cancer risk (HR = 1.05, 95% CI 1.00, 1.11). In stratified analyses, elevated associations were observed only in those who were premenopausal at baseline, as well as those who were past or current smokers. Because all participants were nurses at baseline, the authors also conducted analyses stratified by night shift work status and found that findings were stronger among women who worked night shifts compared to those who had never worked night shifts.

9.4.2.4   Effect Modification

In the studies reviewed above, there were a number of analyses showing that associations between outdoor LAN and breast cancer might be modified by race, BMI, menopausal status, smoking, shift work, and urbanicity [174, 177, 180, 182]. It is not completely clear why these factors might serve as effect modifiers, but they warrant further investigation. For instance, night shift work has been consistently associated with breast cancer within the Nurses' Health Study cohorts, and it has been proposed that this association may be mediated by circadian disruption [165, 183]. Because both outdoor LAN exposure and night shift work are thought to drive circadian disruption, there may be a synergistic relationship between these two factors that combine to increase breast cancer risk above each factor individually.

9.4.3   Summary: Strengths, Limitations, and Future Directions

As described above, there is an emerging body of literature that reveals fairly consistent associations between outdoor LAN and breast cancer. However, the majority of these studies are ecological, and few prospective analyses have been conducted. This places a strong limitation on any statements about causality. In the future, more prospective analyses would make a stronger case for a causal relationship between LAN and breast cancer. In addition, there are a number of shortcomings to the literature on this topic. First, and perhaps foremost, is that exposure assessment for LAN contains a great deal of error. The majority of reviewed studies used satellite images of outdoor LAN to assess exposure, yet it is unclear how well outdoor LAN captures personal LAN exposure. A recent study by Rea et al. demonstrated that satellite images of LAN held very low to no correlations with personal-level measures of exposure, assessed through sensors worn at the eye level [184], due to a person's indoor environments that diminish exposure to outside light (e.g. blinds and curtains). In addition, to accurately capture chronic exposure to LAN, these personal level measures of exposure would be required for long time periods. While time-activity data (e.g., GPS) will assist with knowing the location where a person is located at a given time; sensors to detect the personal exposure to LAN in the indoor environment would still be needed to address measurement error. As with other breast cancer studies of environmental exposures, the LAN studies mentioned here have focused on adult-life exposure to LAN; future studies could also assess early-life exposure to LAN with detailed residential histories during the time when satellite LAN information is available. Future studies should also assess potential mediators of the LAN and breast cancer relationship. For instance, measures of sleep patterns, for instance through accelerometry, might confirm the specific behavioral pathway through which LAN might affect circadian patterns. In addition, temporally-matched melatonin measures would explain how exposure to LAN might affect circadian patterns and breast cancer risk together. But, again it is costly and burdensome to obtain these measures over long time periods. Future analyses should also include information on noise and other spatial factors that can be correlated with LAN and may also explain circadian disruption. As shown in a recent case-control study in Spain [178], more studies should gather information on specific wavelengths of light that might be most active in driving melatonin suppression and circadian disruption.

The literature on outdoor LAN and breast cancer risk is nascent, and the extant studies have limitations, including few prospective analyses, major exposure misclassification, and little exploration of potential mechanisms through which LAN might affect breast cancer risk. In addition, some studies have demonstrated effect modification by race, socioeconomic status, smoking, night shift work, urbanicity, and menopausal status; however, there is currently little understanding as to why LAN might have differential effects across these factors. There is a pressing need for future prospective studies with improved exposure assessment, mediation analyses, and further exploration of mechanisms for effect modification before exposure to outdoor LAN can be classified as a risk factor for breast cancer.

9.5   Overall Conclusions

As an emerging area for breast cancer research, environmental exposures may influence breast cancer development directly and via important energetic factors related to breast cancer risk and survival. These geospatial exposures discussed above play unique roles in the context of energetics of breast cancer development and breast cancer survival. Natural vegetation exposure may influence energy balance by impacting physical activity levels, as well as social engagement and mental health that also may further influence physical activity patterns. Identifying environmental factors to promote physical activity and identifying their barriers is warranted to reduce breast cancer risk and to improve breast cancer survival as physical inactivity is one of few well-established modifiable risk and survival factors and a majority of people in the US do not meet recommended levels of physical activity. One must also consider that outdoor air quality is a ubiquitous ambient exposure, and when performing physical activity outdoors, higher doses of air pollution may be inhaled that might counteract some of the benefits from physical activity. Outdoor light at night exposure may disrupt energy balance by disturbing sleep patterns and circadian rhythms and by influencing diet and physical activity patterns. Optimizing the quality of geospatial environments, such as the novel factors covered in this chapter (natural vegetation, air quality, and outdoor light at night), could inform population-level interventions for breast cancer prevention and survival, given their known or hypothesized roles in energy balance, most notably via physical activity and circadian patterns.

Future epidemiologic studies of geospatial exposures and breast cancer outcomes should focus attention on several features. Improving exposure measurement is a key feature of most environmental epidemiology studies. Global positioning systems (GPS) in concert with accelerometry may aid in classifying movement across space and time to improve upon environmental exposure classification, though it remains uncertain if this is a reliable tool for long-term exposure measurements and indoor exposure to outdoor environmental exposures. Leveraging more recent technologies—such as wearable air pollution sensors [185], smartphone applications that can measure personal exposure to LAN and Google Street View images that have been utilized to capture vegetation on city streets at eye-level [56, 186–188]—may also assist in specifying features of environmental exposures that may better capture measure a person's environment (e.g. types of vegetation, real-time localized air pollution predictions). In addition to exposure measurement improvements, breast cancer research should address environmental exposures across the life course, particularly during early-life when the breast is most vulnerable to exogenous exposures. Epidemiologic studies should gather detailed residential history information and if possible, enroll younger women to allow determination of exposures during adolescence and early adulthood as early-life exposure to modifiable and environmental exposures when the breast is developing is when the breast is most vulnerable to carcinogenesis [1, 135, 189]. In addition, utilizing intermediate markers of breast cancer risk (e.g., mammographic density or benign breast disease) may offer more immediate insight in to whether environmental exposures are related to variation in breast tissue composition. Moreover, geospatial determinants of breast cancer survival outcomes, such as breast cancer mortality, mental health, and quality of life, is an area of research that should be further considered across the continuum of breast health.

References

1. Colditz GA. Epidemiology and prevention of breast cancer. Cancer Epidemiol Biomark Prev Publ Am Assoc Cancer Res Cosponsored Am Soc Prev Oncol. 2005;14(4):768–72.
2. Buell P. Changing incidence of breast cancer in Japanese-American women. J Natl Cancer Inst. 1973;51(5):1479–83.
3. Kolonel LN. Cancer patterns of four ethnic groups in Hawaii. J Natl Cancer Inst. 1980;65(5):1127–39.
4. Reynolds P, Hurley S, Goldberg DE, Anton-Culver H, Bernstein L, Deapen D, et al. Regional variations in breast cancer among California teachers. Epidemiol. 2004;15(6):746–54.
5. Vieira V, Webster T, Weinberg J, Aschengrau A, Ozonoff D. Spatial analysis of lung, colorectal, and breast cancer on Cape Cod: an application of generalized additive models to case-control data. Environ Health Glob Access Sci Source. 2005;4:11.
6. Laden F, Spiegelman D, Neas LM, Colditz GA, Hankinson SE, Manson JE, et al. Geographic variation in breast cancer incidence rates in a cohort of U.S. women. J Natl Cancer Inst. 1997;89(18):1373–8.
7. Tamimi RM, Spiegelman D, Smith-Warner SA, Wang M, Pazaris M, Willett WC, et al. Population attributable risk of modifiable and non modifiable breast cancer risk factors in postmenopausal breast cancer. Am J Epidemiol. 2016;184(12):884–93.
8. Krieger N. Epidemiology and the web of causation: has anyone seen the spider? Soc Sci Med. 1994;39(7):887–903.
9. Breast Cancer and the Environment: Prioritizing Prevention. Report of the Interagency Breast Cancer and Environmental Research Coordinating Committee (IBCERCC). February 2013.
10. Institute of Medicine. Breast cancer and the environment: a life course approach [Internet]. Washington, DC: The National Academies Press; 2012.. Available from: https://www.nap.edu/catalog/13263/breast-cancer-and-the-environment-a-life-course-approach
11. American Cancer Society. Breast cancer facts & figures 2015–2016. Atlanta: American Cancer Society, Inc; 2015.
12. Lynch SM, Rebbeck TR. Bridging the gap between biologic, individual, and macroenvironmental factors in cancer: a multilevel approach. Cancer Epidemiol Biomark Prev Publ Am Assoc Cancer Res Cosponsored Am Soc Prev Oncol. 2013;22(4):485–95.
13. Krieger N. History, biology, and health inequities: emergent embodied phenotypes and the illustrative case of the breast cancer estrogen receptor. Am J Public Health. 2013;103(1):22–7.
14. Krieger N, Jahn JL, Waterman PD, Chen JT. Breast cancer estrogen receptor status according to biological generation: US black and white women born 1915–1979. Am J Epidemiol. 2018;187(5):960–70.
15. Fong KC, Hart JE, James P. A review of epidemiologic studies on greenness and health: updated literature through 2017. Curr Environ Health Rep. 2018;5(1):77–87.
16. James P, Banay RF, Hart JE, Laden F. A review of the health benefits of greenness. Curr Epidemiol Rep. 2015;2(2):131–42.
17. Kondo MC, Fluehr JM, McKeon T, Branas CC. Urban green space and its impact on human health. Int J Environ Res Public Health. 2018;15(3):445.
18. James P, Hart JE, Banay RF, Laden F. Exposure to greenness and mortality in a nationwide prospective cohort study of women. Environ Health Perspect. 2016;124(9):1344–52.

19. Markevych I, Schoierer J, Hartig T, Chudnovsky A, Hystad P, Dzhambov AM, et al. Exploring pathways linking greenspace to health: theoretical and methodological guidance. Environ Res. 2017;158:301–17.
20. Frumkin H, Bratman GN, Breslow SJ, Cochran B, Kahn PH, Lawler JJ, et al. Nature contact and human health: a research agenda. Environ Health Perspect. 2017;125(7):075001.
21. Giovannucci E. An integrative approach for deciphering the causal associations of physical activity and cancer risk: the role of adiposity. J Natl Cancer Inst. 2018;110(9):935–41.
22. Zhong S, Jiang T, Ma T, Zhang X, Tang J, Chen W, et al. Association between physical activity and mortality in breast cancer: a meta-analysis of cohort studies. Eur J Epidemiol. 2014;29(6):391–404.
23. Dean LT, Gehlert S, Neuhouser ML, Oh A, Zanetti K, Goodman M, et al. Social factors matter in cancer risk and survivorship. Cancer Causes Control. 2018;29(7):611–8.
24. Mason C, Alfano CM, Smith AW, Wang C-Y, Neuhouser ML, Duggan C, et al. Long-term physical activity trends in breast cancer survivors. Cancer Epidemiol Biomark Prev Publ Am Assoc Cancer Res Cosponsored Am Soc Prev Oncol. 2013 Jun;22(6):1153–61.
25. Villeneuve PJ, Jerrett M, Su JG, Weichenthal S, Sandler DP. Association of residential greenness with obesity and physical activity in a US cohort of women. Environ Res. 2018;160:372–84.
26. Shariff-Marco S, Von Behren J, Reynolds P, Keegan THM, Hertz A, Kwan ML, et al. Impact of social and built environment factors on body size among breast cancer survivors: the pathways study. Cancer Epidemiol Biomark Prev Publ Am Assoc Cancer Res Cosponsored Am Soc Prev Oncol. 2017;26(4):505–15.
27. Iqbal J, Ginsburg O, Rochon PA, Sun P, Narod SA. Differences in breast cancer stage at diagnosis and cancer-specific survival by race and ethnicity in the United States. JAMA. 2015;313(2):165–73.
28. Kohler BA, Sherman RL, Howlader N, Jemal A, Ryerson AB, Henry KA, et al. Annual report to the nation on the status of cancer, 1975–2011, Featuring incidence of breast cancer subtypes by race/ethnicity, poverty, and state. J Natl Cancer Inst. 2015;107(6):djv048.
29. Coughlin SS, Yoo W, Whitehead MS, Smith SA. Advancing breast cancer survivorship among African-American women. Breast Cancer Res Treat. 2015;153(2):253–61.
30. Hermes GL, Delgado B, Tretiakova M, Cavigelli SA, Krausz T, Conzen SD, et al. Social isolation dysregulates endocrine and behavioral stress while increasing malignant burden of spontaneous mammary tumors. Proc Natl Acad Sci USA. 2009;106(52):22393–8.
31. Lagerlund M, Sontrop JM, Zackrisson S. Psychosocial factors and attendance at a population-based mammography screening program in a cohort of Swedish women. BMC Womens Health. 2014;14(1):33.
32. Dean L, Subramanian SV, Williams DR, Armstrong K, Charles CZ, Kawachi I. The role of social capital in African-American women's use of mammography. Soc Sci Med. 2014;104:148–56.
33. Busch EL, Whitsel EA, Kroenke CH, Yang YC. Social relationships, inflammation markers, and breast cancer incidence in the Women's Health Initiative. Breast Edinb Scotl. 2018;39:63–9.
34. Kroenke CH, Michael YL, Poole EM, Kwan ML, Nechuta S, Leas E, et al. Postdiagnosis social networks and breast cancer mortality in the after breast cancer pooling project. Cancer. 2017;123(7):1228–37.
35. Hinzey A, Gaudier-Diaz MM, Lustberg MB, DeVries AC. Breast cancer and social environment: getting by with a little help from our friends. Breast Cancer Res. 2016;18(1):54.
36. Beasley JM, Newcomb PA, Trentham-Dietz A, Hampton JM, Ceballos RM, Titus-Ernstoff L, et al. Social networks and survival after breast cancer diagnosis. J Cancer Surviv Res Pract. 2010;4(4):372–80.
37. Kroenke CH, Michael YL, Shu X-O, Poole EM, Kwan ML, Nechuta S, et al. Post-diagnosis social networks, and lifestyle and treatment factors in the after breast cancer pooling project. Psychooncology. 2017;26(4):544–52.

38. Kroenke CH, Kubzansky LD, Schernhammer ES, Holmes MD, Kawachi I. Social networks, social support, and survival after breast cancer diagnosis. J Clin Oncol Off J Am Soc Clin Oncol. 2006;24(7):1105–11.
39. Syrowatka A, Motulsky A, Kurteva S, Hanley JA, Dixon WG, Meguerditchian AN, et al. Predictors of distress in female breast cancer survivors: a systematic review. Breast Cancer Res Treat. 2017;165(2):229–45.
40. Kroenke CH, Kwan ML, Neugut AI, Ergas IJ, Wright JD, Caan BJ, et al. Social networks, social support mechanisms, and quality of life after breast cancer diagnosis. Breast Cancer Res Treat. 2013;139(2):515–27.
41. Kroenke CH, Michael Y, Tindle H, Gage E, Chlebowski R, Garcia L, et al. Social networks, social support and burden in relationships, and mortality after breast cancer diagnosis. Breast Cancer Res Treat. 2012;133(1):375–85.
42. Fang F, Fall K, Mittleman MA, Sparén P, Ye W, Adami H-O, et al. Suicide and cardiovascular death after a cancer diagnosis. N Engl J Med. 2012;366(14):1310–8.
43. Jim HSL, Phillips KM, Chait S, Faul LA, Popa MA, Lee Y-H, et al. Meta-analysis of cognitive functioning in breast cancer survivors previously treated with standard-dose chemotherapy. J Clin Oncol Off J Am Soc Clin Oncol. 2012;30(29):3578–87.
44. Berman MG, Jonides J, Kaplan S. The cognitive benefits of interacting with nature. Psychol Sci. 2008;19(12):1207–12.
45. Gascon M, Triguero-Mas M, Martínez D, Dadvand P, Rojas-Rueda D, Plasència A, et al. Residential green spaces and mortality: a systematic review. Environ Int. 2016;86:60–7.
46. Bezold CP, Banay RF, Coull BA, Hart JE, James P, Kubzansky LD, et al. The association between natural environments and depressive symptoms in adolescents living in the United States. J Adolesc Health Off Publ Soc Adolesc Med. 2018;62(4):488–95.
47. Bezold CP, Banay RF, Coull BA, Hart JE, James P, Kubzansky LD, et al. The relationship between surrounding greenness in childhood and adolescence and depressive symptoms in adolescence and early adulthood. Ann Epidemiol. 2018;28(4):213–9.
48. Hartig T, Mitchell R, de Vries S, Frumkin H. Nature and health. Annu Rev Public Health. 2014;35:207–28.
49. Pope CA, Dockery DW. Health effects of fine particulate air pollution: lines that connect. J Air Waste Manag Assoc. 2006;56(6):709–42.
50. James P, Kioumourtzoglou M-A, Hart JE, Banay RF, Kloog I, Laden F. Interrelationships between walkability, air pollution, greenness, and body mass index. Epidemiol. 2017;28(6):780–8.
51. James P. Greenness and breast cancer in a US-based nationwide prospective cohort study. Abstract Number: 562. International Society for Environmental Epidemiology Annual Meeting; 2017.
52. Datzmann T, Markevych I, Trautmann F, Heinrich J, Schmitt J, Tesch F. Outdoor air pollution, green space, and cancer incidence in Saxony: a semi-individual cohort study. BMC Public Health. 2018;18(1):715.
53. O'Callaghan-Gordo C, Kogevinas M, Cirach M, Castaño-Vinyals G, Aragonés N, Delfrade J, et al. Residential proximity to green spaces and breast cancer risk: the multicase-control study in Spain (MCC-Spain). Int J Hyg Environ Health. 2018;221(8):1097–106.
54. Mitchell R, Popham F. Effect of exposure to natural environment on health inequalities: an observational population study. Lancet. 2008;372(9650):1655–60.
55. O'Callaghan Gordo C. Natural outdoors environments and prostate and breast cancer risk: a case-control in Spain. Abstract Number: O-219. International Society for Environmental Epidemiology Annual Meeting; 2016.
56. Larkin A, Hystad P. Evaluating street view exposure measures of visible green space for health research. J Expo Sci Environ Epidemiol. 2018;19
57. James P, Hart JE, Hipp JA, Mitchell JA, Kerr J, Hurvitz PM, et al. GPS-based exposure to greenness and walkability and accelerometry-based physical activity. Cancer Epidemiol Biomark Prev Publ Am Assoc Cancer Res Cosponsored Am Soc Prev Oncol. 2017;26(4):525–32.

58. Dons E, Laeremans M, Orjuela JP, Avila-Palencia I, Carrasco-Turigas G, Cole-Hunter T, et al. Wearable sensors for personal, monitoring and estimation of inhaled traffic-related air pollution: evaluation of methods. Environ Sci Technol. 2017;51(3):1859–67.
59. Chaney RA, Sloan CD, Cooper VC, Robinson DR, Hendrickson NR, McCord TA, et al. Personal exposure to fine particulate air pollution while commuting: an examination of six transport modes on an urban arterial roadway. PloS One. 2017;12(11):e0188053.
60. Zuurbier M, Hoek G, Oldenwening M, Lenters V, Meliefste K, van den Hazel P, et al. Commuters' exposure to particulate matter air pollution is affected by mode of transport, fuel type, and route. Environ Health Perspect. 2010;118(6):783–9.
61. Dewulf B, Neutens T, Van Dyck D, de Bourdeaudhuij I, Int Panis L, Beckx C, et al. Dynamic assessment of inhaled air pollution using GPS and accelerometer data. J Transp Health. 2016;3(1):114–23.
62. Environmental toxins and breast cancer on Long Island. I. Polycyclic aromatic hydrocarbon DNA adducts. Outdoor air pollution. IARC Monogr Eval Carcinog Risk Hum 109: 431–444. [Internet]. Lyon: WHO International Agency for Research on Cancer (IARC); 2015 Dec. Report No.: IARC Monographs on the Evaluation of Carcinogenic Risks to Humans. Volume 109. [Internet]. Available from: http://monographs.iarc.fr/ENG/Monographs/vol109/mono109.pdf
63. National Center for Environmental Assessment. Air quality criteria for particulate matter (Volumes I and II). Research Triangle Park: US Environmental Protection Agency; 2004.
64. Brook RD, Franklin B, Cascio W, Hong Y, Howard G, Lipsett M, et al. Air pollution and cardiovascular disease: a statement for healthcare professionals from the expert panel on population and prevention science of the American heart association. Circulation. 2004;109(21):2655–71.
65. Brook RD, Urch B, Dvonch JT, Bard RL, Speck M, Keeler G, et al. Insights into the mechanisms and mediators of the effects of air pollution exposure on blood pressure and vascular function in healthy humans. Hypertension. 2009;54(3):659–67.
66. Guo L, Byun H-M, Zhong J, Motta V, Barupal J, Zheng Y, et al. Effects of short-term exposure to inhalable particulate matter on DNA methylation of tandem repeats. Environ Mol Mutagen. 2014;55(4):322–35.
67. Panni T, Mehta AJ, Schwartz JD, Baccarelli AA, Just AC, Wolf K, et al. A genome-wide analysis of DNA methylation and fine particulate matter air pollution in three study populations: KORA F3, KORA F4, and the normative aging study. Environ Health Perspect. 2016;5
68. Lodovici M, Bigagli E. Oxidative stress and air pollution exposure. J Toxicol. 2011;2011:487074.
69. Rajagopalan S, Al-Kindi SG, Brook RD. Air pollution and cardiovascular disease: JACC state-of-the-art review. J Am Coll Cardiol. 2018;72(17):2054–70.
70. Coussens LM, Werb Z. Inflammation and cancer. Nature. 2002;420(6917):860–7.
71. De Nardo DG, Coussens LM. Inflammation and breast cancer. Balancing immune response: crosstalk between adaptive and innate immune cells during breast cancer progression. Breast Cancer Res. 2007;9(4):212.
72. Baumgarten SC, Frasor J. Minireview: inflammation: an instigator of more aggressive Estrogen Receptor (ER) positive breast cancers. Mol Endocrinol. 2012;26(3):360–71.
73. Crusz SM, Balkwill FR. Inflammation and cancer: advances and new agents. Nat Rev Clin Oncol. 2015;12(10):584–96.
74. Villaseñor A, Flatt SW, Marinac C, Natarajan L, Pierce JP, Patterson RE. Postdiagnosis C-reactive protein and breast cancer survivorship: findings from the WHEL study. Cancer Epidemiol Biomark Prev Publ Am Assoc Cancer Res Cosponsored Am Soc Prev Oncol. 2014;23(1):189–99.
75. Nelson SH, Brasky TM, Patterson RE, Laughlin GA, Kritz-Silverstein D, Edwards BJ, et al. The association of the C-reactive protein inflammatory biomarker with breast cancer incidence and mortality in the women's health initiative. Cancer Epidemiol Biomark Prev Publ Am Assoc Cancer Res Cosponsored Am Soc Prev Oncol. 2017;26(7):1100–6.

76. Allin KH, Nordestgaard BG, Flyger H, Bojesen SE. Elevated pre-treatment levels of plasma C-reactive protein are associated with poor prognosis after breast cancer: a cohort study. Breast Cancer Res. 2011;13(3):R55.
77. Pierce BL, Ballard-Barbash R, Bernstein L, Baumgartner RN, Neuhouser ML, Wener MH, et al. Elevated biomarkers of inflammation are associated with reduced survival among breast cancer patients. J Clin Oncol Off J Am Soc Clin Oncol. 2009;27(21):3437–44.
78. Wulaningsih W, Holmberg L, Garmo H, Malmstrom H, Lambe M, Hammar N, et al. Prediagnostic serum inflammatory markers in relation to breast cancer risk, severity at diagnosis and survival in breast cancer patients. Carcinogenesis. 2015;36(10):1121–8.
79. Chen WY, Holmes MD. Role of aspirin in breast cancer survival. Curr Oncol Rep. 2017;19(7):48.
80. Zheng J, Tabung FK, Zhang J, Liese AD, Shivappa N, Ockene JK, et al. Association between post-cancer diagnosis dietary inflammatory potential and mortality among invasive breast cancer survivors in the women's health initiative. Cancer Epidemiol Biomark Prev Publ Am Assoc Cancer Res Cosponsored Am Soc Prev Oncol. 2018;27(4):454–63.
81. Fowler ME, Akinyemiju TF. Meta-analysis of the association between dietary inflammatory index (DII) and cancer outcomes. Int J Cancer. 2017;141(11):2215–27.
82. Tabung FK, Steck SE, Liese AD, Zhang J, Ma Y, Caan B, et al. Association between dietary inflammatory potential and breast cancer incidence and death: results from the women's health initiative. Br J Cancer. 2016;114(11):1277–85.
83. Lee K-H, Shu X-O, Gao Y-T, Ji B-T, Yang G, Blair A, et al. Breast cancer and urinary bio-markers of polycyclic aromatic hydrocarbon and oxidative stress in the Shanghai women's health study. Cancer Epidemiol Biomark Prev Publ Am Assoc Cancer Res Cosponsored Am Soc Prev Oncol. 2010;19(3):877–83.
84. Fortner RT, Tworoger SS, Wu T, Eliassen AH. Plasma florescent oxidation products and breast cancer risk: repeated measures in the Nurses' health study. Breast Cancer Res Treat. 2013;141(2):307–16.
85. Sisti JS, Lindström S, Kraft P, Tamimi RM, Rosner BA, Wu T, et al. Premenopausal plasma carotenoids, fluorescent oxidation products, and subsequent breast cancer risk in the nurses' health studies. Breast Cancer Res Treat. 2015;151(2):415–25.
86. Nichols HB, Anderson C, White AJ, Milne GL, Sandler DP. Oxidative stress and breast cancer risk in premenopausal women. Epidemiol. 2017;28(5):667–74.
87. Lee JD, Cai Q, Shu XO, Nechuta SJ. The role of biomarkers of oxidative stress in breast cancer risk and prognosis: a systematic review of the epidemiologic literature. J Women's Health. 2017;26(5):467–82.
88. Tobias DK, Akinkuolie AO, Chandler PD, Lawler PR, Manson JE, Buring JE, et al. Markers of inflammation and incident breast cancer risk in the women's health study. Am J Epidemiol. 2018;187(4):705–16.
89. Agnoli C, Grioni S, Pala V, Allione A, Matullo G, Gaetano CD, et al. Biomarkers of inflammation and breast cancer risk: a case-control study nested in the EPIC-Varese cohort. Sci Rep. 2017;7(1):12708.
90. De Coster S, van Larebeke N. Endocrine-disrupting chemicals: associated disorders and mechanisms of action. J Environ Public Health. 2012;2012:713696.
91. Hamra GB, Laden F, Cohen AJ, Raaschou-Nielsen O, Brauer M, Loomis D. Lung cancer and exposure to nitrogen dioxide and traffic: a systematic review and meta-analysis. Environ Health Perspect. 2015;123(11):1107–12.
92. IARC Working Group on the Evaluation of Carcinogenic Risks to Humans, International Agency for Research on Cancer, editors. Some non-heterocyclic polycyclic aromatic hydro-carbons and some related occupational exposures. Lyon: Geneva: IARC Press; Distributed by World Health Organization; 2010. 853 p. (IARC monographs on the evaluation of carci-nogenic risks to humans).
93. Santodonato J. Review of the estrogenic and antiestrogenic activity of polycyclic aromatic hydrocarbons: relationship to carcinogenicity. Chemosphere. 1997;34(4):835–48.

94. Sievers CK, Shanle EK, Bradfield CA, Xu W. Differential action of monohydroxylated polycyclic aromatic hydrocarbons with estrogen receptors α and β. Toxicol Sci Off J Soc Toxicol. 2013;132(2):359–67.

95. Carré J, Gatimel N, Moreau J, Parinaud J, Léandri R. Does air pollution play a role in infertility?: a systematic review. Environ Health Glob Access Sci Source. 2017;16(1):82.

96. Murray IA, Patterson AD, Perdew GH. Aryl hydrocarbon receptor ligands in cancer: friend and foe. Nat Rev Cancer. 2014;14(12):801–14.

97. Li Z-D, Wang K, Yang X-W, Zhuang Z-G, Wang J-J, Tong X-W. Expression of aryl hydrocarbon receptor in relation to p53 status and clinicopathological parameters in breast cancer. Int J Clin Exp Pathol. 2014;7(11):7931–7.

98. Reding KW, Young MT, Szpiro AA, Han CJ, DeRoo LA, Weinberg C, et al. Breast cancer risk in relation to ambient air pollution exposure at residences in the sister study cohort. Cancer Epidemiol Biomark Prev Publ Am Assoc Cancer Res Cosponsored Am Soc Prev Oncol. 2015;24(12):1907–9.

99. Hart JE, Bertrand KA, DuPre N, James P, Vieira VM, Tamimi RM, et al. Long-term particulate matter exposures during adulthood and risk of breast cancer incidence in the nurses' health study II prospective cohort. Cancer Epidemiol Biomark Prev Publ Am Assoc Cancer Res Cosponsored Am Soc Prev Oncol. 2016;25(8):1274–6.

100. Andersen ZJ, Ravnskjær L, Andersen KK, Loft S, Brandt J, Becker T, et al. Long-term exposure to fine particulate matter and breast cancer incidence in the Danish nurse cohort study. Cancer Epidemiol Biomark Prev Publ Am Assoc Cancer Res Cosponsored Am Soc Prev Oncol. 2017;26(3):428–30.

101. Andersen ZJ, Stafoggia M, Weinmayr G, Pedersen M, Galassi C, Jørgensen JT, et al. Long-term exposure to ambient air pollution and incidence of postmenopausal breast cancer in 15 European cohorts within the ESCAPE project. Environ Health Perspect. 2017;125(10):107005.

102. Yanosky JD, Paciorek CJ, Laden F, Hart JE, Puett RC, Liao D, et al. Spatio-temporal modeling of particulate air pollution in the conterminous United States using geographic and meteorological predictors. Environ Health Glob Access Sci Source. 2014;13:63.

103. McCormack VA, dos Santos Silva I. Breast density and parenchymal patterns as markers of breast cancer risk: a meta-analysis. Cancer Epidemiol Biomarker Prev. 2006;15(6):1159–69.

104. Yaghjyan L, Arao R, Brokamp C, O'Meara ES, Sprague BL, Ghita G, et al. Association between air pollution and mammographic breast density in the breast cancer surveilance consortium. Breast Cancer Res. 2017;19(1):36.

105. DuPre NC, Hart JE, Bertrand KA, Kraft P, Laden F, Tamimi RM. Residential particulate matter and distance to roadways in relation to mammographic density: results from the Nurses' health studies. Breast Cancer Res. 2017;19(1):124.

106. Emaus MJ, Bakker MF, Beelen RMJ, Veldhuis WB, Peeters PHM, van Gils CH. Degree of urbanization and mammographic density in Dutch breast cancer screening participants: results from the EPIC-NL cohort. Breast Cancer Res Treat. 2014;148(3):655–63.

107. Ferlay J, Soerjomataram I, Dikshit R, Eser S, Mathers C, Rebelo M, et al. Cancer incidence and mortality worldwide: sources, methods and major patterns in GLOBOCAN 2012. Int J Cancer. 2015;136(5):E359–86.

108. American Cancer Society. Cancer facts & figures 2017. Atlanta: American Cancer Society; 2017.

109. Bleyer A, Welch HG. Effect of three decades of screening mammography on breast-cancer incidence. N Engl J Med. 2012;367(21):1998–2005.

110. Hu H, Dailey AB, Kan H, Xu X. The effect of atmospheric particulate matter on survival of breast cancer among US females. Breast Cancer Res Treat. 2013;139(1):217–26.

111. Tagliabue G, Borgini A, Tittarelli A, van Donkelaar A, Martin RV, Bertoldi M, et al. Atmospheric fine particulate matter and breast cancer mortality: a population-based cohort study. BMJ Open. 2016;6(11):e012580.

112. DuPre N, Poole EM, Holmes MD, Hart JE, James P, Beck A, et al. Abstract 3278: particulate matter and traffic-related exposures in relation to breast cancer survival. Cancer Res. 2017;77(13 Supplement):3278.
113. Hart JE, Liao X, Hong B, Puett RC, Yanosky JD, Suh H, et al. The association of long-term exposure to PM2.5 on all-cause mortality in the Nurses' health study and the impact of measurement-error correction. Environ Health Glob Access Sci Source. 2015;14:38.
114. White AJ, Bradshaw PT, Hamra GB. Air pollution and breast cancer: a review. Curr Epidemiol Rep. 2018;5(2):92–100.
115. Goldberg MS, Labrèche F, Weichenthal S, Lavigne E, Valois M-F, Hatzopoulou M, et al. The association between the incidence of postmenopausal breast cancer and concentrations at street-level of nitrogen dioxide and ultrafine particles. Environ Res. 2017;158:7–15.
116. Crouse DL, Goldberg MS, Ross NA, Chen H, Labrèche F. Postmenopausal breast cancer is associated with exposure to traffic-related air pollution in Montreal, Canada: a case-control study. Environ Health Perspect. 2010;118(11):1578–83.
117. Hystad P, Villeneuve PJ, Goldberg MS, Crouse DL, Johnson K. Canadian cancer registries epidemiology research group. Exposure to traffic-related air pollution and the risk of developing breast cancer among women in eight Canadian provinces: a case-control study. Environ Int. 2015;74:240–8.
118. Raaschou-Nielsen O, Andersen ZJ, Hvidberg M, Jensen SS, Ketzel M, Sørensen M, et al. Air pollution from traffic and cancer incidence: a Danish cohort study. Environ Health Glob Access Sci Source. 2011;10:67.
119. Huynh S, von Euler-Chelpin M, Raaschou-Nielsen O, Hertel O, Tjønneland A, Lynge E, et al. Long-term exposure to air pollution and mammographic density in the Danish Diet, cancer and health cohort. Environ Health Glob Access Sci Source. 2015;14:31.
120. Shmuel S, White AJ, Sandler DP. Residential exposure to vehicular traffic-related air pollution during childhood and breast cancer risk. Environ Res. 2017;159:257–63.
121. Shen J, Liao Y, Hopper JL, Goldberg M, Santella RM, Terry MB. Dependence of cancer risk from environmental exposures on underlying genetic susceptibility: an illustration with polycyclic aromatic hydrocarbons and breast cancer. Br J Cancer. 2017;116(9):1229–33.
122. Agudo A, Peluso M, Munnia A, Luján-Barroso L, Barricarte A, Amiano P, et al. Aromatic DNA adducts and breast cancer risk: a case-cohort study within the EPIC-Spain. Carcinogenesis. 2017;38(7):691–8.
123. Gammon MD, Sagiv SK, Eng SM, Shantakumar S, Gaudet MM, Teitelbaum SL, et al. Polycyclic aromatic hydrocarbon-DNA adducts and breast cancer: a pooled analysis. Arch Environ Health. 2004;59(12):640–9.
124. Saieva C, Peluso M, Masala G, Munnia A, Ceroti M, Piro S, et al. Bulky DNA adducts and breast cancer risk in the prospective EPIC-Italy study. Breast Cancer Res Treat. 2011;129(2):477–84.
125. Niehoff N, White AJ, McCullough LE, Steck SE, Beyea J, Mordukhovich I, et al. Polycyclic aromatic hydrocarbons and postmenopausal breast cancer: an evaluation of effect measure modification by body mass index and weight change. Environ Res. 2017;152:17–25.
126. Gammon MD, Santella RM. PAH, genetic susceptibility and breast cancer risk: an update from the Long Island Breast Cancer Study Project. Eur J Cancer. 2008;44(5):636–40.
127. Crew KD, Gammon MD, Terry MB, Zhang FF, Zablotska LB, Agrawal M, et al. Polymorphisms in nucleotide excision repair genes, polycyclic aromatic hydrocarbon-DNA adducts, and breast cancer risk. Cancer Epidemiol Biomark Prev Publ Am Assoc Cancer Res Cosponsored Am Soc Prev Oncol. 2007;16(10):2033–41.
128. Shen J, Gammon MD, Terry MB, Teitelbaum SL, Eng SM, Neugut AI, et al. Xeroderma pigmentosum complementation group C genotypes/diplotypes play no independent or interaction role with polycyclic aromatic hydrocarbons-DNA adducts for breast cancer risk. Eur J Cancer. 2008;44(5):710–7.
129. White AJ, Bradshaw PT, Herring AH, Teitelbaum SL, Beyea J, Stellman SD, et al. Exposure to multiple sources of polycyclic aromatic hydrocarbons and breast cancer incidence. Environ Int. 2016;89–90:185–92.

130. Mordukhovich I, Beyea J, Herring AH, Hatch M, Stellman SD, Teitelbaum SL, et al. Vehicular traffic-related polycyclic aromatic hydrocarbon exposure and Breast Cancer incidence: the Long Island Breast Cancer Study Project (LIBCSP). Environ Health Perspect. 2016;124(1):30–8.

131. Mordukhovich I, Beyea J, Herring AH, Hatch M, Stellman SD, Teitelbaum SL, et al. Polymorphisms in DNA repair genes, traffic-related polycyclic aromatic hydrocarbon exposure and Breast Cancer incidence. Int J Cancer. 2016;139(2):310–21.

132. Garcia E, Hurley S, Nelson DO, Hertz A, Reynolds P. Hazardous air pollutants and breast cancer risk in California teachers: a cohort study. Environ Health Glob Access Sci Source. 2015;14:14.

133. Liu R, Nelson DO, Hurley S, Hertz A, Reynolds P. Residential exposure to estrogen disrupting hazardous air pollutants and breast cancer risk: the California Teachers Study. Epidemiol. 2015;26(3):365–73.

134. Hart JE, Bertrand KA, DuPre N, James P, Vieira VM, VoPham T, et al. Exposure to hazardous air pollutants and risk of incident breast cancer in the nurses' health study II. Environ Health Glob Access Sci Source. 2018;17(1):28.

135. Colditz GA, Frazier AL. Models of breast cancer show that risk is set by events of early life: prevention efforts must shift focus. Cancer Epidemiol Biomark Prev Publ Am Assoc Cancer Res Cosponsored Am Soc Prev Oncol. 1995;4(5):567–71.

136. Miller AB, Howe GR, Sherman GJ, Lindsay JP, Yaffe MJ, Dinner PJ, et al. Mortality from breast cancer after irradiation during fluoroscopic examinations in patients being treated for tuberculosis. N Engl J Med. 1989;321(19):1285–9.

137. Tokunaga M, Land CE, Tokuoka S, Nishimori I, Soda M, Akiba S. Incidence of female breast cancer among atomic bomb survivors, 1950–1985. Radiat Res. 1994;138(2):209–23.

138. Bonner MR, Han D, Nie J, Rogerson P, Vena JE, Muti P, et al. Breast cancer risk and exposure in early life to polycyclic aromatic hydrocarbons using total suspended particulates as a proxy measure. Cancer Epidemiol Biomark Prev Publ Am Assoc Cancer Res Cosponsored Am Soc Prev Oncol. 2005;14(1):53–60.

139. Nie J, Beyea J, Bonner MR, Han D, Vena JE, Rogerson P, et al. Exposure to traffic emissions throughout life and risk of breast cancer: the Western New York Exposures and Breast Cancer (WEB) study. Cancer Causes Control. 2007;18(9):947–55.

140. Callahan CL, Bonner MR, Nie J, Han D, Wang Y, Tao M-H, et al. Lifetime exposure to ambient air pollution and methylation of tumor suppressor genes in breast tumors. Environ Res. 2018;161:418–24.

141. White AJ, Chen J, Teitelbaum SL, McCullough LE, Xu X, Hee Cho Y, et al. Sources of polycyclic aromatic hydrocarbons are associated with gene-specific promoter methylation in women with breast cancer. Environ Res. 2016;145:93–100.

142. Willett W. An overview of issues related to the correction of non-differential exposure measurement error in epidemiologic studies. Stat Med. 1989;8(9):1031–40; discussion 1071–1073

143. Kioumourtzoglou M-A, Spiegelman D, Szpiro AA, Sheppard L, Kaufman JD, Yanosky JD, et al. Exposure measurement error in PM2.5 health effects studies: a pooled analysis of eight personal exposure validation studies. Environ Health Glob Access Sci Source. 2014;13(1):2.

144. Boys BL, Martin RV, van Donkelaar A, MacDonell RJ, Hsu NC, Cooper MJ, et al. Fifteen-year global time series of satellite-derived fine particulate matter. Environ Sci Technol. 2014;48(19):11109–18.

145. Bell ML, Dominici F, Ebisu K, Zeger SL, Samet JM. Spatial and temporal variation in PM(2.5) chemical composition in the United States for health effects studies. Environ Health Perspect. 2007;115(7):989–95.

146. Dominici F, Peng RD, Bell ML, Pham L, McDermott A, Zeger SL, et al. Fine particulate air pollution and hospital admission for cardiovascular and respiratory diseases. JAMA. 2006;295(10):1127–34.

147. Lane KJ, Stokes EC, Seto KC, Thanikachalam S, Thanikachalam M, Bell ML. Associations between greenness, impervious surface area, and nighttime lights on biomarkers of vascular aging in Chennai, India. Environ Health Perspect. 2017;125(8):087003.
148. Lunn RM, Blask DE, Coogan AN, Figueiro MG, Gorman MR, Hall JE, et al. Health consequences of electric lighting practices in the modern world: a report on the National Toxicology Program's workshop on shift work at night, artificial light at night, and circadian disruption. Sci Total Environ. 2017;607–608:1073–84.
149. Brainard GC, Rollag MD, Hanifin JP. Photic regulation of melatonin in humans: ocular and neural signal transduction. J Biol Rhythms. 1997;12(6):537–46.
150. Budnick LD, Lerman SE, Nicolich MJ. An evaluation of scheduled bright light and darkness on rotating shiftworkers: trial and limitations. Am J Ind Med. 1995;27(6):771–82.
151. Lewy AJ, Wehr TA, Goodwin FK, Newsome DA, Markey SP. Light suppresses melatonin secretion in humans. Science. 1980;210(4475):1267–9.
152. Czeisler CA, Duffy JF, Shanahan TL, Brown EN, Mitchell JF, Rimmer DW, et al. Stability, precision, and near-24-hour period of the human circadian pacemaker. Science. 1999;284(5423):2177–81.
153. Blask DE. Melatonin, sleep disturbance and cancer risk. Sleep Med Rev. 2009;13(4):257–64.
154. Haus EL, Smolensky MH. Shift work and cancer risk: potential mechanistic roles of circadian disruption, light at night, and sleep deprivation. Sleep Med Rev. 2013;17(4):273–84.
155. Depner CM, Stothard ER, Wright KP. Metabolic consequences of sleep and circadian disorders. Curr Diab Rep. 2014;14(7):507.
156. Blask DE, Dauchy RT, Dauchy EM, Mao L, Hill SM, Greene MW, et al. Light exposure at night disrupts host/cancer circadian regulatory dynamics: impact on the Warburg effect, lipid signaling and tumor growth prevention. PloS One. 2014;9(8):e102776.
157. Haim A, Zubidat AE. Artificial light at night: melatonin as a mediator between the environment and epigenome. Philos Trans R Soc Lond B Biol Sci. 2015;370(1667)
158. Jasser SA, Blask DE, Brainard GC. Light during darkness and cancer: relationships in circadian photoreception and tumor biology. Cancer Causes Control. 2006;17(4):515–23.
159. Blask DE, Dauchy RT, Sauer LA. Putting cancer to sleep at night: the neuroendocrine/circadian melatonin signal. Endocrine. 2005;27(2):179–88.
160. Blask DE, Hill SM, Dauchy RT, Xiang S, Yuan L, Duplessis T, et al. Circadian regulation of molecular, dietary, and metabolic signaling mechanisms of human breast cancer growth by the nocturnal melatonin signal and the consequences of its disruption by light at night. J Pineal Res. 2011;51(3):259–69.
161. Stevens RG, Brainard GC, Blask DE, Lockley SW, Motta ME. Breast cancer and circadian disruption from electric lighting in the modern world. CA Cancer J Clin. 2014;64(3):207–18.
162. Cohen M, Lippman M, Chabner B. Role of pineal gland in aetiology and treatment of breast cancer. Lancet. 1978;2(8094):814–6.
163. Baldwin WS, Barrett JC. Melatonin: receptor-mediated events that may affect breast and other steroid hormone-dependent cancers. Mol Carcinog. 1998;21(3):149–55.
164. Mediavilla MD, Cos S, Sánchez-Barceló EJ. Melatonin increases p53 and p21WAF1 expression in MCF-7 human breast cancer cells in vitro. Life Sci. 1999;65(4):415–20.
165. Schernhammer ES, Kroenke CH, Laden F, Hankinson SE. Night work and risk of Breast Cancer. Epidemiol. 2006;17(1):108–11.
166. Wegrzyn LR, Tamimi RM, Rosner BA, Brown SB, Stevens RG, Eliassen AH, et al. Rotating night-shift work and the risk of Breast Cancer in the nurses' health studies. Am J Epidemiol. 2017;186(5):532–40.
167. Straif K, Baan R, Grosse Y, Secretan B, El Ghissassi F, Bouvard V, et al. Carcinogenicity of shift-work, painting, and fire-fighting. Lancet Oncol. 2007;8(12):1065–6.
168. Stevens RG. Testing the light-at-night (LAN) theory for Breast Cancer causation. Chronobiol Int. 2011;28(8):653–6.
169. Al-Naggar RA, Anil S. Artificial light at night and Cancer: global study. Asian Pac J Cancer Prev. 2016;17(10):4661–4.

170. Keshet-Sitton A, Or-Chen K, Huber E, Haim A. Illuminating a risk for Breast Cancer: a preliminary ecological study on the association between streetlight and Breast Cancer. Integr Cancer Ther. 2017;16(4):451–63.
171. Kim YJ, Lee E, Lee HS, Kim M, Park MS. High prevalence of breast cancer in light polluted areas in urban and rural regions of South Korea: an ecologic study on the treatment prevalence of female cancers based on National Health Insurance data. Chronobiol Int. 2015;32(5):657–67.
172. Kloog I, Haim A, Stevens RG, Barchana M, Portnov BA. Light at night co-distributes with incident breast but not lung cancer in the female population of Israel. Chronobiol Int. 2008;25(1):65–81.
173. Kloog I, Stevens RG, Haim A, Portnov BA. Nighttime light level co-distributes with breast cancer incidence worldwide. Cancer Causes Control. 2010;21(12):2059–68.
174. Portnov BA, Stevens RG, Samociuk H, Wakefield D, Gregorio DI. Light at night and breast cancer incidence in Connecticut: an ecological study of age group effects. Sci Total Environ. 2016;572:1020–4.
175. Rybnikova N, Haim A, Portnov BA. Artificial Light at Night (ALAN) and Breast Cancer incidence worldwide: a revisit of earlier findings with analysis of current trends. Chronobiol Int. 2015;32(6):757–73.
176. Rybnikova N, Portnov BA. Population-level study links short-wavelength nighttime illumination with breast cancer incidence in a major metropolitan area. Chronobiol Int. 2018;16:1–11.
177. Bauer SE, Wagner SE, Burch J, Bayakly R, Vena JE. A case-referent study: light at night and breast cancer risk in Georgia. Int J Health Geogr. 2013;12:23.
178. Keshet-Sitton A, Or-Chen K, Yitzhak S, Tzabary I, Haim A. Can avoiding light at night reduce the risk of Breast Cancer? Integr Cancer Ther. 2016;15(2):145–52.
179. Garcia-Saenz A, Sánchez de Miguel A, Espinosa A, Valentin A, Aragonés N, Llorca J, et al. Evaluating the association between artificial light-at-night exposure and Breast and Prostate Cancer risk in Spain (MCC-Spain Study). Environ Health Perspect. 2018;126(4):047011.
180. Hurley S, Goldberg D, Nelson D, Hertz A, Horn-Ross PL, Bernstein L, et al. Light at night and breast cancer risk among California teachers. Epidemiol. 2014;25(5):697–706.
181. James P, Bertrand KA, Hart JE, Schernhammer ES, Tamimi RM, Laden F. Outdoor light at night and Breast Cancer incidence in the nurses' health study II. Environ Health Perspect. 2017;125(8):087010.
182. Keshet-Sitton A, Or-Chen K, Yitzhak S, Tzabary I, Haim A. Light and the city: breast cancer risk factors differ between urban and rural women in Israel. Integr Cancer Ther. 2017;16(2):176–87.
183. Schernhammer ES, Laden F, Speizer FE, Willett WC, Hunter DJ, Kawachi I, et al. Rotating night shifts and risk of breast cancer in women participating in the nurses' health study. J Natl Cancer Inst. 2001;93(20):1563–8.
184. Rea MS, Brons JA, Figueiro MG. Measurements of light at night (LAN) for a sample of female school teachers. Chronobiol Int. 2011;28(8):673–80.
185. O'Connell SG, Kincl LD, Anderson KA. Silicone wristbands as personal passive samplers. Environ Sci Technol. 2014;48(6):3327–35.
186. Villeneuve PJ, Ysseldyk RL, Root A, Ambrose S, DiMuzio J, Kumar N, et al. Comparing the normalized difference vegetation index with the google street view measure of vegetation to assess associations between greenness, walkability, recreational physical activity, and health in Ottawa, Canada. Int J Environ Res Public Health. 2018;15(8)
187. Lu Y. The association of urban greenness and walking behavior: using google street view and deep learning techniques to estimate residents' exposure to urban greenness. Int J Environ Res Public Health. 2018;15(8)
188. Rzotkiewicz A, Pearson AL, Dougherty BV, Shortridge A, Wilson N. Systematic review of the use of google street view in health research: major themes, strengths, weaknesses and possibilities for future research. Health Place. 2018;52:240–6.
189. Fenton SE, Birnbaum LS. Timing of environmental exposures as a critical element in Breast Cancer risk. J Clin Endocrinol Metab. 2015;100(9):3245–50.

Chapter 10
Neighborhoods and Breast Cancer Survival: The Case for an Archetype Approach

Mindy C. DeRouen, Margaret M. Weden, Juan Yang, Jennifer Jain, Scarlett Lin Gomez, and Salma Shariff-Marco

Abstract Neighborhoods are consistently and independently associated with breast cancer mortality. The majority of studies on neighborhoods and breast cancer mortality have examined neighborhood socioeconomic status (nSES). A small number of studies, on the other hand, have examined individual attributes of the social and/or built environments or composite measures of specific neighborhood dimensions (e.g. walkability or racial/ethnic segregation). However, while examining breast cancer mortality according to specific attributes of neighborhood social and built environments has been useful in determining independent associations between such attributes and breast cancer mortality, this approach cannot inform how the multitude of often highly correlated neighborhood attributes co-exist and likely interact to impact breast cancer outcomes. Appreciating the complex ways that multiple neighborhood dimensions interact to influence health thus necessitates revisiting how neighborhoods are defined in epidemiologic studies. In response, we identified a 9-class neighborhood archetype model for census tracts in California in the decennial year 2000 that considers interactions among a broad range of attributes of neighborhood social and built environments. We have described breast cancer survival disparities according to these neighborhood archetypes. Relative survival differed by neighborhood archetype and associations between neighborhood archetypes and survival varied by stage at diagnosis, race/ethnicity, and nativity. Archetype classes with the highest mortality were defined by lower SES, but also other neighborhood dimensions such as

M. C. DeRouen · S. L. Gomez · S. Shariff-Marco (✉)
Department of Epidemiology and Biostatistics, University of California San Francisco, San Francisco, CA, USA

UCSF Helen Diller Family Comprehensive Cancer Center, San Francisco, CA, USA
e-mail: sshariff@psg.ucsf.edu

M. M. Weden
RAND Corporation, Santa Monica, CA, USA

J. Yang · J. Jain
Department of Epidemiology and Biostatistics, University of California San Francisco, San Francisco, CA, USA

© Springer Nature Switzerland AG 2019
D. Berrigan, N. A. Berger (eds.), *Geospatial Approaches to Energy Balance and Breast Cancer*, Energy Balance and Cancer 15, https://doi.org/10.1007/978-3-030-18408-7_10

rural/urban designation, age and race/ethnicity of residents, commuting and traffic patterns, residential mobility, and food environment. The archetype approach thus yields valuable insights into how multiple neighborhood dimensions work synergistically to impact breast cancer mortality.

Keywords Neighborhood archetypes · Cancer disparities · Breast cancer survival · Race/ethnicity · Nativity

10.1 Neighborhood Effects on Health

Neighborhoods shape individuals' exposure to health-related risks and access to resources; they have an additional and distinct effect on health apart from individual-level characteristics [1–3]. Neighborhoods influence cancer outcomes across the cancer continuum, including outcomes related to prevention, risk, diagnosis, treatment, survivorship, and mortality [4]. The large majority of published studies on associations between neighborhood environments and breast cancer mortality have focused on neighborhood socioeconomic status (nSES) or neighborhood deprivation using single measures or indices of this neighborhood dimension [5–14]. More recent work, including work from our group, has considered additional dimensions of neighborhood built and social environments (e.g., food environment, walkability, and residential racial/ethnic segregation), again measured with single indicators or indices [15–25]. Based on findings from the broader literature on neighborhood conditions and health, however, it is unlikely that any one, single neighborhood attribute or even dimension can account fully for neighborhood determinants of health. Rather, multiple dimensions of neighborhood social and built environments interact to influence health outcomes [2, 3, 26–28]. Hence, effective targeting of neighborhoods for health promotion should consider the multitude of neighborhood dimensions and interactions therein that contribute to what we understand as *the* neighborhood effect.

10.2 Neighborhoods and Breast Cancer Mortality

Breast cancer is the most common cancer and the second-leading cause of cancer deaths among women in the United States (US) [29]. The first study using geospatial data (i.e., census-tract level median household income) to document the association between low nSES and high breast cancer mortality is nearly 50 years old [30]. Since then, many studies have further described associations between indicators of lower nSES and breast cancer mortality within population-based studies [7, 12, 14]. Some have incorporated more complex measures of nSES or deprivation, such as indices that incorporate several Census measures of neighborhood-level education, occupation, and poverty [6, 10, 11, 15, 24]. Furthermore, several multi-level studies have more recently established the independence of nSES from effects due to individual-level sociodemographic, reproductive, and behavioral characteristics and hosptial characteristics [10–12, 15, 21]. However, while composite indices of nSES consider multiple neighorhood attributes (e.g., income, education, occumpation), they do not allow the researcher to observe interactions between those attributes. Moreover, characterizing neighborhoods according to a single dimension such as nSES warrants consideration of other neighborhood dimensions, such as racial/ethnic composition, social cohesion, walkability, food environment, and safety, which are understood to impact health [1, 31–39].

A few studies have identified additional specific dimensions of neighborhood social or built environments that influence breast cancer survival, as summarized in a literature review by our group [4]. These studies used single measures (e.g., racial segregation) or composite measures and indices (e.g., ethnic enclave, food environment indices) to capture a particular neighborhood dimension [4, 13, 17, 18]. Studies of neighborhood racial/ethnic composition and/or racial/ethnic residential segregation, for example, describe independent associations between these measures and breast cancer-specific survival [4, 13, 17, 18]. Neighborhood co-ethnic support or socio-cultural norms related to Asian or Hispanic enclaves have also been studied in the context of breast cancer mortality [40]. Single specific measures (i.e., the proportion of foreign-born residents and linguistically isolated households) were found to have no effect on breast cancer mortality among a racially/ethnically diverse population in the San Francisco Bay Area [16, 21]. Ethnic enclave indices were developed by members of our group for California census tracts and block groups through principal components analysis of several Census measures related to Asian or Hispanic linguistic isolation, ethnic composition, and residents' nativity [19, 22]. No independent associations between residence in Hispanic or Asian ethnic enclave and breast cancer mortality were observed [19, 22]. Among Hispanic women, though, ethnic enclave interacted with nSES to influence mortality. High ethnic enclaves were associated with a greater risk of death within high SES but not low SES neighborhoods, which highlights the importance of considering interactions among neighborhood dimensions [19, 22].

Additional studies in California utilized a suite of neighborhood attributes from the California Neighborhoods Data System (CNDS) to examine numerous dimensions of neighborhood social and built environments, including population density, urban/rural designation, housing/family composition, racial/ethnic composition, immigration, street connectivity, commuting patterns/transportation, recreation, and food outlets [16, 21, 25, 41, 42]. Few of these measures were individually associated with overall or breast cancer-specific survival: increasing population density, proportion of non-single family units, crowding, and an unfavorable restaurant environment were adversely associated with mortality in minimally adjusted models, but were null in models adjusted for individual-level sociodemographic and clinical characteristics [16, 21]. Unexpectedly, increasing number of parks was also adversely associated with mortality in these studies, indicating that there may be unmeasured individual (e.g., income) or contextual-level factors (e.g., safety) that confound or modify the association of parks with mortality and thus obscure true associations. Such a paradoxical observation highlights how any one specific neighborhood attribute may only partially capture a more complex influence of the neighborhood environment and emphasizes the need to characterize neighborhoods across multiple dimensions [16, 21].

Singular measures that capture a particular dimension of the neighborhood social or built environment simplify analyses and present the alluring possibility of attributing specific health outcomes to one or a few neighborhood characteristics. Indices include multiple related measures with the aim to better capture one particular social (e.g., nSES, ethnic enclave) or built (e.g., food environment) environment dimension. However, as single, continuous measures, indices are difficult to interpret since unit increases are dependent on how the composite score is defined, for example, as a simple summation of each component, weighted as in principal components, or some other method. Moreover, indices still fall short of capturing the broad set of dimensions that compose neighborhoods and, importantly, the interactions among those dimensions. It is likely, rather, that pathways through which neighborhoods affect breast cancer mortality include environmental exposures, material deprivation, psychosocial mechanisms (e.g., stress and social support), healthy lifestyle (e.g., physical activity, smoking, and diet), and access to resources, each of which can be influenced jointly by multiple other dimensions of built and social environments [1, 33, 35, 37, 39]. So while examining breast cancer mortality according to specific measures of neighborhood social and built environments has been useful in determining whether specific measures have an independent effect on breast cancer mortality, this approach cannot inform how the multitude of often highly correlated neighborhood dimensions interact to impact breast cancer outcomes. It is likely that these attributes work synergistically to impact health [1, 33, 35, 37, 39]. Thus, appreciating the complex ways in which multiple neighborhood dimensions interact to influence health necessitates revisiting how neighborhoods are defined in research [43].

Furthermore, given their ability to shape individuals' health, neighborhood effects represent a profound influence on health inequities, and in the persistence of disparities in cancer outcomes according to individual-level characteristics, such as race/ethnicity, immigration status, and SES [3, 4]. Disparities in breast cancer survival have been shown for non-Hispanic (NH) Black, American Indian/Alaska Native, and low income women [9, 44, 45]. Research on disparities in cancer survival has, thus, increasingly considered multilevel factors [1, 3, 11, 46–49]. Importantly, available studies have observed that neighborhood-level factors (i.e., nSES and racial/ethnic residential segregation) do not account for racial/ethnic disparities in breast cancer mortality [13, 17, 20, 23]. Moreover, individual-level characteristics have been observed to modify the association between neighborhood factors and breast-cancer mortality, indicating that individuals' experiences within their built and social neighborhood environments vary according to individual-level characteristics, such as race/ethnicity. For example, Cheng et al. found that the proportion of housing units with multiple families and parks were adversely associated, and number of total businesses were favorably associated with overall survival with breast cancer, but only among Hispanic women [25].

10.3   Latent Variable Models to Define Neighborhood Archetypes

Latent variable models provide a statistically rigorous methodological approach to define archetypes; they determine the unobserved (i.e., latent) variable that measures and describes the observed data [50]. The latent variable approach includes both latent class models, in which dichotomous and categorical indicator variables are used to define the archetype, and latent profile models, in which continuous indicator variables are used. Weden et al. summarize the methodological advantages of latent variable models over other statistical methodologies like cluster analysis [43]. In brief, similar to cluster analysis, latent class analysis (LCA) and latent profile analysis (LPA) allow a researcher to assess the potential interactions between many measures and summarize them into a more practical number of inter-relationships, apart from their impact on any given health outcome. This is a critical advantage that extends neighborhood methods in which single indicators or indices are examined independent of one another. For example, standard multivariable regression models that examine interactions between single neighborhood measures (indicators or indices) are restricted by sample power to typically consider, at most, 3-way interactions. This limitation motivates the need for an a priori assessment of the best fitting model for neighborhood archetypes that include more numerous and complex combinations of neighborhood measures. An advantage of the latent variable approach to a priori producing such a neighborhood model is that it allows the researcher to more fully address measurement error, a feature not shared by non-latent measurement methods (e.g., cluster analysis). In other words, it is likely that not all of the characteristics that distinguish one neighborhood archetype from another can be measured, and even if they can be measured it is likely that they will be measured with some error. Latent measurement models are designed to address these concerns [43].

   Latent variable approaches to define neighborhood archetypes have been used to examine select health outcomes (e.g., cardiovascular disease risk and insulin resistance) or health behaviors (e.g., physical activity and BMI); only one study has addressed a cancer outcome [51–58]. Most studies using latent variable approaches to characterize neighborhoods did so with built environment attributes, most commonly with physical activity as the outcome. A study among adolescents in the Minneapolis-St. Paul metro area utilized LCA to define neighborhood archetypes of the built environment to examine associations between neighborhoods and physical activity [55]. Four distinct neighborhood archetypes were identified from ten built environment measures previously shown to be associated with physical activity, but no difference was found in adolescent activity by these archetypes. On the other hand, a study among adolescents in San Diego County found that physical activity, as well as sedentary time and obesity, varied by three neighborhood archetypes based on seven attributes of the built environment [57]. Adams et al. studied the impact of neighborhood archetypes on adult physical activity within Seattle/King County Washington and Baltimore Maryland/Washington DC with LPA of built environment measures (i.e., residential density, land-use mix, retail floor area, intersection density, public transit, parks, and recreational facilities) yielding four neighborhood archetypes that explained differences in adult physical activity better than a single index of walkability [52]. The International Prevalence Study examined neighborhood features across 11 countries to identify international neighborhood typologies hypothesized to correlate with walkability, including residential density, access to shops/services, recreational facilities, public transportation, presence of sidewalks and bike paths, and personal safety. The result was five meaningful neighborhood types that correlated with differences in physical activity as measured through an International Physical Activity Questionnaire across countries [51]. The Coronary Artery Risk Development in Young Adults (CARDIA) study is a multicenter, longitudinal study of cardiometabolic risk [56]. Meyer et al. used LCA to characterize neighborhoods by population density-specific indicators: road connectivity, activity, parks and physical activity facilities, and food stores and restaurants [56]. They examined associations between neighborhood archetypes and diet, physical activity, body mass index, and insulin resistance, but did not observe consistent associations [56].

Two studies using latent variable models to characterize neighborhoods considered social environment attributes. A study by Alves, et al. identified three socioeconomic classes of neighborhoods in the city of Porto, Portugal using LCA and census variables on neighborhood age, education, occupation, and housing characteristics [53]. Among a random sample of 2081 adult residents, the authors found that neighborhood deprivation had a small effect on physical activity and fruit and vegetable consumption. In addition, Jones, et al. used LPA with measures of neighborhood social status (i.e., racial/ethnic composition, employment, poverty, and housing) to identify three neighborhood archetypes in Los Angeles that predicted excess weight [54]. To our knowledge, only one article has used LCA to define neighborhood archetypes to examine a cancer outcome. Palumbo et al. identified two archetypes from two dozen zip-code level indicators of nSES that correlated with race and breast cancer prognostic factors (i.e., tumor stage and size at diagnosis) among African-American and White women at an academic medical center in Pennsylvania [58].

While the aforementioned studies demonstrate neighborhood archetypes as an emerging approach to characterize neighborhoods, they do not fully capture its advantages. In particular, they include only small subsets of social and built environment attributes, often representing a single neighborhood dimension, and thus cannot identify important interactions across dimensions that distinguish neighborhoods. In response, two studies used broader sets of social and built environment attributes. Arcaya et al. used LCA to describe ten neighborhood archetypes in Massachusetts according to six neighborhood dimensions (i.e., health behaviors and outcomes, housing and land use, transportation, retail environment, socioeconomics, and demographic composition) as a tool for evaluating community-based wellness initiatives [59]. These archetypes, however, are not used to examine disparities in health outcomes, but rather to assess the effectiveness of health interventions, and as such include health behaviors and health outcomes as neighborhood attributes in LCA models. A second study from Weden et al. developed neighborhood archetypes for studies of population health and health disparities [43]. Six archetypes were identified with measures of socioeconomic composition, demographics, the built environment, migration and commuting, and household composition for 1990 and 2000 census tracts across the US. Developing archetypes for multiple periods additionally allowed for observations of neighborhood change from 1990 to 2000. However, these archetypes have not been applied to studies of health behaviors or outcomes.

Given that the approach described by Weden et al. included the most comprehensive set of social and built environment attributes to date to define neighborhood archetypes with LCA, we used this approach to develop neighborhood archetypes in California. We characterized year 2000 and 2010 census tracts as well as year 2000 and 2010 census block groups. Here we describe year 2000 census tract archetypes and examine survival among breast cancer cases. Examination of associations between year 2000 archetypes and breast cancer survival provided for a more robust analysis, given the longer follow-up time from the date of diagnosis.

10.4   Defining Neighborhood Archetypes to Examine Cancer Outcomes in California

We developed neighborhood archetypes for California census tracts using a broad suite of social and built environment data for the year 2000. We examined these archetypes according race/ethnicity, stage at diagnosis, and relative survival among women diagnosed with breast cancer using population-based cancer registry data. This work advances current neighborhood research by including additional neighborhood dimensions (e.g., businesses, food environment, traffic density, and ethnic enclaves) that have been shown to be associated with health outcomes in longitudinal studies [31, 32, 34, 36, 38, 60]. It provides a resource for a single neighborhood measure for population health studies that accounts for a large number of neighborhood dimensions.

10.4.1   Neighborhood Data

Neighborhood data were derived from the CNDS, a comprehensive geospatial database compiled to characterize social and built environments for neighborhoods of small geographic areas (i.e., tracts and block groups) in California [41]. Thirty-nine variables measuring attributes of social and built environments of individual census tracts and characterizing five dimensions of social and built environments (i.e., demographics and household composition, immigration, neighborhood SES, walkability, and migration and commuting, see Table 10.1) were included in the LCA. We drew upon published standards to re-categorize these neighborhood indicator variables for LCA models [43]. Education was classified as (1): mid-low, % less

Table 10.1 Descriptions and sources of data for neighborhood characteristics used to fit neighborhood archetype models

Neighborhood characteristic	Data source	Description
Demographics and household composition		
Racial/ethnic composition	Census 2000, 2010 [1, 2]	Tract-level measures of % of each racial/ethnic group (NH White, NH Black, Hispanic, and NH Asian/Pacific Islander)
Age	Census 2000, 2010 [1, 2]	Tract-level measures of residential composition by % age groups (0–17, 18–34, 35–64, 65–79, and 80+ years).
Household composition	Census 2000 [2]; 2008–2012 American Community Survey [3]	Tract-level measures of % single households, % large households, and % female-headed households
Immigration		
Foreign born	Census 2000 [2]; 2008–2012 American Community Survey [3]	Tract-level measures of residential composition on % foreign-born
Linguistic characteristics	Census 2000 [2]; 2008–2012 American Community Survey [3]	Tract-level measures of residential composition on % Asian/Pacific Islander-language and Spanish-speaking households
Socioeconomic status		
Neighborhood socioeconomic status	Census 2000 [2]; 2008–2012 American Community Survey [3]	Tract-level measures of income, education composition, % poverty, % unemployment, % blue collar occupation types, housing and rent values
Home ownership	Census 2000 [2]; 2008–2012 American Community Survey [3]	Tract-level measures of % owner-occupied households and % vacant dwellings
Crime	ESRI 2014 [4]	Tract-level crime indices. Crime data are only available for 2014, so are only utilized to develop 2010 archetypes
Built environment/walkability		
Rural/urban	Census 2000, 2010 [1, 2]	Tract-level combined measure based on census defined % rural and population density
Street connectivity	NAVTEQ [5]	Tract-level alpha measure (ratio of the actual number of complete loops to the maximum number of possible loops given the number of intersections)
Traffic count and density	California Dept of Transportation [6]	Tract-level measures of volume of traffic
Greenspace	California Protected Areas Data Portal [7]	Tract-level measure of % greenspace
Businesses	Dun & Bradstreet annual business listings (1990–2015), via Walls & Associates [8], California Department of Food and Agriculture [9]	Tract-level measures of total businesses, retail food environment index (the ratio of the number of convenience stores, liquor stores, and fast-food restaurants to supermarkets and farmers' markets), restaurant environment index (the ratio of the number of fast-food restaurants to other restaurants), and density of recreational facilities

(continued)

Table 10.1 (continued)

Neighborhood characteristic	Data source	Description
Migration and commuting		
Residential mobility	Census 2000 [2]; 2008–2012 American Community Survey [3]	Tract-level measures of % residents who resided in a different county 5 years ago
Commuting	Census 2000 [2]; 2008–2012 American Community Survey [3]	Tract-level measures of % of residents commuting various times to work (<30 m, 30–44 m, 45–59 m, 60 m+), % traveling by car or motorcycle, public transportation, walking or biking, other, work from home

high school > median and/or % high school > median; (2): mid-high, % high school > median and/or % some college > median and/or %BA and over > median; and (3): stratified, all other patterns. Income composition was classified as (1): mid-low, % income <30,000 > median and/or % income 30,000–59,000 > median; (2): mid-high, % income 30,000–59,000 > median and/or % income 60,000–74,000 > median; (3): high, % income 60,000–74,000 > median and/or % income >75,000 > median; and (4): stratified, all other patterns. The rural/urban distinction is based on tract-level Census-defined urbanized areas [61, 62] and population density. Rural/urban was classified as (1): Rural, % Rural >0%; (2): Urban/less populated, % Rural = 0%, population density < median; and (3): Urban/more populated, %Rural = 0%, population density > = median. The retail food environment index is the ratio of the number of convenience stores, liquor stores, and fast-food restaurants to supermarkets and farmers' markets [16, 21]. The restaurant environment index is the ratio of the number of fast-food restaurants to other restaurants [16, 21]. The ratios of the restaurant environment index, retail food environment index, and recreational facility density, were grouped as (1): numerator = 0; and (2): numerator >0. All other variables were dichotomized using the median value for the state of California as the cut point. Census tracts with missing values (n = 41) were excluded from LCA models.

10.4.2   Latent Class Models to Develop Neighborhood Archetypes

LCA modeling was implemented using R package poLCA (R Foundation for Statistical Computing, Vienna, Austria) and SAS procedure PROC LCA (SAS Institute, Cary, North Carolina). We estimated a latent class model with L classes from a set of M categorical items. Let the vector $Y_i = (Y_{i1}, \ldots, Y_{iM})$ denote the ith subject with responses to the M items, where variable Y_{iM} has possible values 1, 2, $\ldots, r_m$. Let $L_i = 1, 2, \ldots, L$ be the latent class membership of the ith subject, and let $I(y = k)$ be the indicator function that equals to 1 if $y = k$ and 0 otherwise. If the l_i

latent class is observed, the joint probability that the ith subject belong to class l given responses $y_i = (y_{i1}, \ldots y_{iM})$ would be:

$$\Pr\left(Y_i = y_i, L_i = l\right) = \gamma_l \, \Pi_{m=1}^{M} \Pi_{k=1}^{r_m} \rho_{mk|l}^{I\left(y_{im}=k\right)},$$

where $\gamma_l = \Pr(l_i = l)$ denotes the marginal probability of the lth class membership in the population, and $\rho_{mk|l} = \Pr(Y_{iM} = k| \, l_i = l)$ represents the probability of response k to the mth item given the lth class membership.

Several LCA models, ranging from those yielding three, five, six, nine, and twelve classes, were considered to assess the best fit for the data. Goodness of fit criteria including percentage of seeds associated with best fitted model, the log-likelihood ratio test statistics, deviance statistics, the Akaike Information Criterion (AIC), the normal and adjusted Schwarz Bayesian Information Criterion (BIC), and the raw and scaled entropy of class partitioning were compared across models [50, 63–66]. In addition, we considered the interpretability of the classes via qualitative review of the definitions and neighborhood classifications for familiar counties (e.g., San Francisco, Alameda, Los Angeles, and San Diego). As detailed below, we employed these quantitative and qualitative criteria to determine that two class measurement models (a 5-class and 9-class model) best fit the neighborhood data. Class-conditional probabilities for all 39 variables in the 5-class and 9-class neighborhood archetypes are available from authors upon request.

After identifying the best fitting models for the 5-class and 9-class neighborhood archetypes, we then defined a 5 category and 9 category neighborhood archetype variable for census tracts in California. The posterior class membership was assigned to each census tract according to the posterior class membership probability from the LCA model. The matrices containing class-conditional response probabilities and associated standard errors were output for each level of the characteristics variable for a given latent class membership.

10.4.3   Neighborhood Archetypes for California

Descriptions and labels for classes of the 5-class and 9-class neighborhood archetypes are shown in Table 10.2. Classes are described according to their strongest dimensions (i.e., class-conditional probabilities greater than 0.6 or less than 0.4, or the highest across the archetype classes). For example, within the 5-class archetype model, the High status/Status fringe neighborhoods (25.0% of California tracts) are characterized by older NH White residents, high SES, healthy food, and plentiful recreational facilities while the New urban/Pedestrian neighborhoods (16.2% of California tracts) are in downtown areas with high mixed land use and characterized by racially/ethnically diverse residents that are relatively young and mostly single. According to the 5-class archetype model, approximately one-third of California census tracts (30.8%) and population (33.3%) reside in Inner city/Urban sprawl neighborhoods that are densely populated and of lower SES, with more

Table 10.2 Comparison of neighborhood characteristics of 5 and 9 class neighborhood archetype models: description, census tract frequency, and population coverage, 2000

		Census tracts[a]		Population[b]	
5-class Archetype	Description	N	(%)	N	(%)
High status/ Status fringe	'McMansions' and golf-course communities, high SES, older NH White (baby boomer) residents, healthy food outlets, and more recreational facilities	1753	25.0%	7,992,521	23.6%
New urban/ Pedestrian	Downtown, highly mixed-land use, high racial/ethnic diversity (except Hispanic), predominantly young, single millennials, and gen-Xers	1137	16.2%	5,129,029	15.2%
Metropolitan pioneer	Mixed land-use (sometimes 'up-and-coming') neighborhoods within a city but not right downtown, middle-class working families, high diversity in race/ethnicity, immigration, and languages	904	12.9%	4,659,633	13.8%
Rural/ Micropolitan	Lower SES, older NH White residents, single headed households	1055	15.1%	4,757,304	14.1%
Inner city/ Urban sprawl	Densely populated, lower SES, with more racial/ethnic minority (especially NH Black and Hispanic) residents, working-class families, rentals/vacant housing, and unhealthy food outlets	2159	30.8%	11, 269,388	33.3%
9-class Archetype	Description	N	(%)	N	(%)
Upper middle-class suburb	High SES, more NH White, API, and midlife residents, fewer female headed households, low residential mobility, more green space and recreational facilities	846	12.1%	4,172,910	12.3%
High status	'McMansions' and golf-course communities, high SES, older NH White (baby boomer) residents, healthy food outlets, and more recreational facilities	814	11.6%	3,542,270	10.5%
New urban/ Pedestrian	Downtown, highly mixed land use, high racial/ethnic diversity (except Hispanic), predominantly young, single millennials and gen-Xers	926	13.2%	4,205,539	12.4%
Mixed SES-class suburb	Middle class working families with some mixed land use, no unhealthy food outlets, more recreational facilities, low racial/ethnic diversity, more commuting, less street connectivity, and lower traffic density	553	7.9%	2,602,528	7.7%
Suburban pioneer	Mixed land-use (sometimes 'up-and-coming') neighborhoods within a city but not right downtown, high diversity in race/ethnicity, immigration status, and languages— distinguished from City pioneer neighborhoods by middle-class working families with children and homeowners	699	10.0%	3,639,948	10.8%

(continued)

Table 10.2 (continued)

5-class Archetype	Description	Census tracts[a] N	(%)	Population[b] N	(%)
Rural/ Micropolitan	Rural, lower SES, older and NH White residents, single headed households	537	7.7%	2,368,327	7.0%
City pioneer	Mixed land-use (sometimes 'up-and-coming') neighborhoods within a city but not right downtown, high diversity in race/ethnicity, immigration status, and languages—distinguished from Suburban pioneer neighborhoods by more single and female-headed households, older residents, more lower-middle class residents, and residential mobility	781	11.1%	3,669,614	10.9%
Hispanic small towns	Lower-middle SES, more Hispanic residents (not more foreign-born), some mixed land-use, unhealthy food outlets, short commute, low traffic density, and less green space	706	10.1%	3,660,385	10.8%
Inner city	Densely populated, lower SES, more racial/ethnic minority (especially NH Black and Hispanic) and working-class residents, rentals/vacant housing, and unhealthy food outlets	1146	16.4%	5,946,354	17.6%

[a]The total number of California census tracts represented in 2000 was 7008
[b]The total California population represented in 2000 was 33,807,875

racial/ethnic minority residents, working-class families, and have relatively high numbers of rentals and vacant housing and unhealthy food outlets (Table 10.2). On the other hand, the smallest proportion of census tracts (12.9%) and population (13.8%) reside in Metropolitan pioneer neighborhoods that are near, but not in, downtown areas and have modern mixed-land use, middle-class working families, and relatively high diversity according to race/ethnicity, immigration status, and language. According to the 9-class model, the largest proportion of census tracts (16.4%), representing the largest proportion of the California population (17.6%), comprise Inner city neighborhoods, which are densely populated, lower SES neighborhoods with greater populations of NH Black and Hispanic residents, working class households, rentals and vacant housing, and unhealthy food outlets. The smallest proportion of census tracts (7.7%), and the smallest proportion of the population (7.0%) are represented by Rural/Micropolitan neighborhoods, which are rural, lower SES neighborhoods with older NH White residents and single-headed households.

The 5- and 9-class archetypes have some overlapping classes, making the 9-class archetype seem an extension of the 5-class (Table 10.3). Two archetypes in the 9-class model are represented in the 5-class model (i.e., Rural/Micropolitan, and New Urban/Pedestrian), while the remainder represent extensions of archetypes in

Table 10.3 Frequencies and proportions of California census tracts (2000) according to 5-class and 9-class archetypes

	5-class Archetype									
	High status/Status fringe		New urban/Pedestrian		Metropolitan pioneer		Rural/Micropolitan		Inner city/Urban sprawl	
	N	(Row %)	N	(Row %)	N	(Row %)	N	(Row %)	N	(Row %)
9-class Archetype										
Upper middle-class suburb	688	(81%)	6	(1%)	152	(18%)	0	(0%)	0	(0%)
High status	784	(96%)	11	(1%)	0	(0%)	19	(2%)	0	(0%)
New urban/Pedestrian	54	(6%)	865	(93%)	4	(0%)	3	(0%)	0	(0%)
Mixed SES-class suburb	227	(41%)	3	(1%)	157	(28%)	166	(30%)	0	(0%)
Suburban pioneer	0	(0%)	7	(1%)	558	(80%)	0	(0%)	134	(19%)
Rural/Micropolitan	0	(0%)	8	(1%)	0	(0%)	529	(99%)	0	(0%)
City pioneer	0	(0%)	237	(30%)	12	(2%)	111	(14%)	421	(54%)
Hispanic small town	0	(0%)	0	(0%)	21	(3%)	227	(32%)	458	(65%)
Inner city	0	(0%)	0	(0%)	0	(0%)	0	(0%)	1146	(100%)

the 5-class model. For example, the High status/Status fringe archetype of the 5-class model was split into High status and Upper middle-class suburb types in the 9-class model; while both of these neighborhoods are high SES neighborhoods with more green space and recreational facilities, the Upper middle-class neighborhoods are distinguished by fewer older residents and female-headed households and more Asian and Pacific Islander (API) and foreign-born residents. The Metropolitan pioneer type of the 5-class model was split further into City Pioneer and Suburban Pioneer in the 9-class model; both are 'up-and-coming' neighborhoods with mixed land-use and high diversity right outside of downtown areas, but City pioneer neighborhoods have comparatively more single and female-headed households, older residents, more lower-middle class (as opposed to higher-middle class) residents, and greater residential mobility. Additionally, Mixed SES-class suburbs and Hispanic small towns emerged as new types of neighborhoods within the 9-class model. Interestingly the Hispanic small town neighborhoods of the 9-class model seemed to pull mostly from Rural/Microplitan neighborhoods and the Inner city/ Urban sprawl neighborhoods, which are highly divergent types of the 5-class model. Given the greater granularity of the 9-class model, and thus greater representation of interacting neighborhood dimensions, we present our observations on breast cancer survival using this model.

Figure 10.1 maps California census tracts according to the 9-class model and, in more detail, the metropolitan areas of San Francisco, Oakland, Los Angeles, and San Diego. The preponderance of Rural/Micropolitan communities is apparent in Northern and Eastern California, as is the concentration of more densely populated neighborhoods along the coastline. San Francisco has a large number of New urban/ Pedestrian neighborhoods, with diverse (although non-Hispanic) residents that are relatively young and single. The Oakland metropolitan area shows Inner city, City pioneer, and New urban/Pedestrian neighborhoods along the San Francisco Bay and High status and Upper middle-class suburb neighborhoods towards the east. Los Angeles and San Diego likewise show concentrations of Inner city, City and Suburban pioneer, and New urban/Pedestrian neighborhoods surrounded by Upper middle-class suburb and High status suburb neighborhoods; these Southern California metropolitan areas have a greater number of Hispanic small town neighborhoods compared to San Francisco and Oakland. Hispanic small towns, though, can be found both in the less populated areas of greater California in addition to areas adjacent to Inner cities.

10.5   Neighborhood Archetypes and Breast Cancer Survival

To describe preliminary associations between neighborhood archetypes and breast cancer survival, we identified 179,495 first primary invasive breast cancer cases [International Classification of Disease for Oncology, 3rd Edition, (ICD-O-3) site codes C50.0–50.9] from the California Cancer Registry (CCR) diagnosed among females from 1996 through 2005. These diagnosis years were selected because they

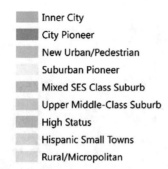

Inner City
City Pioneer
New Urban/Pedestrian
Suburban Pioneer
Mixed SES Class Suburb
Upper Middle-Class Suburb
High Status
Hispanic Small Towns
Rural/Micropolitan

(a)

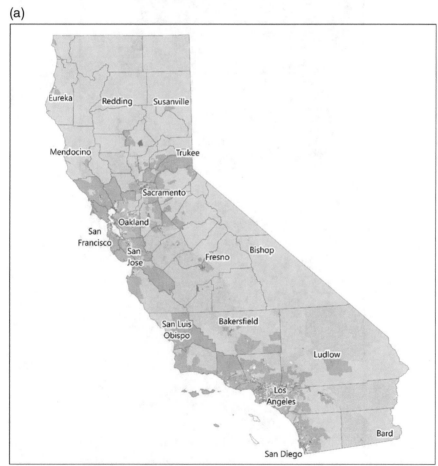

Fig. 10.1 Map of distribution of neighborhood archetypes across census tracts in (**a**) California and the counties surrounding (**b**) San Francisco, (**c**) Oakland, (**d**) Los Angeles, and (**e**) San Diego, California 2000. Black lines indicate county boundaries

(b)

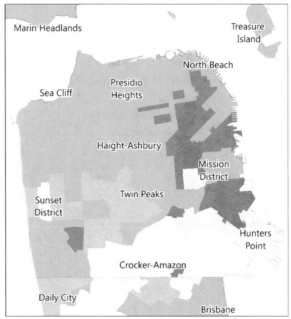

(c)

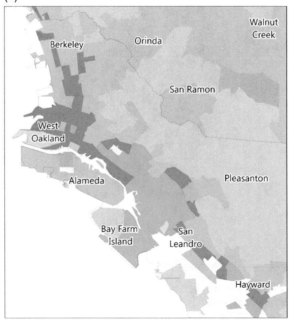

Fig. 10.1 (continued)

(d)

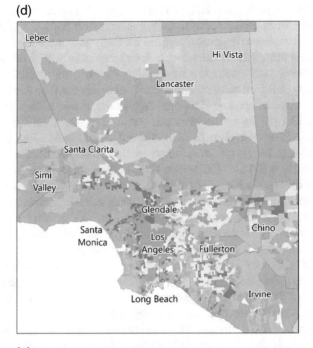

(e)

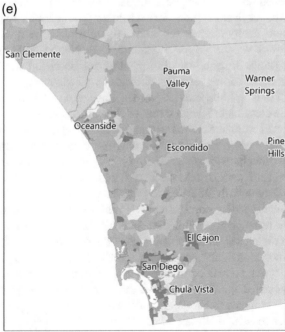

Fig. 10.1 (continued)

comprise a 10 year period around the 2000 Census and provide at least 10 years of follow-up time for assessing survival. CCR data on race/ethnicity, age at diagnosis, and tumor and treatment characteristics are routinely abstracted from the medical record. Data on birthplace are incomplete for approximately 30% of Hispanic and API cancer cases, so we utilized a previously developed and validated method to impute nativity based on cases' social security numbers for Hispanics and 6 Asian subgroups (Chinese, Japanese, Filipino, Vietnamese, Asian Indian, and Koreans) [22, 67, 68]. Underlying causes of death, coded in International Classification of Diseases, 9th edition (ICD-9) before December 31, 1998, and in 10th edition (ICD-10) after January 1st, 1999, were obtained from death certificates, and deaths assigned codes 174.0–174.9 (ICD-9) or C50.0-C50.9 (ICD-10) were identified as due to breast cancer. Each case was assigned to a 2000 census on basis of the geocodes obtained from their residential address at diagnosis (available from the CCR) and then linked to neighborhood archetypes based on 2000 census tract ID to examine breast cancer-specific survival patterns by neighborhood archetypes.

Survival time was computed as the number of months between the date of diagnosis and the end of follow up, which was defined as the first occurrence of the following dates: date of death, date of last known contact, or study end date (December 31, 2013). For breast cancer-specific survival analyses, patients who died from non-breast cancer causes were right censored at the time of death. The average 10 year survival estimates for overall or breast cancer-specific survival were computed using the life-table method. Kaplan-Meier survival curves were calculated to depict the survival functions for each archetypes class: the log-rank test was used to test homogeneity of these functions. All survival analyses were carried out using SAS software version 9.3 (SAS Institute, Cary, North Carolina).

Figure 10.2 shows distributions of the 9-class neighborhood archetypes at time of diagnosis for breast cancer cases in California by race/ethnicity and stage at diagnosis. Over half of NH White and API women diagnosed with breast cancer resided in Upper middle-class suburb, High status, or New urban/Pedestrian neighborhoods. NH White and API women were not distributed identically, however, as the proportion of NH White women residing in Rural/Micropolitan (12.6%) and High status (22.0%) neighborhoods was greater than the proportion of API women in these neighborhoods (1.8% and 6.6%, respectively) and the proportion of API women in Upper middle-class suburb (28.0%) and Suburban pioneer (19.1%) neighborhoods were much greater than the proportion of NH White women in these neighborhoods (16.0% and 6%, respectively). While less than 20% of NH White and less than 25% of API women diagnosed with breast cancer resided in Inner City, Hispanic small town, or City pioneer neighborhoods, nearly 60% of NH Black and approximately half of Hispanic women resided in these neighborhood types. A higher proportion of NH Black women diagnosed with breast cancer resided in City pioneer neighborhoods (18.5%), compared to Hispanic women (10.1%), while a higher proportion of Hispanic women resided in Hispanic small towns (15.2%), compared to the proportion of NH Black women in this neighborhood type (10.7%).

In addition, stage at breast cancer diagnosis was not distributed equally across neighborhoods (Fig. 10.2b). Nearly 50% of all cases diagnosed were among residents of Upper middle-class suburb, High status, and New urban/Pedestrian neighborhoods.

(a)

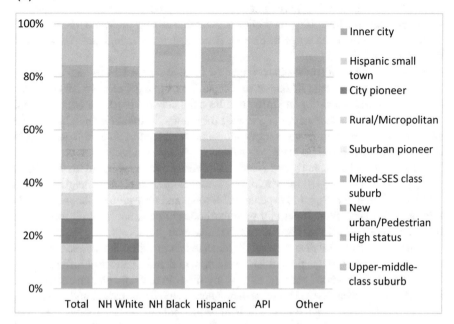

(b)

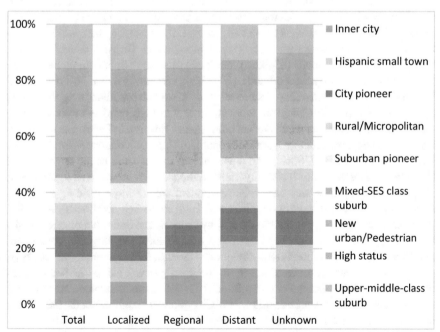

Fig. 10.2 Distribution of breast cancer cases across 9-class neighborhood archetypes according to (**a**) race/ethnicity and (**b**) stage at diagnosis, California 1996–2005

However, cases among residents of these neighborhoods represent only 40% of late stage (distant) disease. It is particularly evident that proportions of cases diagnosed among residents of Inner city, Hispanic small town, and City pioneer neighborhoods increase with advancing stage of disease (localized, 24.6%; regional, 28.4%; and distant 34.5%).

Figure 10.3 presents breast cancer-specific relative survival for 9-class neighborhood archetypes by stage of diagnosis. Regardless of stage, relative survival was highest for women residing in Upper middle-class suburbs (91% for localized and 66% for regional distant stage) and lowest for women in Inner city neighborhoods (83% for localized and 49% for regional/distant stage). More favorable survival is apparent for Upper middle-class suburb and High status neighborhoods, followed by Mixed SES-class suburb and New urban/Pedestrian neighborhoods that have similar survival curves, Rural/Micropolitan and Suburban pioneer neighborhoods that have similar curves, and Hispanic small town and City pioneer neighborhoods that have similar curves. Inner city neighborhoods are distinct from all others and have the lowest relative survival across the follow-up period.

Figure 10.4 shows relative survival for localized disease stratified by race/ethnicity and nativity (among Hispanic and API women) and demonstrates that differences in survival by neighborhood archetypes vary by these individual-level characteristics. For localized disease, NH White women diagnosed with breast cancer and residing in Upper middle-class, High status, and Rural/Micropolitan neighborhoods had high relative survival (89–91%); those residing in New urban/Pedestrian, City pioneer, and Mixed SES-class suburban neighborhoods had moderate relative survival (87–89%); and those residing in Hispanic small town, Suburban pioneer, and Inner city neighborhoods had low relative survival (85–87%). For NH Black women, there was high relative survival among those residing in Upper middle-class, Hispanic small town, and City pioneer neighborhoods (83–92%); moderate survival in Suburban pioneer, High status, and Inner city neighborhoods (79–82%); and low survival in New urban/ Pedestrian, Mixed SES-class suburban, and Rural/Micropolitan neighborhoods (74–79%). For US-born Hispanic women, there was high relative survival among those residing in High status, Suburban pioneer, and New urban/Pedestrian neighborhoods (89–92%); moderate in Rural/Micropolitan, Upper middle-class, and City pioneer neighborhoods (87–88%); and low survival in Hispanic small town, Mixed SES-class suburban, and Inner city neighborhoods (81–86%). For foreign-born Hispanic women, there was high relative survival among those residing in Mixed SES-class suburban, Rural/Micropolitan, and High status neighborhoods (90–93%); moderate survival in Upper middle-class, City pioneer, and Suburban pioneer neighborhoods (88–89%); and low survival in New urban/Pedestrian, Hispanic small town, and Inner city neighborhoods (82–88%). For US-born API women, there was high relative survival among those residing in Suburban pioneer, Mixed SES-class suburb, and Rural/Micropolitan neighborhoods (93–94%); moderate survival in Upper middle-class, New urban/Pedestrian, and City pioneer neighborhoods (92–93%); and low relative survival in Inner city, Hispanic small town, and High status neighborhoods (90–92%). For foreign-born API women, there was high relative survival among those residing in Upper middle class, High status, New urban/Pedestrian, and City pioneer neighborhoods (91–92%); moderate survival in Rural/Micropolitan and

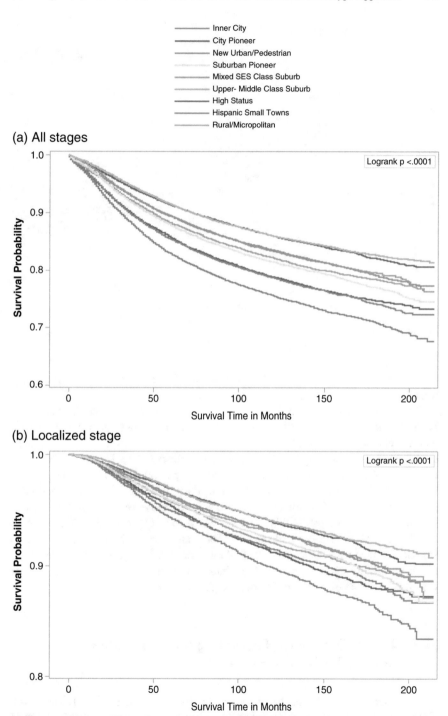

Fig. 10.3 Kaplan Meier curves for breast cancer-specific relative survival according to 9-class neighborhood archetypes for (**a**) all stages, (**b**) localized stage, and (**c**) regional and distant stages at diagnosis

(c) Regional/Distant stage

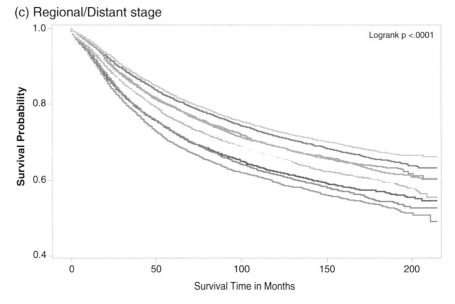

Fig. 10.3 (continued)

Hispanic small town neighborhoods (88–89%); and low relative survival in Inner city, Mixed SES-class suburban, and Suburban pioneer neighborhoods (82–88%).

Patterns of relative survival for women diagnosed with regional/distant stage breast cancer were more consistent across racial/ethnic groups (data not shown), with women residing in Upper middle-class neighborhoods more likely to have the highest relative survival among NH White (67%), NH Black (54%), US-born API (80%), and foreign-born API (65%) women. Among foreign-born Hispanic women highest relative survival was observed for those residing in High status neighborhoods (65%); and among US-born Hispanic women for those residing in New urban/Pedestrian neighborhoods (65%). Residents of Inner city among NH White (52%), NH Black (41%), US-born Hispanic (50%), and foreign-born Hispanic (49%) women had the lowest relative survival of these racial/ethnic groups, while residents of Rural/Micropolitan neighborhoods had the lowest relative survival among US-born API (54%) and foreign-born API (55%) women.

10.6   Future Directions: Expanding the Application of Neighborhood Archetypes

First, we demonstrated that the archetype approach can be applied to develop a single classification system for neighborhoods drawing on a comprehensive suite of social and built environment attributes. Second, we demonstrated place-based

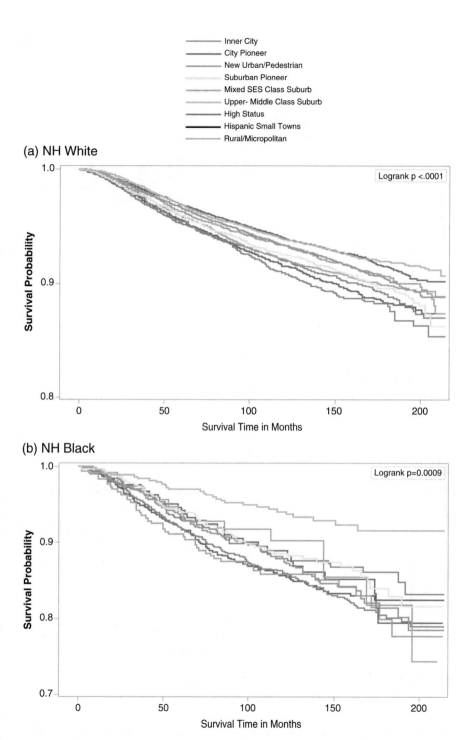

Fig. 10.4 Kaplan Meier curves for breast cancer-specific relative survival localized disease at diagnosis according to 9-class neighborhood archetypes for (**a**) non-Hispanic (NH) White, (**b**) NH Black, (**c**) US-born NH Asians/Pacific Islander (API), (**d**) foreign-born API, (**e**) US-born Hispanic, and (**f**) foreign-born Hispanic women

(c) U.S. born API

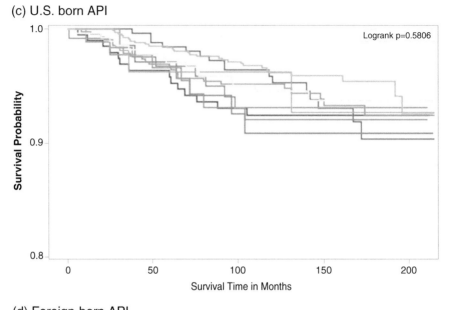

(d) Foreign-born API

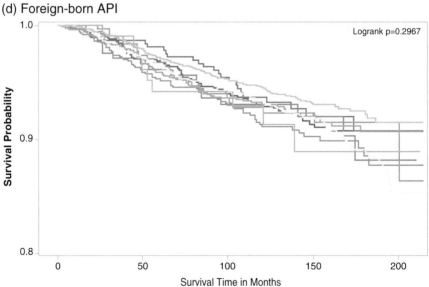

Fig. 10.4 (continued)

disparities in breast cancer-specific relative survival in California, which vary by race/ethnicity and nativity. The neighborhood archetypes developed and these preliminary analyses help illustrate the complexities of the influence of neighborhoods on cancer outcomes.

(e) U.S.-born Hispanic

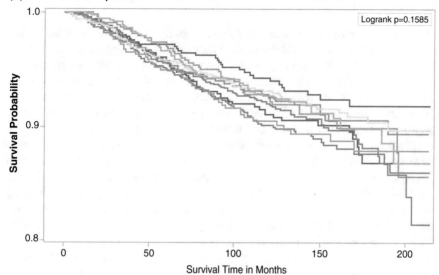

(f) Foreign-born Hispanic

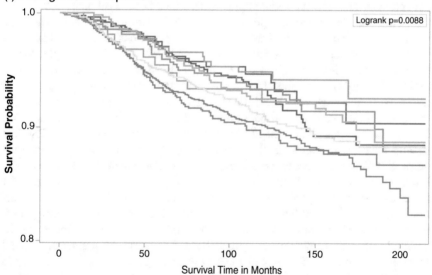

Fig. 10.4 (continued)

10.6.1   The Strength of Neighborhood Archetypes

With our small area-level neighborhood data from the CNDS, we identified 5-class and 9-class archetypes for 2000 and 2010 California census tracts that can be readily used in studies of place and health. Furthermore, while developed specifically with California data, the approach may be applied to other states to develop state-specific archetypes, or even a national set of archetypes as previously demonstrated by Weden et al. {Weden 2011 #37}. With this type of summary measure capturing synergistic relationships of attributes across multiple neighborhood dimensions, research questions on the direct and interaction effects of neighborhood and individual-level factors on cancer, or other health, outcomes can be better addressed. Moreover, as a single, summary measure that can be used across studies to illuminate how (i.e., by identifying which features are working synergistically) and where (i.e., by identifying which types of neighborhoods experience worse outcomes) to apply interventions, this neighborhood archetype measure is a highly significant addition to population health studies and studies of cancer disparities.

As expected, these preliminary results demonstrate the complexity of the influence of place on breast cancer survival. Unlike prior studies, however, we were able to characterize neighborhoods beyond nSES, ethnic/immigrant enclaves, or built environment, and observe the complex interactions between dimensions. In this way, our neighborhood archetypes provide a mechanism to efficiently synthesize and parameterize the most consistently observed interactions across social and built environment attributes that together define neighborhoods. For example, longer breast cancer survival among women residing in Mixed SES-class suburb compared to Suburban pioneer neighborhoods illustrates the power of the neighborhood archetype to illuminate the multi-dimensional effect of neighborhoods on health outcomes; these two neighborhoods are both characterized by middle-class suburban families, but are distinguished by racial/ethnic diversity (i.e., Mixed SES-class suburbs have low racial/ethnic diversity and a higher proportion of NH White residents while Suburban pioneer neighborhoods have high racial/ethnic diversity and a lower proportion of NH White residents). Likewise, relative survival is higher for residents of Suburban pioneer neighborhoods compared to City pioneer neighborhoods, and while both of these neighborhoods have high racial/ethnic diversity, they are distinguished by household characteristics and nSES (i.e., City pioneer neighborhoods have more single and female-headed households, greater residential mobility, and lower SES than Suburban pioneer neighborhoods). This ability to observe the effects of many interactions with a single, summary measure is a benefit of the archetype approach. For this reason, we also favor the 9-class model over the 5-class model, although the most appropriate model may frequently be dictated by available sample sizes.

10.6.2   Intersections Between Neighborhood Archetypes and Individual Social Status

Similar to prior studies characterizing neighborhoods by race/ethnicity, we observed that the neighborhoods where women diagnosed with breast cancer reside vary by race/ethnicity. In addition, while breast cancer survivors residing in Inner city or Rural/Micropolitan neighborhoods generally had the worst survival and those residing in High status or Upper middle-class neighborhoods generally had the best survival, results varied across racial/ethnic groups, especially for localized disease compared to regional/distant disease. For example, for localized breast cancer, Suburban pioneer neighborhoods showed the highest relative survival for US-born API women, but the lowest for foreign-born API women. Similarly, for women in High status neighborhoods, the highest relative survival was observed for US-born Hispanic women, while the lowest was observed for US-born API women. For every archetype, except Upper middle-class, survival probabilities among NH Black women were worse than among any other racial/ethnic group. Place-based disparities among Hispanic and NH Black women showed the largest disparity across archetypes, with a difference of 10% and 17%, respectively for localized disease. More striking place-based disparities for regional/distant breast cancer were observed for US-born API women; however, this likely reflects small sample sizes. Disparities for other groups were more similar with a range of 12–15% differences in relative survival.

Our observations are reflected in emerging frameworks to understand health disparities, including those that recognize the potential affects of intersectionality of multiple axes of social oppression (e.g., social class, gender, and race/ethnicity) on optimal health [69–71]. A growing collection of cancer studies demonstrate the importance of multiple social vulnerabilities on health, and calls have been made for cancer studies to routinely consider all available measures of social status in pursuit of a more complete understanding of the roles of social determinants of health [8, 11, 14, 15, 22, 46–48, 69, 72, 73]. Moreover, our results indicate that individual social status moderates neighborhood effects on breast cancer survival, even with the multitude of neighborhood dimensions represented within our neighborhood archetypes. This highlights the importance of individuals' lived experiences within their neighborhood environments and that access to health-promoting neighborhood built and social resources may depend on residents' individual social status. Mediators of differential neighborhood effects on cancer outcomes by race/ethnicity and nativity likely include racial/ethnic and cultural discrimination [74–78]. Discrimination has been studied independently in regards to general health outcomes, but continued efforts to develop more accurate measures and to examine them alongside neighborhood archetypes within cancer studies are warranted [78–81].

10.6.3 Additional Considerations

Neighborhood archetypes characterize neighborhoods by distinguishing them across modifiable attributes that can be addressed through policy and/or community interventions to promote health. However, methodological studies to validate these neighborhood archetypes and further understand associations between archetypes and breast cancer survival are needed. Using mixed methods approaches, validation of the defining attributes of archetypes among residents will inform quantitative data used in LCA to develop this system [82]. For example, information from residents on the quality or usefulness of parks and food retailers likely differ across neighborhoods in ways that could differentiate their health-promoting capacity, but our secondary data does not capture these aspects of neighborhood amenities. Mapping or application of geospatial methods may be useful to further explain these findings. For example, it may be determined whether spatial clustering of archetypes is meaningful to breast cancer outcomes. Additionally, outlier neighborhoods that are defined by poor social and built environment attributes yet facilitate positive health outcomes for all residents—or alternatively, neighborhoods defined by positive social and built environments yet fail to facilitate positive health outcomes—warrant further study. Groundtruthing neighborhood archetypes in this way is important to identify how these factors may function to promote or deter good health, so that, ultimately, modifiable factors can be identified that offer opportunities to increase a community's health-promoting capacity [83–89].

Our findings also warrant further investigation into the potential pathways through which neighborhoods are differentially impacting survival for women diagnosed with breast cancer in California. For example, a key potential mediator of associations between neighborhood archetypes and breast cancer-specific survival is healthcare access and context. Health care context or geographic accessibility to healthcare has been shown to explain associations between nSES and cancer outcomes [90–93]. Thus, accounting for access to and quality of healthcare resources and facilities within these neighborhood archetypes will be helpful in understanding observed disparities. Other neighborhood dimensions that might be at play are those factors associated with spatial concentration of disadvantage, that is, discriminatory patterns to accessibility of material resources and availability of commercial infrastructure. For example, recently, Krieger et al., developed a measure of the concentration of extremes identifying neighborhoods experiencing high levels of poverty and segregation and comparing them to those that are experiencing low levels of poverty and segregation [94]. They found the greatest effects on health outcomes for infant and premature mortality within areas experiencing both socioeconomic deprivation and racial/ethnic segregation [94]. In addition, overlaying enclave status may help us better understand which types of enclave neighborhoods are protective to which subpopulations (e.g., US-born or foreign-born residents) likely to reside there.

Lastly, these findings should be replicated in other geographies, with other outcomes, and with other cancer sites. Such replication would inform as to how robust these archetypes are for understanding place-based health disparities and the potential pathways through which they impact health and contribute to disparities.

References

1. Diez Roux AV, Mair C. Neighborhoods and health. Ann NY Acad Sci. 2010;1186:125–45.
2. Kawachi I, Berkman LF. Neighborhoods and health. New York: Oxford University Press; 2003.
3. Warnecke RB, Oh A, Breen N, Gehlert S, Paskett E, Tucker KL, et al. Approaching health disparities from a population perspective: the national institutes of health centers for population health and health disparities. Am J Public Health. 2008;98:1608–15.
4. Gomez SL, Shariff-Marco S, DeRouen M, Keegan TH, Yen IH, Mujahid M, et al. The impact of neighborhood social and built environment factors across the cancer continuum: current research, methodological considerations, and future directions. Cancer. 2015;121:2314–30.
5. Banegas MP, Tao L, Altekruse S, Anderson WF, John EM, Clarke CA, et al. Heterogeneity of breast cancer subtypes and survival among Hispanic women with invasive breast cancer in California. Breast Cancer Res Treat. 2014;144:625–34.
6. Bassett MT, Krieger N. Social class and black-white differences in breast cancer survival. Am J Public Health. 1986;76:1400–3.
7. Byers TE, Wolf HJ, Bauer KR, Bolick-Aldrich S, Chen VW, Finch JL, et al. The impact of socioeconomic status on survival after cancer in the United States: findings from the National Program of Cancer Registries Patterns of Care Study. Cancer. 2008;113:582–91.
8. Chang CM, Su YC, Lai NS, Huang KY, Chien SH, Chang YH, et al. The combined effect of individual and neighborhood socioeconomic status on cancer survival rates. PloS one. 2012;7:e44325.
9. Harper S, Lynch J, Meersman SC, Breen N, Davis WW, Reichman MC. Trends in area-socioeconomic and race-ethnic disparities in Breast Cancer incidence, stage at diagnosis, screening, mortality, and survival among women ages 50 years and over (1987–2005). Cancer Epidemiol Biomark Prev. 2009;18:121–31.
10. Lian M, Perez M, Liu Y, Schootman M, Frisse A, Foldes E, et al. Neighborhood socioeconomic deprivation, tumor subtypes, and causes of death after non-metastatic invasive breast cancer diagnosis: a multilevel competing-risk analysis. Breast Cancer Res Treat. 2014;147:661–70.
11. Shariff-Marco S, Yang J, John EM, Sangaramoorthy M, Hertz A, Koo J, et al. Impact of neighborhood and individual socioeconomic status on survival after breast cancer varies by race/ethnicity: the Neighborhood and Breast Cancer Study. Cancer Epidemiol Biomark Prev. 2014;23:793–811.
12. Sprague BL, Trentham-Dietz A, Gangnon RE, Ramchandani R, Hampton JM, Robert SA, et al. Socioeconomic status and survival after an invasive breast cancer diagnosis. Cancer. 2011;117:1542–51.
13. Warner ET, Gomez SL. Impact of neighborhood racial composition and metropolitan residential segregation on disparities in breast cancer stage at diagnosis and survival between black and white women in California. J Community Health. 2010;35:398–408.
14. Yu XQ. Socioeconomic disparities in breast cancer survival: relation to stage at diagnosis, treatment and race. BMC Cancer. 2009;9:364.
15. Shariff-Marco S, Yang J, John EM, Kurian AW, Cheng I, Leung R, et al. Intersection of race/ethnicity and socioeconomic status in mortality after Breast Cancer. J Community Health. 2015;40:1287–99.
16. Shariff-Marco S, Gomez SL, Sangaramoorthy M, Yang J, Koo J, Hertz A, et al. Impact of neighborhoods and body size on survival after breast cancer diagnosis. Health Place. 2015;36:162–72.
17. Russell EF, Kramer MR, Cooper HL, Gabram-Mendola S, Senior-Crosby D, Jacob Arriola KR. Metropolitan area racial residential segregation, neighborhood racial composition, and breast cancer mortality. Cancer Causes Control. 2012;23:1519–27.
18. Russell E, Kramer MR, Cooper HLF, Thompson WW, Arriola KRJ. Residential racial composition, spatial access to care, and Breast Cancer mortality among women in Georgia. J Urban Health Bull NY Acad Med. 2011;88:1117–29.

19. Keegan THM, Quach T, Shema S, Glaser SL, Gomez SL. The influence of nativity and neighborhoods on breast cancer stage at diagnosis and survival among California Hispanic women. BMC Cancer. 2010;10:603.
20. Pruitt SL, Lee SJ, Tiro JA, Xuan L, Ruiz JM, Inrig S. Residential racial segregation and mortality among black, white, and Hispanic urban breast cancer patients in Texas, 1995–2009. Cancer. 2015;121:1845–55.
21. Keegan TH, Shariff-Marco S, Sangaramoorthy M, Koo J, Hertz A, Schupp CW, et al. Neighborhood influences on recreational physical activity and survival after breast cancer. Cancer Causes Control. 2014;25:1295–308.
22. Gomez SL, Clarke CA, Shema SJ, Chang ET, Keegan THM, Glaser SL. Disparities in Breast Cancer survival among Asian women by ethnicity and immigrant status: a population-based study. Am J Public Health. 2010;100:861–9.
23. Bemanian A, Beyer KM. Measures matter: the local exposure/isolation (LEx/Is) metrics and relationships between local-level segregation and breast cancer survival. AACR; 2017.
24. Dasgupta P, Baade PD, Aitken JF, Turrell G. Multilevel determinants of breast cancer survival: association with geographic remoteness and area-level socioeconomic disadvantage. Breast Cancer Res Treat. 2012;132:701–10.
25. Cheng I, Shariff-Marco S, Koo J, Monroe KR, Yang J, John EM, et al. Contribution of the neighborhood environment and obesity to breast cancer survival: the California Breast Cancer Survivorship Consortium. Cancer Epidemiol Biomark Prev. 2015;24:1282–90.
26. Diez Roux AV. Investigating neighborhood and area effects on health. Am J Public Health. 2001;91:1783–9.
27. Sampson RJ, Morenoff JD, Gannon-Rowley T. Assessing "neighborhood effects": social processes and new directions in research. Annual Rev Sociol. 2002;28:443–78.
28. Cummins S, Curtis S, Diez-Roux AV, Macintyre S. Understanding and representing 'place' in health research: a relational approach. Soc Sci Med. 2007;65:1825–38.
29. American Cancer Society. Cancer Facts and Figures 2018. Atlanta: American Cancer Society; 2018.
30. Lipworth L, Abelin T, Connelly RR. Socio-economic factors in the prognosis of cancer patients. J Chronic Dis. 1970;23:105–15.
31. An R, Sturm R. School and residential neighborhood food environment and diet among California youth. Am J Prev Med. 2012;42:129–35.
32. Boone-Heinonen J, Gordon-Larsen P, Kiefe CI, Shikany JM, Lewis CE, Popkin BM. Fast food restaurants and food stores: longitudinal associations with diet in young to middle-aged adults: the CARDIA study. Arch Intern Med. 2011;171:1162–70.
33. Gallo LC, Penedo FJ. Espinosa de los Monteros K, Arguelles W. Resiliency in the face of disadvantage: do Hispanic cultural characteristics protect health outcomes? J Pers. 2009;77:1707–46.
34. Jerrett M, McConnell R, Chang CC, Wolch J, Reynolds K, Lurmann F, et al. Automobile traffic around the home and attained body mass index: a longitudinal cohort study of children aged 10–18 years. Prev Med. 2010;50(Suppl 1):S50–8.
35. Krieger N. Theories for social epidemiology in the 21st century: an ecosocial perspective. Int J Epidemiol. 2001;30:668–77.
36. Lee H. The role of local food availability in explaining obesity risk among young school-aged children. Soc Sci Med. 2012;74:1193–203.
37. Meijer M, Rohl J, Bloomfield K, Grittner U. Do neighborhoods affect individual mortality? A systematic review and meta-analysis of multilevel studies. Social Sci Med. 2012;74:1204–12.
38. Osypuk TL, Diez Roux AV, Hadley C, Kandula NR. Are immigrant enclaves healthy places to live? The multi-ethnic study of Atherosclerosis. Social Sci Med. 2009;69:110–20.
39. Yen IH, Michael YL, Perdue L. Neighborhood environment in studies of health of older adults: a systematic review. Am J Prev Med. 2009;37:455–63.
40. Fang CY, Tseng M. Ethnic density and cancer: a review of the evidence. Cancer. 2018;124:1877–903.

41. Gomez SL, Glaser SL, McClure LA, Shema SJ, Kealey M, Keegan TH, et al. The California neighborhoods data system: a new resource for examining the impact of neighborhood characteristics on cancer incidence and outcomes in populations. Cancer Causes Control. 2011;22:631–47.
42. Shariff-Marco S, Von Behren J, Reynolds P, Keegan THM, Hertz A, Kwan ML, et al. Impact of social and built environment factors on body size among breast cancer survivors: the pathways study. Cancer Epidemiol Biomark Prev. 2017;26:505–15.
43. Weden MM, Bird CE, Escarce JJ, Lurie N. Neighborhood archetypes for population health research: is there no place like home? Health Place. 2011;17:289–99.
44. Klassen AC, Smith KC. The enduring and evolving relationship between social class and breast cancer burden: a review of the literature. Cancer Epidemiol. 2011;35:217–34.
45. McKenzie F, Jeffreys M. Do lifestyle or social factors explain ethnic/racial inequalities in breast cancer survival? Epidemiol Rev. 2009;31:52–66.
46. Danos DM, Ferguson TF, Simonsen NR, Leonardi C, Yu Q, Wu X-C, et al. Neighborhood disadvantage and racial disparities in colorectal cancer incidence: a population-based study in Louisiana. Ann Epidemiol. 2018;28:316–21. e2
47. DeRouen MC, Schupp CW, Koo J, Yang J, Hertz A, Shariff-Marco S, et al. Impact of individual and neighborhood factors on disparities in prostate cancer survival. Cancer Epidemiol. 2018;53:1–11.
48. Ellis L, Canchola AJ, Spiegel D, Ladabaum U, Haile R, Gomez SL. Racial and ethnic disparities in cancer survival: the contribution of tumor, sociodemographic, institutional, and neighborhood characteristics. J Clin Oncol. 2017;36:25–33.
49. Singh GK, Jemal A. Socioeconomic and racial/ethnic disparities in cancer mortality, incidence, and survival in the United States, 1950–2014: over six decades of changing patterns and widening inequalities. J Environ Public Health. 2017;2017
50. Hagenaars JA, Halman LC. Searching for ideal types: the potentialities of latent class analysis. Eur Sociol Rev. 1989;5:81–96.
51. Adams MA, Ding D, Sallis JF, Bowles HR, Ainsworth BE, Bergman P, et al. Patterns of neighborhood environment attributes related to physical activity across 11 countries: a latent class analysis. Int J Behav Nutr Phys Act. 2013;10:34.
52. Adams MA, Todd M, Kurka J, Conway TL, Cain KL, Frank LD, et al. Patterns of walkability, transit, and recreation environment for physical activity. Am J Prev Med. 2015;49:878–87.
53. Alves L, Silva S, Severo M, Costa D, Pina MF, Barros H, et al. Association between neighborhood deprivation and fruits and vegetables consumption and leisure-time physical activity: a cross-sectional multilevel analysis. BMC Public Health. 2013;13:1103.
54. Jones M, Huh J. Toward a multidimensional understanding of residential neighborhood: a latent profile analysis of Los Angeles neighborhoods and longitudinal adult excess weight. Health Place. 2014;27:134–41.
55. McDonald K, Hearst M, Farbakhsh K, Patnode C, Forsyth A, Sirard J, et al. Adolescent physical activity and the built environment: a latent class analysis approach. Health Place. 2012;18:191–8.
56. Meyer KA, Boone-Heinonen J, Duffey KJ, Rodriguez DA, Kiefe CI, Lewis CE, et al. Combined measure of neighborhood food and physical activity environments and weight-related outcomes: The CARDIA study. Health Place. 2015;33:9–18.
57. Norman GJ, Adams MA, Kerr J, Ryan S, Frank LD, Roesch SC. A latent profile analysis of neighborhood recreation environments in relation to adolescent physical activity, sedentary time, and obesity. J Public Health Manag Pract. 2010;16:411–9.
58. Palumbo A, Michael Y, Hyslop T. Latent class model characterization of neighborhood socioeconomic status. Cancer Causes Control. 2016;27:445–52.
59. Arcaya M, Reardon T, Vogel J, Andrews BK, Li W, Land T. Peer reviewed: tailoring community-based wellness initiatives with latent class analysis—Massachusetts community transformation grant projects. Prev Chronic Dis. 2014;11
60. Brownson RC, Hoehner CM, Day K, Forsyth A, Sallis JF. Measuring the built environment for physical activity: state of the science. Am J Prev Med. 2009;36:S99–123.. e12

61. Collins FS, Varmus H. A new initiative on precision medicine. N Engl J Med. 2015;372:793–5.
62. US Census Bureau. Census 2000 Summary File 3 Technical Documentation. 2002.
63. Celeux G, Soromenho G. An entropy criterion for assessing the number of clusters in a mixture model. J Classif. 1996;13:195–212.
64. Hagenaars JA, AL MC. Applied latent class analysis. Cambridge: Cambridge University Press; 2002.
65. Lanza ST, Dziak JJ, Huang L, Xu S, Collins LM. Proc LCA & Proc LTA users' guide (Version 1.3.2). Penn State: University Park, The Methodology Center; 2011.
66. Lanza ST, Rhoades BL. Latent class analysis: an alternative perspective on subgroup analysis in prevention and treatment. Prev Sci Off J Soc Prev Res. 2013;14:157–68.
67. Gomez SL, Quach T, Horn-Ross PL, Pham JT, Cockburn M, Chang ET, et al. Hidden breast cancer disparities in Asian women: disaggregating incidence rates by ethnicity and migrant status. Am J Public Health. 2010;100(Suppl 1):S125–31.
68. Keegan TH, John EM, Fish KM, Alfaro-Velcamp T, Clarke CA, Gomez SL. Breast cancer incidence patterns among California Hispanic women: differences by nativity and residence in an enclave. Cancer Epidemiol Biomark Prev. 2010;19:1208–18.
69. Williams DR, Kontos EZ, Viswanath K, Haas JS, Lathan CS, Mac Conaill LE, et al. Integrating multiple social statuses in health disparities research: the case of lung cancer. Health Serv Res. 2012;47:1255–77.
70. Williams DR, Sternthal M. Understanding racial-ethnic disparities in health: sociological contributions. J Health Soc Behav. 2010;51:S15–27.
71. Schulz AJ, Mullings LE. Gender, race, class, & health: intersectional approaches. San Francisco: Jossey-Bass; 2006.
72. Braveman PA, Cubbin C, Egerter S, Chideya S, Marchi KS, Metzler M, et al. Socioeconomic status in health research: one size does not fit all. JAMA. 2005;294:2879–88.
73. Warren Andersen S, Blot WJ, Shu XO, Sonderman JS, Steinwandel M, Hargreaves MK, et al. Associations between neighborhood environment, health behaviors, and mortality. Am J Prev Med. 2018;54:87–95.
74. Clark R, Anderson NB, Clark VR, Williams DR. Racism as a stressor for African Americans: a biopsychosocial model. Am Psychol. 1999;54:805.
75. Krieger N. Embodying inequality: a review of concepts, measures, and methods for studying health consequences of discrimination. Int J Health Serv. 1999;29:295–352.
76. Williams DR. Racial/ethnic variations in women's health: the social embeddedness of health. Am J Public Health. 2002;92:588–97.
77. Williams DR, Jackson PB. Social sources of racial disparities in health. Health Aff. 2005;24:325–34.
78. Shavers VL, Shavers BS. Racism and health inequity among Americans. J Natl Med Assoc. 2006;98:386.
79. Quach T, Nuru-Jeter A, Morris P, Allen L, Shema SJ, Winters JK, et al. Experiences and perceptions of medical discrimination among a multiethnic sample of breast cancer patients in the Greater San Francisco Bay Area, California. Am J Public Health. 2012;102:1027–34.
80. Sellers SL, Bonham V, Neighbors HW, Amell JW. Effects of racial discrimination and health behaviors on mental and physical health of middle-class African American men. Health Educ Behav. 2009;36:31–44.
81. Williams DR, Mohammed SA. Discrimination and racial disparities in health: evidence and needed research. J Behav Med. 2009;32:20–47.
82. Pluye P, Hong QN. Combining the power of stories and the power of numbers: mixed methods research and mixed studies reviews. Annu Rev Public Health. 2014;35:29–45.
83. Appleyard B. Sustainable and healthy travel choices and the built environment: analyses of green and active access to rail transit stations along individual corridors. Transp Res Rec J Transp Res Board. 2012:38–45.
84. Appleyard B. The meaning of livable streets to schoolchildren: an image mapping study of the effects of traffic on children's cognitive development of spatial knowledge. J Transp Health. 2017;5:27–41.

85. Appleyard B, Ferrell C, Carroll M, Taecker M. Toward livability ethics: a framework to guide planning, design, and engineering decisions. Transp Res Rec J Transp Res Board. 2014:62–71.
86. Appleyard B, Ferrell CE, Taecker M. Toward a typology of transit corridor livability: the transportation/land use/livability connection. Transportation Research Board 95th Annual Meeting; 2016.
87. Appleyard B, Ferrell CE, Taecker M. Transit corridor livability: realizing the potential of transportation and land use integration. Transp Res Rec. 2017;2671(1):20–30.
88. Ferrell C, Appleyard B, Taecker M, Armusewicz C, Schroder C, Casey E, et al. A Handbook for Building Livable Transit Corridors: Methods, Metrics, and Strategies (No. TCRP H-45): Transit Cooperative Research Program; 2016.
89. Kwan M-P. The limits of the neighborhood effect: contextual uncertainties in geographic, environmental health, and social science research. Ann Am Assoc Geogr. 2018:1–9.
90. Wang F, McLafferty S, Escamilla V, Luo L. Late-stage breast cancer diagnosis and health care access in Illinois. Prof Geogr. 2008;60:54–69.
91. Dai D. Black residential segregation, disparities in spatial access to health care facilities, and late-stage breast cancer diagnosis in metropolitan Detroit. Health Place. 2010;16:1038–52.
92. Onega T, Duell EJ, Shi X, Wang D, Demidenko E, Goodman D. Geographic access to cancer care in the US. Cancer. 2008;112:909–18.
93. Weaver KE, Rowland JH, Bellizzi KM, Aziz NM. Forgoing medical care because of cost: assessing disparities in healthcare access among cancer survivors living in the United States. Cancer. 2010;116:3493–504.
94. Krieger N, Waterman PD, Spasojevic J, Li W, Maduro G, Van Wye G. Public health monitoring of privilege and deprivation with the index of concentration at the extremes. Am J Public Health. 2016;106:256–63.

Chapter 11
Environmental Modification of Adult Weight Loss, Physical Activity, and Diet Intervention Effects

Shannon N. Zenk, Elizabeth Tarlov, and Amber N. Kraft

Abstract Evolving understanding of the epidemiology of breast and other cancers suggests increased body mass index (BMI) is a major risk factor. Unfortunately, more than two-thirds of US adults are overweight or obese. Despite tremendous investment by individuals, the federal government, and other groups, weight loss interventions are ineffective in achieving sustained weight loss for most individuals. Environmental factors may play a role. In this chapter, we review evidence for whether people's environments modify the effectiveness of interventions to reduce weight and improve related behavioral determinants, physical activity and diet. We identified a total of 13 studies testing environmental modification of intervention effects: two for weight loss, eight for physical activity, and three for diet interventions. We found little evidence suggesting effectiveness of interventions varied between people living in different environments. However, given the small number of studies and even smaller number of studies testing any particular environmental feature, our understanding of environmental modification of weight loss and related behavioral interventions is incomplete. We discuss limitations of the research conducted to date and next steps for research.

Keywords Environment · Neighborhood · Weight loss · Obesity · Intervention · Clinical trial · Diet · Physical activity

S. N. Zenk (✉) · A. N. Kraft
University of Illinois at Chicago, Chicago, IL, USA
e-mail: szenk@uic.edu; akraft3@uic.edu

E. Tarlov
University of Illinois at Chicago, Chicago, IL, USA

Edward Hines Jr. VA Hospital, Chicago, IL, USA
e-mail: elizabeth.tarlov@va.gov

© Springer Nature Switzerland AG 2019   255
D. Berrigan, N. A. Berger (eds.), *Geospatial Approaches to Energy Balance and Breast Cancer*, Energy Balance and Cancer 15, https://doi.org/10.1007/978-3-030-18408-7_11

11.1   Introduction

Overweight and obesity remain major threats to the public's health. Over the past decade the age-standardized prevalence of obesity [body mass index (BMI) $\geq$ 30] in U.S. adults rose from 33.7% in 2007–2008 to 39.6% in 2015–2016 [14]. The increase was particularly pronounced in women. In 2015–2016, 41.1% of women and 37.9% of men were obese. Evolving understanding of the epidemiology of breast and other cancers suggests increased body mass index (BMI) is a key risk factor. Evidence of a causal relationship is strong for many types of cancer, including post-menopausal breast cancer [26, 51]. Increased BMI is also associated with second primary cancers and poorer survival and quality of life after breast cancer diagnosis [3, 5, 7, 8, 38].

Growing research suggests that limitation of weight gain and intentional weight loss can reduce cancer risk [26]. This has been demonstrated for breast cancer as well as endometrial cancer and is buttressed by results of animal studies which have provided strong evidence that calorie restriction reduces risk of mammary gland, colon, liver, pancreas, skin, and pituitary gland cancers, with less conclusive but consistent evidence for prostate cancer, lymphoma, and leukemia. Little evidence is available regarding effects of weight reduction and weight management interventions on recurrence, survival, and other outcomes in cancer survivors [25, 52]. Several recently completed or ongoing clinical trials will help to fill those gaps [6]. Based on evidence relating obesity to risk of second primary tumors and recurrence as well as known benefits of weight loss for diabetes prevention and quality of life, current survivorship care guidelines advocate lifestyle modification and weight reduction for cancer survivors with obesity [42]. Thus, given high rates of obesity in populations at risk for cancer, strong evidence that obesity confers risk for many cancers, and known benefits of weight loss for health generally, weight management is an important goal in cancer control.

Physical activity and diet are also important targets for intervention to reduce cancer risk and improve outcomes. The 2018 Physical Activity Guidelines Advisory Committee [40] concluded that evidence is strong that physical activity is protective against bladder, colon, endometrium, esophageal adenocarcinomas, stomach, kidney, and breast cancers. Moreover, for breast cancer, a dose-response relationship between greater amounts of physical activity and lower cancer risk was supported by strong evidence. The bulk of the evidence for specific dietary components and different cancer types is suggestive of risk or protective effects, rather than strong [51]. The strongest evidence is for colorectal cancer; whole grain, dairy, and fiber intakes decrease risk while processed meat and red meat intakes increase risk. Nonetheless, research suggests that consumption of non-starchy vegetables, dairy products, and foods containing carotenoids, as well as diets high in calcium may reduce risk of pre- and/or post-menopausal breast cancer.

Because high BMI, weight gain, insufficient physical activity, and certain dietary components are important contributors to breast cancer, identifying effective approaches to decrease BMI and change behaviors that contribute to risk could help to reduce the burden of breast cancer and other cancers. Unfortunately, while behavioral interventions designed to help people lose weight can have some short-term effect, they tend to be ineffective in the long term [2, 30]. And people's responses to these weight loss interventions vary considerably [29]. Some people lose weight initially, but most begin to gain the weight back after 6–12 months [4, 30]. Other people do not lose weight or at least are unable to lose a clinically significant amount of weight, or 5–10% of their body weight [1, 9]. Weight loss interventions focused on cancer survivors and interventions to increase physical activity and improve diets observe similar heterogeneity in individual outcomes [6, 7].

What factors contribute to these variations in people's success? A variety of biological, behavioral, and psychosocial factors likely contribute [29, 49]. Less commonly recognized, or at least studied to date, is the possibility that people's environments contribute to differential response to weight loss and behavioral interventions [43]. People exposed to environments that are less conducive to physical activity and healthy eating may be less likely to initiate and sustain behaviors that support initial weight loss and longer-term weight loss maintenance. Many aspects of a neighborhood's built and social environments may be relevant, including its walkability, crime- and traffic-related safety, the accessibility of places such as parks and fitness facilities to engage in physical activity, the accessibility of different food sources such as supermarkets and fast food restaurants, and the availability, prices, and marketing of foods encountered in all these food outlets.

In this chapter, we review the evidence on environmental modification of adult weight loss, physical activity, and diet intervention effects, with a particular focus on behavioral weight loss interventions. We begin by describing two studies that compared the effectiveness of weight loss interventions for people living in different environments: EMPOWER and the Department of Veterans Affairs MOVE! Program. Because studies of weight loss interventions are sparse, and physical activity and diet are major determinants of obesity, we also provide an overview of studies examining whether the effects of physical activity and diet intervention effects on non-weight loss outcomes differed depending on characteristics of participants' environments (e.g., through stratified analyses or interaction terms in regression analyses). Because the primary interest is the interaction between intervention and environment, these do not include studies of the direct effects of environmental characteristics on body weight outcomes, physical activity, and diet, but rather the moderating effect of environmental factors on these intervention outcomes. We then discuss the state of the science and next steps for research.

11.2   Environmental Modification of Adult Weight Loss Interventions

We identified two studies that examined whether people's success in weight loss interventions differed depending on their environment. Because it is the largest and most comprehensive study to date, we describe our study of the US Department of

Veterans Affairs (VA) weight management program, MOVE!, in more detail. Table 11.1 provides an overview of these two studies' key features and findings. We begin by describing the EMPOWER study.

11.2.1 Empower

Mendez and colleagues investigated 127 participants in the EMPOWER study [32]. EMPOWER was a group-delivered weight loss intervention that involved participants setting daily goals for diet and weekly goals for physical activity, self-monitoring their diet and physical activity using a smartphone application, and weighing themselves daily. Most participants were female (90.6%) and white (81.1%); the mean age was 51.3 years (SD 10.2); and over one in three participants had an annual household income over $100,000. On average, participants weighed 201.8 lbs. at baseline (SD 32.7). Using a one-group pre-post design, Mendez and colleagues found that participants, on average, lost 17.7 lbs. (+/− 12.6), or 8.8% (+/− 6%) of their baseline body weight, by 6 months after starting the program. The study found no significant differences in weight loss by levels of neighborhood per capita grocery store/supermarket density or restaurant density, Participants living in neighborhoods (census tracts) with 25–75% black residents had the greatest weight reduction (mean = −11.84%, SD = 5.26) compared to those living in neighborhoods with <25% black residents (mean = −8.66, SD = 5.91) and those with >75% black residents (mean = −2.42, SD = 6.63). Neighborhood socioeconomic indicators (e.g., poverty rate, percentage low income) did not modify intervention effectiveness. Thus, evidence of environmental modification of intervention effects on weight loss were confined to neighborhood racial composition alone.

11.2.2 VA MOVE! Program

With colleagues, we are studying environmental modification of the behavioral weight management program, MOVE!, in the VA healthcare system. MOVE! began in 2006 and is based on an updated Diabetes Prevention Program [15, 19, 24]. VA clinical guidelines call for universal screening for obesity and referral to MOVE! or another weight management program for patients who are obese or overweight with at least one obesity-related comorbidity, unless weight loss is contraindicated. MOVE! participants receive an individualized plan to support change in diet and physical activity behaviors. Through individual or group counseling sessions and behavioral strategies including goal setting, problem solving, and relapse prevention, MOVE! addresses dietary and physical activity modifications [20, 24, 27]. Multiple evaluations have been conducted of MOVE! weight loss outcomes. A recent summary and review of these studies pointed out that weight change resulting from any MOVE! participation was between 0.95–1.84 kg at 6 months and

Table 11.1 Overview of characteristics and findings of studies testing environmental modification of weight loss interventions

Study/ Intervention	First Author	Year	Study design					Objective or self-reported	Outcome	Timepoint(s) for moderation test	Analytic Sample	Age	Environmental moderators		Objective or perceived	Findings
			Design										Construct			
EMPOWER	Mendez	2016	Pre/post					Objective	% body weight change	6 months	127	Mean = 51.2	Grocery stores		Objective	No significant associations
													Restaurants		Objective	No significant associations
													Census tract proportion black residents		Objective	Participants who lived in racially mixed neighborhoods (25–75% black) lost more weight compared to those who lived in more segregated neighborhoods (0– < 25% black).
													Census tract education		Objective	No significant associations
													Census tract annual household income		Objective	No significant associations
													Census tract household poverty rate		Objective	No significant associations
													Census tract socioeconomic disadvantage index		Objective	No significant association
													Grocery stores		Objective	No significant associations

(continued)

Table 11.1 (continued)

Study/ Intervention	First Author	Year	Study design Design	Age	Analytic Sample	Timepoint(s) for moderation test	Outcome	Objective or self-reported	Environmental moderators Construct	Objective or perceived	Findings
Weight and veterans' environments study (WAVES)	Tarlov	2018	Pre/post nonequivalent groups design	20–80	1,946,992 men; 157,402 women	6 months	BMI	Objective	Supermarkets	Objective	Compared to participants who lived closer to supermarkets, female participants who lived at least 1 mile from the nearest supermarket lost more weight, and female participants who lived at least 1.8 miles from the nearest supermarket lost the most weight. No significant associations were found for men.
									Fast-food restaurants	Objective	Male participants living near the highest number of fast-food restaurants (>76 stores within 3 miles) lost less weight than the reference group (0–13 stores). No significant associations were found for women.
									Convenience stores	Objective	Male participants who lived at least 2/3 mile from the nearest convenience store (compared to <1/3 mile) lost more weight, as did men with >6 convenience stores within 1 mile (compared to no convenience stores). No significant associations were found for women.

Zenk	2018	Pre/post nonequivalent groups design	20–80	560,173 men; 52,577 women	12, 18, and 24 months	BMI	Objective	Share of healthy food outlets (proportion of supermarkets relative to supermarkets, convenience stores, and fast-food restaurants)	Objective	No significant associations
								Supermarkets	Objective	No significant associations
								Fast food restaurants	Objective	No significant associations
								Convenience stores	Objective	No significant associations
Zenk	Under review	Pre/post nonequivalent groups design	20–80	612,750 men; 461,302 women	6, 12, 18, and 24 months	BMI	Objective	Walkability	Objective	No significant associations
								Parks	Objective	No significant associations
								Fitness facilities	Objective	No significant associations

0.13–3.3 kg at 12 months and that less than 15% of participants lost a clinically significant amount of weight [28]. Thus, MOVE! outcomes are similar to those from other evaluations of DPP-like interventions, including in regard to wide inter-individual variation in benefits obtained [28, 35].

We evaluated environmental modification of MOVE! effects using a nationwide metropolitan sample to determine whether the inter-individual variation in short- and longer-term weight loss effects was partially due to differences in people's environments. Our goal was to estimate short- and longer-term causal effects of MOVE! for subgroups of people living in different environments. We derived the sample from a cohort of males (n = 3,035,525) and females (225,590) aged 20–80 years [56]. Cohort inclusion criteria included: receipt of primary healthcare in the VA (i.e., had at least one VA healthcare encounter in the 2 years prior to baseline) between 2009 and 2014; community-dwelling (i.e., no long-stay nursing home residence at baseline) in the continental US; at least one home address geocode; and valid, clinically plausible height (at least one) and weight (at least two) measurements. We restricted the study to those living in a metropolitan county in the continental US, defined as large central metro, large fringe metro, medium metro, or small metro by the National Center for Health Statistics urban-rural classification scheme [17]. MOVE! participants were cohort members who had at least two MOVE! visits within a 6 month period and who also had no MOVE! visits within the 12 months prior to the first MOVE! visit. In addition, each MOVE! participant had to have at least one weight measurement taken around the time of his/her first MOVE! visit (e.g., +/− 30 days) and at least one weight measurement taken after that time. We created a comparison group from the remaining cohort members who did not participate in MOVE!. Propensity score analysis was used to match the comparison group to the MOVE! group on over 120 covariates [56].

Information on patients in the MOVE! and comparison groups came from the 2009–2014 VA Corporate Data Warehouse and VA/CMS data repository. These sources contain patient-level clinical and administrative data from electronic health records and other sources. Thus, we had access to clinically measured patient height and weight data. Information on patients' environments were based on their home geocodes as of September 30 of each year, obtained from VA records. Environmental measures were derived for four different neighborhood definitions, ranging from 0.25 mile to 5 miles, using an adapted "smartmap" approach [16, 56]. Using secondary data, we constructed a wide variety of environmental measures including density and proximity of supermarkets, grocery stores, fast food restaurants, convenience stores, general merchandise stores (and the relative density of "healthier" to less healthy food outlets); multiple indicators of walkability such as density of destinations, street intersection density, population density, employment density, and housing unit density; and density of recreational places such as parks and fitness facilities. Census tract and block group demographic and socioeconomic indicators (e.g., median household income, percentage of residents below the federal poverty line) are available and were used to address neighborhood-level confounding, although interpretation of independent neighborhood effects based on these compositional variables is not possible because patient-level socioeconomic indicators are not available. That is, because there is a correlation between neighborhood and individual socioeconomic factors, associations between neighborhood socioeconomic indicators and weight loss may be confounded by individual socioeconomic status [10].

We studied environmental modification using a quasi-experimental pre-post, control group design. Because we were evaluating effects of MOVE! as implemented in a real-world setting, randomization to either the intervention or control group was not possible. However, our use of a generalized difference-in-differences design with an inverse propensity score weighted comparison group lessens threats to validity associated with a cross-sectional design comparing MOVE! participants and comparisons and with a longitudinal pre-post design of only MOVE! participants. The inverse propensity score weights help ensure that MOVE! participants and comparison group members have similar characteristics at baseline. The generalized difference-in-differences regressions account for unmeasured, time-invariant confounders that may have survived the matching procedure. We examined MOVE! effects at four timepoints: 6 months, 12 months, 18 months, and 24 months after program initiation. Consistent with prior studies, we considered effects at 6 months initial or short-term program effect and used 12, 18, and 24 months as longer-term program effects. Analytic samples differ somewhat across analyses, particularly for studies of short-term and longer-term MOVE! effects. Because males in the sample tended to be older and less racially/ethnically diverse than the females, all analyses were conducted separately for males and females, and we caution that results for males and females should not be directly compared.

With regard to sample characteristics [56], most of the sample was male (over 90%). Among males, the largest share (47.1%) of MOVE! participants were aged 60–69 years; 65.4% were non-Hispanic white and 22.0% were non-Hispanic black; and the mean BMI was 35.3 (SD 6.6). Hypertension (61.8%) and hyperlipidemia (49.2%) were among the most common medical diagnoses. Among females, the largest share (34.9%) of MOVE! participants were aged 50–59; 51.8% were non-Hispanic white and 36.1% were non-Hispanic black; and the mean BMI was 34.4 (SD 6.5). Depression (40.3%), hypertension (35.3%), and hyperlipidemia (28.4%) were among the most common medical diagnoses.

Overall, we found that the MOVE! program was associated with an approximate 0.7-unit BMI reduction at 6 months in both males and females [48]. Weight regain began by 12 months in both males and females [53, 57]. Males continued to regain weight at 18 months and 24 months, while females' weight regain leveled off at 12 months. However, for both males and females, the MOVE! group had significantly lower BMI relative to baseline at all four follow-up points—even at 24 months— suggesting that participants were maintaining a healthier weight than they were at program initiation.

In our examination of the neighborhood food environment—specifically the accessibility of different types of food outlets—we found that at 6 months the MOVE! program was less effective for males living near a high number of convenience stores and fast food restaurants [48]. Specifically, at 6 months, male MOVE! participants living by the highest number of convenience stores (> = 6) within one mile reduced their BMI, on average, by 0.15 fewer units than those with no convenience store within one mile. This result was consistent when examining distance to the nearest convenience store. Furthermore, at 6 months, male MOVE! participants living by the highest number of fast food restaurants (>75) within 3 miles reduced their BMI, on average, by 0.10 fewer units than those with the fewest fast food restaurants (<14). No difference in the MOVE! effect was found by fast food restaurant proximity. In males, we also found no difference in the MOVE! effect by neighborhood supermarket availability or the relative share of supermarkets among nearby food outlets. In females, MOVE! participants living 1.0–1.79 miles and 1.80 miles or further from the nearest supermarket reduced their BMI, on average, by an additional 0.16 units and 0.20 units, respectively, than those living 0.55 mile or less from the nearest supermarket. We found no evidence that the MOVE! effect on BMI change at 6 months in females differed depending on fast food restaurant or convenience store density or proximity. We also studied whether convenience store, fast food restaurant, or supermarket density and the relative mix of supermarkets and fast food restaurants moderated the effect of MOVE! participation on BMI change at 12, 18, or 24 months [57]. We found no evidence of environmental modification of MOVE! program effectiveness at any of these time points for any of these food environment features for either males or females. These findings held when we examined food outlet density within 0.5 mile and 3 miles, proximity to the nearest food outlet, and alternative operational definitions of food outlets.

In our examination of the physical activity-related built environment, we studied whether neighborhood walkability and accessibility of parks and fitness facilities modified the effectiveness of the MOVE! program at 6, 12, 18, and 24 months [53]. We tested these effects for alternative distances (e.g., 0.25 and 1 mile for walkability, 1 mile and 3 miles for parks and fitness facilities). We also examined both density and acreage of neighborhood parks. We found no evidence that MOVE!-associated BMI change differed between those with different neighborhood environments.

11.3   Environmental Modification of Adult Physical Activity and Diet Interventions

We identified eight studies testing environmental modification of adult physical activity intervention effects and three studies focused on environmental modification of diet intervention effects. In the eight studies of physical activity interventions (summarized in Table 11.2) [21–23, 33, 34, 37, 39, 45, 54], sample sizes ranged from 94 to 423. Two of the eight studies examined environmental modification beyond 12 months. Indicators of walkability (n = 8 studies) and safety (n = 7 studies) were most commonly examined. Among the multiple environmental factors tested, little evidence of moderation effects emerges. Kerr and colleagues found larger intervention effects for men living in less walkable neighborhoods [21]. Perez and colleagues found larger intervention effects among those living in

Table 11.2 Overview of characteristics and findings of studies testing environmental modification of physical activity interventions

Study/Intervention	First author	Year	Study design			Analytic sample	Timepoint(s) for moderation test	Outcome	Objective or self-reported	Environmental moderators		Findings
			Design	Age						Construct	Objective or perceived	
Behavior change consortium NIH-funded physical activity trials	King	2006	Three independent RCTs (analyzed separately)	Means (by trial) = 61.1; 44.4; 63.0		94; 122; 256	6, 12, and 24 months (separate time periods for each of three study sites)	MVPA	Self-report	Safety	Perceived	Participants who strongly agreed that crosswalks helped walkers feel safe showed greater increases in MVPA than participants who did not strongly agree at 12 months for one study, and at 24 months for another study. For one study, participants who strongly agreed that their neighborhood was generally safe showed larger increases in MVPA at 2 years than participants who did not strongly agree. In the same study, results were consistent for the statement "my neighborhood is safe enough that I would let a 10-year old boy walk around my block alone in the daytime." for one study, participants who reported speeding drivers showed smaller increases in MVPA at 6 months than participants reporting less concern over speeding drivers.

(continued)

Table 11.2 (continued)

Study/Intervention	First author	Year	Study design					Environmental moderators		
			Design	Age	Analytic sample	Timepoint(s) for moderation test	Outcome	Objective or self-reported	Construct	Objective or perceived	Findings
Fe en Accion/faith in action	Perez	2017	Two-group cluster RCT	18–65 years	319	12 months	MVPA	Objective (MVPA) and self-report (leisure time MVPA)	Land use mix	Perceived	No significant associations
									Aesthetics	Perceived	No significant associations
									Street connectivity	Perceived	No significant associations
									Residential density	Perceived	No significant associations
									Sidewalk maintenance	Perceived	No significant associations
									Safety from traffic	Perceived	No significant associations
									Safety from crime	Perceived	No significant associations
									Neighborhood esthetics	Perceived	Participants reporting favorable neighborhood esthetics showed higher levels of MVPA (both total MVPA and leisure-time MVPA) than participants rating neighborhood esthetics less favorable.
									Neighborhood social cohesion	Perceived	No significant associations
									Access to destinations near the home	Perceived	No significant associations
									Access to recreational facilities	Perceived	No significant associations

Study	Author	Year	Design	Age	Sample	Duration	Physical activity measure	Self-report	Walkability index	Objective	Results
Lifestyle interventions and Independence for elders pilot (LIFE-P) study	King	2017	RCT	70–89 years	400	12 months	Walking for exercise/leisure, walking for errands, and gardening	Self-report		Objective	No significant associations
Patient-centered assessment and counseling for exercise and nutrition via the internet (PACEi)	Kerr	2010	RCT	Women: 18–55; men: 25–55	309 men; 286 women	12 months	Walking	Self-report	Aesthetics	Perceived	No significant associations
									Trees	Perceived	No significant associations
									Hills	Perceived	No significant associations
									Traffic safety	Perceived	No significant associations
									Speed safety	Perceived	No significant associations
									Seeing others exercising	Perceived	No significant associations
									Crime safety	Perceived	No significant associations
									Pedestrian facilities	Perceived	No significant associations
									Walkability index (calculated from residential density, street connectivity, land use mix, retail floor area ratio)	Objective	Men living in low walkable neighborhoods increased their daily walking time, while men in high walkable neighborhoods decreased their daily walking time. (no change in control group) no significant associations were found for women.

(continued)

Table 11.2 (continued)

Study/Intervention	First author	Year	Design	Age	Analytic sample	Timepoint(s) for moderation test	Outcome	Objective or self-reported	Construct	Objective or perceived	Findings
			Study design						Environmental moderators		
SHAPE	Michael	2009	Nonequivalent groups pre-post design (neighborhood-level RCT)	Mean: 74	423	3 and 6 months	Weekly minutes brisk walking	Self-report	Walkability (sidewalk coverage, connectivity, public transportation access, distribution of parks/green space, and level of automobile traffic volume)	Objective	No significant associations
Step by step study	Merom	2009	RCT	30–65; mean = 49.2	314	3 months	Weekly minutes walking	Self-report	Lighting	Perceived	No significant associations
									Close-by destinations	Perceived	No significant associations
									Access to recreational facilities	Perceived	No significant associations
									Safety	Perceived	No significant associations
									Traffic	Perceived	No significant associations
									Connectivity	Perceived	No significant associations
									Hills	Perceived	No significant associations
									Aesthetics	Perceived	Participants who rated their neighborhood's aesthetics lower increased total walking time more than participants who rated their neighborhood's aesthetics higher

Program	Author	Year	Design	Age	N	Duration	Outcomes	Objective and self-report	Walkability (composite of variables listed above)	Perceived / Objective	Findings
Women's lifestyle PA program	Schoeny	2017	RCT	40–65	288	24 and 48 weeks	Daily step counts; weekly minutes of moderate-to-vigorous physical activity (overall, leisure); weekly minutes walking	Objective and self-report	Walkability	Perceived	No significant associations
									Aggravated assault/battery rate	Objective	Intervention effects differed by neighborhood assault/battery ($p < 0.10$). Among those living in neighborhoods with high assault/battery, participants receiving group meetings had greater increases in daily steps than those in receiving group meetings plus motivated automated calls.
Women's walking program	Oh	2010	Nonequivalent groups posttest only (neighborhood-level RCT)	40–65	148	24 weeks	% of prescribed walks completed	Objective and self-report	Violent crimes	Perceived and objective	No significant associations
									Disorder crimes	Perceived and objective	No significant associations
									Gun violence	Perceived and objective	No significant associations

(continued)

Table 11.2 (continued)

Study/Intervention	Study design								Environmental moderators			
	First author	Year	Design	Age	Analytic sample	Timepoint(s) for moderation test	Outcome	Objective or self-reported	Construct	Objective or perceived	Findings
	Zenk	2009	Nonequivalent groups posttest only (neighborhood-level RCT)	40–65	252	24 weeks	% of prescribed walks completed	Objective and self-report	Crime safety	Perceived	No significant associations
									Walkability (land use mix, street intersection density, housing unit density, public transit stop density)	Objective	No significant associations
									Aesthetics	Objective	No significant associations
									Walking facilities (i.e., recreational open space; recreation centers; shopping malls)	Objective	No significant associations
									Safety (violent crime)	Objective	No significant associations

neighborhoods with better neighborhood aesthetics [39], while Merom and colleagues found larger intervention effects among those with poorer neighborhood aesthetics [33]. Intervention effects were larger in safer neighborhoods in one study [23] and in less safe neighborhoods in another study [45].

As summarized in Table 11.3, environmental modification of diet intervention effects was assessed up to 12 months after intervention initiation [13, 18, 50]. Sample sizes ranged from 156 to 249. Two studies included measures of in-store food availability. Two studies examined accessibility of food outlets. One study included perceived measures of nutrition-related neighborhood barriers (e.g., not enough restaurants with healthy choices). Jilcott Pitts and colleagues found no evidence that the density or proximity of food outlets (i.e., supermarkets, supercenters, farmers' markets, fast food restaurants, convenience/corner stores) or perceived nutrition-related neighborhood barriers moderated intervention effectiveness on blood carotenoids or self-reported diet [18]. Gustafson and colleagues found that an intervention had a greater effect on those with less supermarket access and who perceived less healthy food availability [13]. Wedick and colleagues found no evidence that the intervention had different effects depending on participants' healthy food availability [50].

11.3.1 Results for Secondary Outcomes

There is also evidence for environmental modification of intervention effects on outcomes beyond those primarily targeted by the intervention. Specifically, while diet counseling was 75% of intervention content and time, Jilcott Pitts and colleagues assessed 6 month weight change and physical activity change following a lifestyle intervention. They found that participants living in a neighborhood with a higher proportion of food outlets that tend to offer a wider selection of healthy foods (supermarkets, supercenters, farmers' markets) lost less weight on average by 6 months after program initiation than other participants [18]. In other words, participants with a less healthy mix of food outlets near their home lost more weight. The study found no evidence for a number of other environmental features: density or proximity of food outlets (supermarkets, supercenters, farmers' markets, fast food restaurants, convenience/corner stores), walkability, crime, density or proximity of physical activity venues (parks, trails, gyms/fitness facilities), or perceived physical activity-related neighborhood barriers (e.g., no street lights, speeding drivers). Few associations indicative of environmental modification of intervention effects on physical activity outcomes (pedometer measured steps, self-reported physical activity) were found. Exceptions were that increased distance to the closest private gym was associated with a greater increase in physical activity time and having a lower density of private gyms was associated with a greater increase in pedometer-measured daily steps.

Table 11.3 Overview of characteristics and findings of studies testing environmental modification of diet interventions

Study/Intervention	Study design					Timepoint(s) for moderation test	Outcome	Objective or self-reported	Environmental moderators		Findings
	First author	Year	Design	Age	Analytic aample				Construct	Objective or perceived	
Heart healthy Lenoir project	Jilcott Pitts	2017	Pre/post	Mean = 56.5	249	6 months	Body weight	Objective (blood carotenoids) and self-report	Supermarkets	Objective	No significant associations
									Fast food restaurants	Objective	No significant associations
									Farmers' markets	Objective	No significant associations
									Convenience/corner stores	Objective	No significant associations
									Share of healthy food outlets (proportion of supermarkets and farmers' markets relative to all outlets)	Objective	No significant associations
									Nutrition barriers	Perceived	No significant associations
Weightwise study	Gustafson	2012	RCT	40–64	156	16 weeks	Fruit and vegetable	Self-report	Supermarkets	Objective	Participants who lived in neighborhoods with low supermarket density increased fruit and vegetable intake more than participants living in neighborhoods with high supermarket density.

								In-store healthy food availability	Perceived	Participants who perceived lower in-store availability of healthy foods and low-fat foods increased fruit and vegetable intake more than participants who perceived high in-store availability.
Wedick	2015	RCT	Mean = 52	204	3, 6, and 12 months	Fiber, fruit and vegetable, whole grain, and overall dietary quality	Self-report	In-store healthy food availability	Objective	No significant associations
NA										

(continued)

11.4   How Do We Make Sense of the State of the Science?

As reviewed above, few studies examined environmental modification of interventions targeting adult weight loss and its proximate behavioral determinants, physical activity and diet. We identified a total of 13 studies: two weight loss interventions, eight physical activity interventions, and three diet interventions. This may be surprising given the large U.S. investment in obesity and lifestyle intervention research, our $59.8 billion weight loss industry, overall modest weight loss outcomes in interventions, and our failure to make a dent in adult obesity rates [31, 36, 47]. Many aspects of the environment including insufficient or inaccessible (e.g., due to safety concerns) pedestrian and recreational infrastructure and easy availability of energy-dense, nutrient-poor foods can make it difficult to engage in active living and healthy eating [44, 46]. Yet, as shown in Table 11.4, the number of studies testing any given environmental feature is small. Thus, understanding what features of the environment might be targeted for improvement to boost people's ability to succeed in weight loss interventions in the short- and long-term is an area ripe for research.

Studies to date provide some evidence that weight loss intervention outcomes vary for people with different residential environments, with additional corroboration of environmental modification coming from physical activity and diet interventions. In an earlier paper, we proposed that the concept of complements and substitutes from Grossman's health production theory provides a useful perspective for thinking about environmental modification of weight loss and other lifestyle interventions [12, 53]. The idea of complements and substitutes leads to competing hypotheses. On the one hand, interventions may complement environmental supports (e.g., walkable infrastructure, high availability of nutritious foods, low availability

Table 11.4 Number of environmental modification studies examining various environmental features by intervention type: weight loss, physical activity, and diet

Environmental feature	Outcome			
	Weight loss	Physical activity	Diet	Total
Supermarkets/grocery stores	2		2	4
Fast food restaurants	2		1	3
Convenience stores	2		1	3
Share of healthy food outlets	1		1	2
Food availability			2	2
Other food environment	1		2	3
Walkability	1	8		9
Recreational venues	1	3		4
Aesthetics		4		4
Other built environment		3		3
Safety		7		7
Other social environment	1	2		3
Physical environment		2		2

of energy-dense foods), leading to larger intervention effects for people living in environments with more supports. On the other hand, interventions may substitute for environmental deficits (e.g., lack of parks, high availability of unhealthy food), leading to larger intervention effects for people living in environments with more deficits. Given that racial/ethnic minorities and low SES individuals are more likely to live in neighborhoods with environmental deficits, substitution could help to reduce disparities.

As reviewed above, Mendez found participants (90% of whom were female) living in more integrated neighborhoods (25–75% black residents) lost the most weight at 6 months. As a secondary outcome in a lifestyle intervention focused primarily on diet change, Jilcott Pitts found participants (80% of whom were female) with a less healthy mix of food outlets near their home lost the most weight at 6 months. In the MOVE! program, we found that male intervention participants with low numbers of convenience stores and fast food restaurants near their home lost more weight at 6 months; and we found that female intervention participants living farther from the nearest supermarket lost the most weight. These results provide mixed support for the competing hypotheses of complementarity and substitution. Our results for men and Mendez's results are consistent with a complementarity hypothesis: intervention participants with more environmental supports lost more weight in the intervention. Our results for women and Jilcott Pitts's results are consistent with a substitution hypothesis: intervention participants facing more environmental deficits lost more weight in the intervention. Results from physical activity and diet interventions are similarly mixed in terms of their support for complementarity or substitution. If future work supports complementarity, then environmental supports may be a necessary precondition for people to succeed in their weight loss efforts. This would suggest the need for policies and other environmental changes to enhance environmental supports. If future work supports substitution, this would suggest weight loss interventions may be a beneficial strategy for those living in environments deficient in resources and could help to reduce disparities.

11.5   Next Steps for Research

The small number of studies and even smaller number of studies investigating any particular environmental feature severely limits our understanding of environmental modification of weight loss, physical activity, or diet interventions. More research is needed to address pressing questions and methodological limitations of research to date.

Critical questions include those related to the influence of "micro-scale" environmental features and the social environment on people's weight loss efforts. These more qualitative aspects of people's environments may be more influential on weight and related behaviors than the macro-level environmental features typically studied to date such as the density of supermarkets or distance to the nearest fitness facility. On the "energy in" side, studies are needed to test whether the availability, pricing, and marketing of foods encountered at point of purchase alter intervention effectiveness. While food outlet type (e.g., supermarket, convenience store, fast food restaurant) is a reasonable proxy of food availability, these features do vary within food outlet types. On the "energy out" side, features of recreational venues such as sports courts and fields and pedestrian infrastructure such as sidewalk availability may be relevant, as may their quality or maintenance. Beyond crime-related safety, little is known about how the social environment such as traffic safety, disorder, social norms, and social cohesion or other social dynamics might alter intervention effectiveness. Built environment effects on outcomes may also depend on these and other aspects of the social environment.

It remains unclear for whom the environment matters in regard to intervention success. How environmental conditions affect intervention effectiveness of subpopulations disproportionately affected by obesity, including women, racial/ethnic minorities, low SES groups, and persons with physical disabilities, is an important question. Most of these groups tend to live in environments with fewer supports for physical activity and healthy eating. If interventions are less effective for those living in poorer environments, interventions may exacerbate health disparities. To inform weight loss interventions to reduce breast cancer risk and improve survivorship outcomes, studies of pre- and post-menopausal women with longer term follow-up are needed. Ongoing breast cancer trials could add environmental measures post hoc as an initial step in this direction. Environmental features may affect weight management efforts differently in those populations, whether owing to differences in specific dietary needs, food shopping patterns, distribution of responsibilities within the family, or other factors.

Whether the environment moderates the effectiveness of other weight loss interventions is another question for future research. Efforts to test environmental modification of weight loss interventions so far have focused on behavioral/lifestyle interventions. Yet, environmental modification is also possible for other types of weight loss interventions such as bariatric surgery and should be tested [41].

Another question for future research, which we are currently studying, is how the "fit" between the environment and components of weight loss interventions affect outcomes [56]. This research is funded by the U.S. Department of Veterans Affairs. We propose that participants will lose more weight if weight loss interventions are matched to, or aligned with, environmental features. Failure to consider through intervention design and implementation the environmental contexts in which participants live, work, and play may curb intervention effectiveness. Our hypothesis is that weight loss interventions such as MOVE! will be more effective when intervention components complement environmental resources and substitute for environmental deficits. For example, participants living in neighborhoods lacking healthy foods and recreational places may benefit from intervention components (e.g., healthy food provision, on-site physical activity space) that substitute for these environmental limitations. Likewise, intervention components (e.g., pedometers or Fitbits, concentrated nutrition counseling) can complement environmental supports in participants' neighborhoods (e.g., walkability, healthy food availability), triggering or enhancing their positive effects on weight loss. To test these possibilities, our ongoing study exploits variation in four categories of intervention components (i.e., nutrition, physical activity, behavioral health, and distance supports) across the 140 facilities that deliver the VA MOVE! Program. The findings could inform intervention strategies that are tailored to participants' environments, hopefully improving weight loss outcomes.

Research is also needed to address methodological limitations of research to date. Extant studies were all secondary analyses – conducted later using available data. Most research was likely underpowered in terms of the number of study subjects and/or distinct neighborhood settings, limiting ability to detect environmental modification. Research was also typically limited to follow up of 12 months or less, and focused exclusively on residential environments. Research explicitly designed to test environmental modification is needed. This means studies that are adequately powered in terms of sample size, have sufficient environmental variation across participants, and collect environmental measures at baseline and at each follow-up point including long term. These studies could also measure other environments that may be influential such as workplaces and broader "activity spaces," or the individualized area where a person conducts activities and spends time including workplaces, schools, and locations of socialization and the routes a person travels between locations [11, 55]. Still, secondary analyses of weight loss interventions will continue to be useful, especially given that sufficient sample sizes and environmental variability may only be achieved if data are pooled across intervention studies.

The need for more research on environmental modification of weight loss interventions is highlighted in the Accumulating Data to Optimally Predict obesity Treatment (ADOPT) Core Measures Project, a recent initiative of the National Institutes of Health. The long-term goal of ADOPT is to advance knowledge of individual variability in response to weight loss interventions in order to inform more effective, tailored interventions [29]. As a first step, ADOPT proposed a conceptual framework and a core list of high-priority constructs and measures to include in weight loss interventions. In addition to biological, behavioral, and psychosocial factors that have been most commonly studied as predictors or moderators of weight loss interventions, ADOPT also proposed key environmental constructs and measures for inclusion [43]. A limitation of ADOPT's recommended environmental measures is that feasibility in terms of required expertise and resources for using the measure in a clinical trial weighed heavily into the recommendations. As a result, arguably measures that best capture the quality of people's environments and that may be most influential on intervention outcomes were ultimately not recommended.

11.6 Concluding Thoughts

Weight loss and weight loss maintenance is an important strategy to reduce breast cancer risk in postmenopausal and perhaps premenopausal women. It will also reduce risk of a dozen more cancers in both women and men. Increasing physical activity and, for some cancers, improving diet may also reduce cancer risk directly and indirectly by inducing weight loss. Identifying factors that contribute to disappointing longer-term outcomes of weight loss and related lifestyle interventions for many could help to improve or tailor these interventions. It may also help to identify necessary complementary policy or environmental interventions. Research to date on environmental modification of weight loss, physical activity, and diet interventions is limited. But extant research indicates the environment could play a role and should be explored in future studies.

Acknowledgments We thank the National Cancer Institute for supporting the writing of this chapter (R01CA172726). Funding for the Weight and Veterans' Environments Study (WAVES) was provided by the National Cancer Institute (R01CA172726) and the U.S. Department of Veterans Affairs (IIR 13-085).

References

1. Batsis JA, Gill LE, Masutani RK, et al. Weight loss interventions in older adults with obesity: a systematic review of randomized controlled trials since 2005. J Am Geriatr Soc. 2017;65(2):257–68. https://doi.org/10.1111/jgs.14514.
2. Bray GA, Frühbeck G, Ryan DH, et al. Management of obesity. Lancet. 2016;387(10031):1947–56. https://doi.org/10.1016/S0140-6736(16)00271-3.
3. Brooks JD, John EM, Mellemkjaer L, et al. Body mass index, weight change, and risk of second primary breast cancer in the WECARE study: influence of estrogen receptor status of the first breast cancer. Cancer Med. 2016;5(11):3282–91. https://doi.org/10.1002/cam4.890.
4. Brownell K. The humbling experience of treating obesity: should we persist or desist? Behav Res Ther. 2010;48:717–9. https://doi.org/10.1016/j.brat.2010.05.018.
5. Chan DSM, Vieira AR, Aune D, et al. Body mass index and survival in women with breast cancer-systematic literature review and meta-analysis of 82 follow-up studies. Ann Oncol. 2014;25(10):1901–14. https://doi.org/10.1093/annonc/mdu042.
6. Chlebowski RT, Reeves MM. Weight loss randomized intervention trials in female Cancer survivors. J Clin Oncol. 2016;34(35):4238–48. https://doi.org/10.1200/JCO.2016.69.4026.
7. Demark Wahnefried W, Schmitz KH, Alfano CM, et al. Weight management and physical activity throughout the cancer care continuum. CA-Cancer J Clin. 2018;68(1):64–89. https://doi.org/10.3322/caac.21441.
8. Druesne-Pecollo N, Touvier M, Barrandon E, Chan DS, et al. Excess body weight and second primary cancer risk after breast cancer: a systematic review and meta-analysis of prospective studies. Breast Cancer Res Treat. 2012;135(3):647–54. https://doi.org/10.1007/s10549-012-2187-1.
9. Franz MJ, Van Wormer JJ, Crain AL, et al. Weight-loss outcomes: a systematic review and meta-analysis of weight-loss clinical trials with a minimum 1-year follow-up. J Am Diet Assoc. 2007;107(10):1755–67. https://doi.org/10.1016/j.jada.2007.07.017.
10. Geronimus AT, Bound J. Use of census-based aggregate variables to proxy for socioeconomic group: evidence from national samples. Am J Epidemiol. 1998;148(5):475–86. https://doi.org/10.1093/oxfordjournals.aje.a009673.
11. Golledge RG, Stimson RJ. Spatial behavior: a geographic perspective. New York: Guilford Press; 1997.
12. Grossman M. On the concept of health capital and the demand for health. J Polit Econ. 1972;80(2):223–55. https://doi.org/10.1086/259880.
13. Gustafson AA, Sharkey J, Samuel-Hodge CD, et al. Food store environment modifies intervention effect on fruit and vegetable intake among low-income women in North Carolina. J Nutr Metab. 2012;2012:1–8. https://doi.org/10.1155/2012/932653.

14. Hales CM, Fryar CD, Carroll MD, et al. Trends in obesity and severe obesity prevalence in US youth and adults by sex and age, 2007-2008 to 2015-2016. JAMA. 2018;319(16):1723–5. https://doi.org/10.1001/jama.2018.3060.
15. Hamman RF, Wing RR, Edelstein SL, et al. Effect of weight loss with lifestyle intervention on risk of diabetes. Diabetes Care. 2006;29(9):2102–7. https://doi.org/10.2337/dc06-0560.
16. Hurvitz PM, Moudon AV. Home versus nonhome neighborhood: quantifying differences in exposure to the built environment. Am J Prev Med. 2012;42(4):411–7. https://doi.org/10.1016/j.amepre.2011.11.015.
17. Ingram DD, Franco SJ. 2013 NCHS urban-rural classification scheme for counties. U.S. Department of Health and Human Services, Centers for Disease Control and Prevention, National Center for Health Statistics, Hyattsville, Maryland; 2014.
18. Jilcott Pitts SB, Keyserling TC, Johnston LF et al. Examining the association between intervention-related changes in diet, physical activity, and weight as moderated by the food and physical activity environments among rural, southern adults. J Acad Nutr Diet 117(10):1618–1627. S2212-2672(17)30352-0; 2017.
19. Jones K. MOVE! Weight management program for veterans. 05/22 National Center for health promotion and disease prevention, U.S. Department of Veterans Affairs; (2012).
20. Kahwati LC, Lance TX, Jones KR, et al. RE-AIM evaluation of the veterans health Administration's MOVE! Weight management program. Transl Behav Med. 2011;1(4):551–60. https://doi.org/10.1007/s13142-011-0077-4.
21. Kerr J, Norman GJ, Adams MA, et al. Do neighborhood environments moderate the effect of physical activity lifestyle interventions in adults? Health Place. 2010;16(5):903–8. https://doi.org/10.1016/j.healthplace.2010.05.002.
22. King AC, Salvo D, Banda JA, et al. Preserving older adults' routine outdoor activities in contrasting neighborhood environments through a physical activity intervention. Prev Med. 2017;96:87–93. https://doi.org/10.1016/j.ypmed.2016.12.049.
23. King AC, Marcus B, Ahn D, et al. Identifying subgroups that succeed or fail with three levels of physical activity intervention: the activity counseling trial. Health Psychol. 2006;25(3):336–47. https://doi.org/10.1037/0278-6133.25.3.336.
24. Kinsinger LS, Jones KR, Kahwati L, et al. Design and dissemination of the MOVE! Weight-management program for veterans. Prev Chronic Dis. 2009;6(3):A98.
25. Kitson S, Ryan N, Mac Kintosh ML, et al. Interventions for weight reduction in obesity to improve survival in women with endometrial cancer. Cochrane Database Syst Rev. 2018;1:2. https://doi.org/10.1002/14651858.CD012513.pub2.
26. Lauby-Secretan B, Scoccianti C, Loomis D, et al. Body fatness and cancer—viewpoint of the IARC working group. N Engl J Med. 2016;375(8):794–8. https://doi.org/10.1056/NEJMsr1606602.
27. Littman AJ, Damschroder LJ, Verchinina L, et al. National evaluation of obesity screening and treatment among veterans with and without mental health disorders. Gen Hosp Psychiatry. 2015;37(1):7–13. https://doi.org/10.1016/j.genhosppsych.2014.11.005.
28. Maciejewski ML, Shepherd-Banigan M, Raffa SD, et al. Systematic review of behavioral weight management program MOVE! For veterans. Am J Prev Med. 2018;54(5):704–14. https://doi.org/10.1016/j.amepre.2018.01.029.
29. Mac Lean PS, Rothman AJ, Nicastro HL, et al. The accumulating data to optimally predict obesity treatment (ADOPT) core measures project: rationale and approach. Obesity. 2018;26:S6–S15. https://doi.org/10.1002/oby.22154.
30. MacLean PS, Wing RR, Davidso T, et al. NIH working group report: innovative research to improve maintenance of weight loss. Obesity. 2015;23(1):7–15. https://doi.org/10.1002/oby.20967.
31. Marketdata Enterprises (2017) The US weight loss & diet control market. http://www.market-dataenterprises.com/diet-market-our-specialty.
32. Mendez DD, Gary-Webb TL, Goode R, et al. Neighborhood factors and six-month weight change among overweight individuals in a weight loss intervention. Prev Med Rep. 2016;4:569–73. https://doi.org/10.1016/j.pmedr.2016.10.004.

33. Merom D, Bauman A, Phongsavan P, et al. Can a motivational intervention overcome an unsupportive environment for walking—findings from the step-by-step study. Ann Behav Med. 2009;38(2):137–46. https://doi.org/10.1007/s12160-009-9138-z.
34. Michael YL, Carlson NE. Analysis of individual social-ecological mediators and moderators and their ability to explain effect of a randomized neighborhood walking intervention. Int J Behav Nutr Phys Act. 2009;6(1):49. https://doi.org/10.1186/1479-5868-6-49.
35. Moin T, Damschroder LJ, AuYoung M, et al. Diabetes prevention program translation in the veterans health administration. Am J Prev Med. 2017;53(1):70–7. https://doi.org/10.1016/j.amepre.2016.
36. Ogden CL, Carroll MD, Flegal KM. Prevalence of obesity in the United States. JAMA. 2014;312(2):189–90. https://doi.org/10.1001/jama.2014.6228.
37. Oh AY, Zenk SN, Wilbur J, et al. Effects of perceived and objective neighborhood crime on walking frequency among midlife African American women in a home-based walking intervention. J Phys Act Health. 2010;7(4):432–41. https://doi.org/10.1123/jpah.7.4.432.
38. Park SM, Yun YH, Kim YA, et al. Prediagnosis body mass index and risk of secondary primary Cancer in male Cancer survivors: a large cohort study. J Clin Oncol. 2017;34(34):4116–24. https://doi.org/10.1200/JCO.2016.66.4920.
39. Perez LG, Kerr J, Sallis JF, et al. Perceived neighborhood environmental factors that maximize the effectiveness of a multilevel intervention promoting physical activity among Latinas. Am J Health Promot. 2018;32(2):334–43. https://doi.org/10.1177/0890117117742999.
40. Physical Activity Guidelines Advisory Committee. Physical activity guidelines advisory committee report. Washington, DC: US Department of Health and Human Services; 2008. p. A1–H14.
41. Reid RER, Carver TE, Reid TGR, et al. Effects of neighborhood walkability on physical activity and sedentary behavior long-term post-bariatric surgery. Obes Surg. 2017;27(6):1589–94. https://doi.org/10.1007/s11695-016-2494-4.
42. Runowicz CD, Leach CR, Henry NL, et al. American cancer society/American society of clinical oncology breast cancer survivorship care guidelines. J Clin Oncol. 2016;34(6):611–35. https://doi.org/10.1200/JCO.2015.64.3809.
43. Saelens BE, Arteaga SS, Berrigan D, et al. Accumulating Data to Optimally Predict Obesity Treatment (ADOPT) core measures: environmental domain. Obesity. 2018;26:S35–44. https://doi.org/10.1002/oby.22159.
44. Sallis JF, Cervero RB, Ascher W, et al. An ecological approach to creating active living communities. Annu Rev Public Health. 2006;27(1):297–322. https://doi.org/10.1146/annurev.publhealth.27.021405.102100.
45. Schoeny ME, Fogg L, Buchholz SW, et al. Barriers to physical activity as moderators of intervention effects. Prev Med Rep. 2017;5:57–64. https://doi.org/10.1016/j.pmedr.2016.11.008.
46. Story M, Kaphingst KM, Robinson-O'Brien R, et al. Creating healthy food and eating environments: policy and environmental approaches. Annu Rev Public Health. 2008;29(1):253–72. https://doi.org/10.1146/annurev.publhealth.29.020907.090926.
47. Swift A (2016) Fewer Americans in this decade want to lose weight. http://www.gallup.com/poll/198074/fewer-americans-lose-weight-past-decade.aspx2017.
48. Tarlov E, Wing C, Gordon H et al. Does effectiveness of weight management programs depend on the food environment? Evidence from a nationwide program. Health Serv Res. 2018;53:4268–4290.
49. Teixeira PJ, Carraça EV, Marques MM, et al. Successful behavior change in obesity interventions in 622 adults: a systematic review of self-regulation mediators. BMC Med. 2015;13(1):84. https://doi.org/10.1186/s12916-015-0323-6.
50. Wedick NM, Ma Y, Olendzki BC, et al. Access to healthy food stores modifies effect of a dietary intervention. Am J Prev Med. 2015;48(3):309–17. https://doi.org/10.1016/j.amepre.2014.08.020.
51. World Cancer Research Fund/American Institute for Cancer Research (2018) Diet, nutrition, physical activity and cancer: a global perspective. Continuous update project expert report. https://www.wcrf.org/dietandcancer

52. Yeganeh L, Harrison C, Vincent AJ, et al. Effects of lifestyle modification on cancer recurrence, overall survival and quality of life in gynaecological cancer survivors: a systematic review and meta-analysis. Maturitas. 2018;111:82–9. https://doi.org/10.1016/j.maturitas.2018.03.001.
53. Zenk SN, Tarlov E, Wing C et al. (Under review) Does the built environment influence the effectiveness of a nationwide behavioral weight management program?
54. Zenk SN, Wilbur J, Wang E, et al. Neighborhood environment and adherence to a walking intervention in African American women. Health Educ Behav. 2009;36(1):167–81. https://doi.org/10.1177/1090198108321249.
55. Zenk SN, Schulz AJ, Matthews SA, et al. Activity space environment and dietary and physical activity behaviors: a pilot study. Health Place. 2011;17(5):1150–61. https://doi.org/10.1016/j.healthplace.2011.05.001.
56. Zenk SN, Tarlov E, Powell LM, et al. Weight and Veterans' Environments Study (WAVES) I and II: rationale, methods, and cohort characteristics. Am J Health Promot. 2018a;32(3):779–94. https://doi.org/10.1177/0890117117694448.
57. Zenk SN, Tarlov E, Wing CM, et al. Long-term weight loss effects of a behavioral weight management program: does the community food environment matter? Int J Environ Res Public Health. 2018b;15(2):211. https://doi.org/10.3390/ijerph15020211.

Part III
Screening, Diagnosis and Beyond

Chapter 12
Geographic Influences on Screening Mammography

Elena B. Elkin

Abstract Screening mammography is generally recommended for women in their 50s and 60s and may also be appropriate for many women in their 40s and 70s. Federal regulation of mammography facilities in the 1990s, prompted by growing use and increased insurance coverage of screening, raised concerns about women's access to mammography. Since that time, a number of investigators have studied the relationship between geographic access to mammography and the use and outcomes of screening. A review of this literature finds some association between geographic access and use of screening mammography. There is less evidence for an association between geographic access to mammography and breast cancer stage at diagnosis. Despite methodologic challenges to studying these relationships and interpreting findings, results of such studies can help identify areas where geographic access to mammography can be improved. Targeted efforts to enhance geographic access to mammography may increase screening uptake in women for whom it is recommended and reduce disparities in screening use and outcomes.

Keywords Screening mammography · Geography · Access · MQSA

12.1 Introduction

Geographic influences on screening mammography have been the subject of both academic investigations and federal monitoring for at least three decades. Since the early 1990s, researchers and public health officials have studied disparities in the use of screening mammography, including geographic variation and neighborhood characteristics that may impede or facilitate access to screening. Since the early 2000s, academic and federal investigators have been analyzing geographic access,

E. B. Elkin (✉)
Department of Epidemiology and Biostatistics, Memorial Sloan Kettering Cancer Center, New York, NY, USA
e-mail: elkine@mskcc.org

© Springer Nature Switzerland AG 2019   285
D. Berrigan, N. A. Berger (eds.), *Geospatial Approaches to Energy Balance and Breast Cancer*, Energy Balance and Cancer 15, https://doi.org/10.1007/978-3-030-18408-7_12

specifically using federal and local datasets and geographic information systems to explore whether and how geography affects the use and outcomes of screening mammography.

This chapter provides an overview of the literature addressing geographic influences on screening mammography. It begins with a review of screening mammography recommendations, essential for understanding changes over time in the population eligible for and encouraged to pursue routine screening. It also provides a brief review of non-geographic factors associated the use of screening mammography. The literature on geography and mammography is subsequently reviewed in two sections: (1) studies of the relationship between geographic factors and use of mammography, and (2) studies of the relationship between geographic factors and breast cancer stage at diagnosis, a putative outcome of screening mammography. Literature on the role of mobile mammography facilities and of human resources for mammography is also addressed. Finally, the chapter considers methodologic challenges to the study of geography and mammography, as well as recommendations for future research and translations of results.

12.2 Screening Mammography Trials, Tribulations, and Recommendations

The efficacy of mammography as a breast cancer screening modality was first demonstrated in the 1970s, with the results of the Health Insurance Plan (HIP) randomized trial showing a reduction in breast cancer mortality [1]. Extended follow-up of this trial [2–4] and the results of subsequent randomized trials have shown 10%–30% relative reductions in breast cancer-specific mortality associated with mammography screening among women ages 50 and older [5–9], although not all results achieved statistical significance. Despite debate regarding methods and results of the randomized trials [10–15], international consensus emerged on the merits of routine screening mammography for women ages 50–69 [16, 17], with most industrialized countries recommending at least biennial screening mammograms for women in this age group [17–21].

Screening recommendations for women outside this age group have been much more controversial and have fluctuated over time and varied across professional organizations and expert groups, particularly in the U.S. The efficacy of routine screening is somewhat attenuated in women 40–49 compared with their older peers, with an estimated relative reduction in breast cancer mortality of about 15% [22]. Moreover, the ratio of benefit to harm may also be less favorable among women in their 40s, who have a lower absolute risk of developing cancer [23]. Through the 1990s and the first decade of the twenty-first century, women were generally encouraged to begin routine screening mammography at age 40. Population-based surveys such as the National Health Interview Survey and Behavioral Risk Factor Surveillance System Survey (BRFSS) addressed questions about screening mammography to women age 40 and older [24–27]. However, in 2009 the U.S. Preventive Services Taskforce (USPSTF) recommended *against* routine screening mammograms for women in their 40s, advising them instead to make individual decisions about screening, in collaboration with their physicians, in the context of their personal breast cancer risk, values, and preferences [28]. The USPSTF reaffirmed this recommendation in 2016 following an updated review of the evidence [29]. The American Medical Association, American College of Physicians, American Academy of Family Physicians and the American College of Preventive Medicine supported the panel's 2009 recommendation. The American College of Obstetricians and Gynecologists (ACOG) and the American College of Radiology (ACR) expressed opposition and recommended annual screening mammography starting at age 40. ACOG subsequently modified its statement, recommending that women at average risk of breast cancer be *offered* screening mammography starting at age 40 years and start no later than age 50, and explicitly stating that the decision about when to begin routine screening should be made through a shared decision-making process that includes discussion of benefits, harms, values, and preferences [30]. In 2015, following its own evidence review and analysis of population data, the American Cancer Society (ACS) recommended annual screening beginning at age 45, with an opportunity to begin screening at age 40 [31]. In 2014, the National Committee for Quality Assurance changed the breast cancer screening quality metric in the Healthcare Effectiveness Data and Information Set (HEDIS), removing women in their 40s from the denominator [32].

Experts have also disagreed on the value of screening mammography in women ages 70 and older. Of the eight original randomized trials of screening mammography, only one included women over age 70, finding a 24–27% relative reduction in breast cancer mortality among women ages 70–74, although this result was not statistically significant [33]. Non-randomized studies of screening mammography in women ages 70 and older have found cancer-specific mortality reductions between 6% and 40% [34–36]. Compared with their younger counterparts, older women face a greater risk of developing breast cancer, but also face a greater risk of death from other causes. Although regular screening mammography for older women may reduce the risk of diagnosis with late-stage disease and thereby improve prognosis [37–39], the resulting average gain in life expectancy may be small compared with the potential benefits of screening women under age 70 and with the costs and potential harms of screening [40]. Given the lack of conclusive evidence on the value of screening mammography in women age 70 and older, recommendations for this age group have been mixed. In 1992, a panel convened by the NCI recommended that screening mammography decisions for women 75 and older be based on clinical judgment [18]. The USPSTF concluded in 1996 that there was insufficient evidence for or against routine screening mammography in women 70 and older [21], and the 2002 update of these guidelines did little to clarify an upper age limit for screening [41]. In 2009, and again in 2016, the USPSTF recommended screening until age 74 [28, 29]. The ACS has not specified an age at which routine screening mammography should be terminated, so long as a woman is in generally good health with a remaining life expectancy of at least 10 years [19, 31, 42]. In the

HEDIS measure for breast cancer screening, the denominator included women up to age 69 until 2014, when it was expanded to age 74 [32]. Medicare has covered biennial screening mammography since 1991 and annual screening since 1998 [43].

12.3 Non-Geographic Correlates of Screening Mammography

Despite much debate about the value of screening in women under age 50 and over age 70, routine screening was generally recommended for women age 40 and older throughout the 1990s and 2000s. During this time, in an effort to increase screening rates and to reduce disparities in screening, numerous studies investigated factors associated with recent screening and with adherence to screening guidelines.

At the individual level, mammography utilization has been associated with demographic, economic, and psychosocial characteristics. Women who are black, Hispanic, Asian, or Native American [44–52], women with less education and lower income [48, 51, 53–61], and women living in rural areas [62] are less likely than their peers to receive screening mammography. Lack of health insurance has also been associated with lower screening mammography utilization [44, 48, 51, 52, 57, 58, 61, 63–65]. Among women with Medicare, having supplemental insurance has been correlated with a higher rate of screening mammography [45, 66, 67]. Among insured women under age 65, membership in a health maintenance organization (HMO) or in a health insurance plan with primary care gatekeeping has been associated with a greater rate of screening mammography, compared with traditional indemnity insurance plans [67–69]. In addition to demographic and economic characteristics, psychosocial factors play a role in use of screening mammography. A woman's knowledge, attitudes, beliefs and fears about cancer, screening, illness, and self-efficacy may affect her likelihood of receiving a mammogram [48, 53, 65, 70–82], and may also interact with racial differences in mammography utilization [83–85]. Lack of social support and greater caregiving responsibilities are correlated with less use of mammography [86]. Use of other preventive health services and prior receipt of a mammogram are associated with greater use of mammography [44, 55, 87].

Among the strongest predictors of screening mammography are physician factors, especially having a regular source of care [45, 57, 60, 64, 66, 88, 89] and receiving a doctor's recommendation for a mammogram [61, 70, 73, 76, 90–96]. Use of screening mammography has also been associated with physician specialty, gender, and training. Women who see a gynecologist are more likely to receive a screening mammogram than those who only see a general internist or family practitioner [48, 60, 61, 65, 68, 93, 97]. Patients of female or more experienced physicians have higher rates of screening mammography than patients of male or less experienced physicians [93, 98, 99]. In studies addressing health care market characteristics, screening mammography rates have been higher in areas with greater HMO penetration [55, 100, 101] and greater reimbursement for mammography [55]. At least two studies found that the supply of primary care physicians in an area was positively correlated with the rate of mammography utilization [55, 102].

12.4   Early Concerns About Geographic Access to Mammography

Concerns about geographic access to mammography in the U.S. emerged in the 1990s, following passage of the Mammography Quality Standards Act (MQSA). Enacted in 1992, this federal law established national uniform quality standards for mammography [103]. The MQSA mandated that all facilities providing screening or diagnostic mammography meet specific requirements for equipment and personnel as well as quality assurance and control programs. Per MQSA, all mammography facilities must be accredited by one of four approved accrediting bodies and pass an annual inspection. Facilities that meet all standards and receive accreditation are eligible for certification by the FDA, a requirement for legal operation of the facility. The FDA has authority to impose sanctions on facilities that fail to meet MQSA standards, including immediate suspension of certification. The MQSA was reauthorized by Congress in 1997 and again in 2004 [104, 105].

Since the MQSA took effect in 1994, its impact has been monitored in a series of federal reports [106–110]. In the first year of FDA inspections, two-thirds of mammography facilities were cited for one or more violations of the standards [107]. Since then compliance has increased consistently, and the MQSA is credited with substantial improvements in mammography quality [107–109]. While apparently successful in meeting its original objective of improving the quality of mammography services, at the time of its passage some observers raised concerns that MQSA-related facility closures could have the unintended consequence of reducing access to mammography. In several reports, federal analysts concluded that the MQSA did not affect access to services. From 1994 to 1997, facility closures were nearly offset by new facility openings or re-openings, and almost all facilities that closed were located within 25 miles of another certified mammography facility [108, 109]. Between 1998 and 2001, the number of certified facilities declined by about 5%, but the total number of mammography machines and radiologic technologists increased 11% and 21% respectively [110]. However, this overall increase in mammography capacity was not equally distributed across the country. A survey of selected counties found that in some metropolitan areas, demand for mammography grew while capacity declined, leading to long waiting times and temporary interruptions in mammography availability [110]. An impact assessment in Minnesota found no appreciable change in the statewide distribution of facilities in the months following implementation of the MQSA, although one rural county lost its only facility [111]. A national survey of facility closures found that 43% of closed facilities were located in minority areas [112].

As federal analysts tracked the location of mammography facilities, academic researchers began studying geographic access to screening mammography and its association with utilization and outcomes. These studies have generally fallen into two categories: (1) those that examine the relationship between geography and use of screening, and (2) those that examine the relationship between geography and stage at diagnosis. Literature in both of these areas is reviewed below. Studies published prior to 2014 were also nicely summarized in a systematic review by Khan-Gates and colleagues [113].

12.5 Geographic Access and Use of Screening Mammography

The earliest published studies examining geographic access to screening mammography generally addressed individual states, cities or metropolitan areas. For example, one of the most frequently cited early studies, published in 2002 by Engleman and colleagues, looked at the availability of mammography in Kansas, a largely rural state, and the use of screening mammography by Kansas Medicare beneficiaries in 1997 and 1998 [114]. The authors examined the distribution of fixed and mobile facilities across the state, finding that most women lived near a facility. Using Medicare claims, they found substantial variation in mammography utilization across counties, and that living further from a facility was associated with lower odds of receiving a mammogram during the 2 year period, although the magnitude of the association was small.

Subsequent studies examined the relationship between geography and mammography use in other regions of the country, including three studies published in 2009 of women in California. With self-reported mammography utilization information from the 2001 California Health Interview Survey, Meersman and colleagues found some evidence of a relationship between the number of nearby mammography facilities and the likelihood of reporting a mammogram within the past 2 years, in particular among women with one or no facilities within two miles of home, compared with women who had 11 or more facilities within two miles of home [115]. Using data from the same statewide survey conducted in 2003 and 2005, Jackson and colleagues found that the number of facilities within a three-mile radius of home was not a significant predictor of recent mammography use among women in urban areas. In rural areas, however, women who had no mammography facilities within a 12 mile radius of home were significantly less likely to report a recent mammogram than women with at least 1 facility within that distance [116]. Of some concern, both of these studies included women who reported a personal history of breast cancer. While such women represented a minority of the study cohorts, the endpoint of each analysis necessarily reflects self-reported mammography use for any reason, rather than screening mammography specifically. The third California study, by Mobley and colleagues, examined mammography use among Medicare beneficiaries in 2002–2003 [117]. By design, more than 30% of the study cohort had a diagnosis of breast cancer. Using Medicare claims to identify receipt of a mammogram, the investigators found a very small effect of distance from the nearest mammography facility on the probability of having a mammogram. The number of facilities per 1000 women age 65 and older in a woman's county of residence was not significantly associated with use of mammography.

Rahman and colleagues examined geographic access and mammography use in the six-county metropolitan area of Denver, Colorado [118]. Data were obtained from 46 facilities participating in the NCI-funded Colorado Mammography Project; these sites represented about half of all mammography facilities in the area at the time. Geographic access was measured using the two-step floating catchment area (2SFCA) method, which assigns an accessibility "score" to each woman as a function of the number of facilities and potential users of those facilities within a specified threshold travel time or distance, or catchment area [119]. The dependent variable in statistical analysis was self-report of a prior mammogram, presumably at the time of a visit for a current mammogram, in 1999–2001. Like the studies of women in California, this one also included women with a history of breast cancer. For both of these reasons, the analysis does not assess the impact of geographic accessibility on screening mammography specifically. Interestingly, the authors found that greater geographic access was associated with lower odds of having had a prior mammogram. In interpreting these findings, the authors noted limitations of the analytic methods and the absence of individual-level information on important demographic, socioeconomic, health insurance, health care, and health status characteristics.

Elting and colleagues studied the location of mammography facilities in Texas between 2002 and 2004, and use of screening mammography reported in the 2004 Behavioral Risk Factor Surveillance System (BRFSS) survey [120]. The BRFSS, a nationwide, state-based, phone survey, asks about the use of mammography for breast cancer screening within the past 2 years. The authors found that half of the 254 counties in Texas had no mammography facility, and that living in a county with at least one facility was associated with more than triple the odds of reporting a recent screening mammogram, compared with residence in a county with no facility. Not surprisingly, counties with no mammography facility tended be more sparsely populated, and their populations were less affluent, less likely to have health insurance, to speak English, and to graduate high school.

Jewett and colleagues used data from a series of population-based case-control studies to examine the relationship between geographic access and frequency of screening mammography among women in Wisconsin [121]. The study cohort included almost 6000 women aged 50–74, with no history of breast cancer, who participated in the Wisconsin Women's Health Study in 1995–2007. Measures of access included driving times to the nearest mammography facility and the number of facilities within 10 km of a woman's residence, and the primary endpoint was self-reported number of screening mammograms in the past 5 years, translated to an annual frequency. Among urban women, the effect of resource availability was non-linear: having one or two facilities within 10 km was significantly associated with more frequent screening, and with the odds of at least one screening mammogram in 2 years, but having additional facilities nearby was associated with little or no increase in screening. Among women in rural areas, the number of facilities within 10 km was not associated with frequency of screening. Driving time to the nearest mammography facility was not associated with frequency of screening among women in urban areas, and appeared to have a mixed relationship with screening among rural women.

As a result of the MQSA, a federal repository of information about screening mammography facilities grew over time. Researchers capitalized on this unique information source, and studies expanded to address the role of geography on mammography use across the country. A report prepared in 2001 for the Food and Drug Administration (FDA) found that within each state, changes over time in the number of mammography facilities per female population did not correlate with changes in estimated mammography utilization [122]. Coughlin and colleagues studied the relationship between geographic access and screening mammography using national mammography facility information, summarized at the county level in the Area Resource File, and 2002 BRFSS data from 49 states and the District of Columbia [123]. In unadjusted analyses, both number of mammography facilities per female population and number of facilities per land area were associated with report of a recent screening mammogram, though neither was statistically significant in multivariable analysis controlling for important demographic, socioeconomic, and health characteristics.

Elkin and colleagues also studied the relationship between mammography capacity and use of screening mammography nationwide. Unlike prior studies, they estimated the number of mammography machines available to women in each county, not just the number of facilities [124]. They defined "inadequate" capacity as <1.2 machines per 10,000 women age 40 and older, based on the assumption that capacity above this threshold would be required to meet the *Healthy People 2010* goal of a 70% screening rate. In separate analyses, machine capacity in 2004 was evaluated as a predictor of a screening mammogram in the past 2 years reported by respondents to the 2006 BRFSS survey, and of a claim for a mammogram in 2004–2005 in a 5% random sample of female Medicare beneficiaries with no prior diagnosis of breast cancer. In the BRFSS cohort, residence in a county with inadequate mammography capacity was associated with 11% lower odds of a mammogram in the past 2 years, and in the Medicare cohort with 14% lower odds of a mammogram for any reason, controlling for demographic, socioeconomic, and health characteristics.

The aforementioned studies all examined the relationship between some aspect of geographic access – travel distance or time, resource availability or capacity – and utilization of mammography. Others have examined access based on the location of resources relative to the population eligible for screening, without assessing actual use of screening. While these analyses cannot demonstrate a relationship between geographic access and outcomes, their characterization of potential access may be useful for public health programs and policy makers responsible for resource allocation decisions. For example, Zenk and colleagues examined the spatial distribution of facilities offering free or low-cost mammograms to women in Chicago in 2004. Estimating minimum street network distance, public transportation travel time, and shortest driving time, they found that mean and median distance and time to the nearest no- or low-cost facility decreased with increasing neighborhood poverty, suggesting that these facilities were well located for their target populations [125]. However, this effect was attenuated in neighborhoods with a high proportion of African-American residents. Peipins and colleagues conducted a similar study, examining expected public and private transportation times to the nearest mammography facility and nearest facility serving uninsured and underinsured women in 2008, among women in each census tract of the two-county metropolitan area of Atlanta, GA [126]. They found that public transportation travel times increased as the neighborhood-level measure of access to a private vehicle increased, suggesting that facilities were well located for women most likely to depend on public transit. However, census tracts with a majority of African-American residents had the longest travel times, independent of private vehicle access. Looking at potential access across the country, based on 2004–2008 Medicare claims to identify facilities and 2010 census data to identify the adult female population in each census block group, Onega and colleagues found that 67% of women lived within 10 min of the nearest mammography facility, and 85% had a travel time of 20 min of less [127]. These authors also investigated potential geographic access to breast MRI, which is still only recommended for screening in high-risk women. They found greater potential barriers to MRI, with almost 20% of women living more than 30 min from the nearest facility performing breast MRI.

Other studies of potential access have examined changes over time and characteristics of areas with no mammography capacity. Elkin and colleagues looked at changes in the number of mammography facilities and machines per population at the county level from 2000 through 2010. They found that both total facilities and machines declined by 10% over that decade, and median county capacity decreased from 1.77 machines to 1.42 machines per 10,000 women age 40 and older [128]. Interestingly, capacity increased in rural areas, but declined in counties with high initial capacity or with increasing managed care penetration, growth in the proportion of residents age 65 and older, or proportion of residents living in poverty. During that decade, 25% of all U.S. counties never had a mammography facility. In a separate study, Peipins and colleagues examined the characteristics of counties with no mammography capacity from 2003 through 2009. Compared with other counties, those with no mammography facilities had lower population density, fewer primary care physicians per population, and a lower percentage of uninsured residents [129]. Thus, while some evidence suggested improvements in access for rural populations, women in rural areas were still the most likely to face geographic barriers to mammography.

Several studies have explored the possible mechanisms by which geography influences access. Trying to understand the role of distance, Alford-Teaster and colleagues asked whether the nearest mammography facility was the one used by women who had a mammogram for any reason. Analyzing data on more than

640,000 mammography exams in the Breast Cancer Surveillance Consortium (BCSC) between 2004 and 2010, supplemented with FDA mammography facility data to account for all facilities in each BCSC registry catchment area, they found that only 35% of exams occurred at a woman's nearest facility, but more than 70% of all exams were performed at a facility within a few minutes' drive of the closest facility [130]. Based on the observation that women living in rural areas were more likely to use the closest facility than their urban peers, the investigators posited that women in areas with greater service abundance were better able or more likely to exercise choice in facilities. Although this study did not directly assess reasons for the use of a facility other than the closest one, the investigators suggested that travel time and job location may also play role, with women possibly choosing to be screened at a facility nearer their work than their residence if that choice aligns with a daily commute.

In another study using BCSC data, limited specifically to screening examinations between 2005 and 2012, Onega and colleagues found that more than 75% of women had a screening mammogram at their nearest facility, but almost of half of women who had a screening MRI did not use the nearest facility [131]. The likelihood of using the nearest facility for mammography or for MRI was influenced by race and by residence in a small town or rural area.

In order to assess the relationship between mammography capacity and appointment wait times, Elkin and colleagues surveyed all mammography facilities in 2008 in California, Connecticut, Georgia, Iowa, New Mexico, and New York. Using a simulated-patient format, a member of the research team called each facility to schedule a baseline screening mammogram at age 40, requesting the next available appointment. There was a statistically significant inverse relationship between county mammography capacity and appointment wait time: each one-unit increase in capacity (analyzed as machines per 10,000 women age 40 and older) was associated with 21% lower odds of a facility reporting a wait time greater than 1 month for the next available appointment [132].

12.6   Geography and Stage at Breast Cancer Diagnosis

As the goal of screening is to detect breast cancers before they would naturally present with symptoms, a number of investigators have studied the relationship between geographic access to screening and stage at breast cancer diagnosis. Few of these studies examine actual use of screening mammography. Rather, they implicitly or explicitly posit that areas with more mammography facilities or shorter distances to mammography facilities will have lower rates of late-stage disease. Evidence supporting these associations, reviewed below, has been mixed.

Several studies have found statistically significant or marginally significant relationships between geographic access to mammography and stage at diagnosis in women age 40 and older. In a study by Mandelblatt and colleagues of breast cancer cases diagnosed in New York City in the early 1980s, greater area mammography capacity was significantly associated with a lower risk of late-stage disease [133]. In nearly 25,000 breast cancer cases in Los Angeles diagnosed 1992–1996, Gumpertz and colleagues found that distance to the nearest mammography facility was a significant predictor of advanced disease (distant metastases or regional disease with a tumor >10 cm) for Hispanic and white women, controlling for individual and area characteristics, even though more than 95% of women lived within 5 km (about 3 miles) of a facility [134]. The authors also noted a sharply increased rate of advanced disease in the few cases living more than 15 km from a facility (~15% vs. 6% overall).

In women diagnosed with breast cancer in Kentucky in 1999–2003, Huang and colleagues found that compared with women who lived within 5 miles of the nearest mammography facility, those who lived 15 miles or more from the nearest facility had 50% higher odds of stage III (regional) or IV (distant) disease, controlling for demographic and health characteristics, health insurance, and area-level factors (adjusted OR 1.50, 95% confidence interval 1.25–1.80, p < 0.0002) [135]. Notably, compared with the aforementioned study of women in predominantly urban Los Angeles county, where nearly all women lived within 3 miles of the nearest mammography facility, in the Kentucky cohort the average travel distance to the nearest facility was 6 miles, and 15% of women diagnosed with breast cancer lived more than 15 miles from the nearest facility.

Examining breast cancer cases diagnosed 1998–2002 in the Detroit tri-county metropolitan area, and using the 2SFCA measure of spatial accessibility, Dai found that mammography access was negatively correlated with late-stage cancer diagnosis, while black residential segregation had a positive correlation [136]. Studying more than 1400 breast cancer cases diagnosed 2002–2008 in a tertiary care system in Wisconsin, Onitilo and colleagues found a trend in the relationship between distance and stage, with median travel time increasing with more advanced stage (p < 0.06) [137]. However, odds ratios for the risk of late-stage (stage III-IV) disease across different categories of travel time were not significant in multivariable analysis, likely due to the limited sample size and event rates within travel time categories.

At least eight studies have found no statistically significant relationship between geographic access to mammography and stage at breast cancer diagnosis in specific cities, states, or regions. Tarlov and colleagues examined breast cancers diagnosed 1996 through 1998 among women age 45 and older living in Chicago [138]. Neither mean distance to the five nearest mammography facilities nor proximity to public transit was associated with diagnosis at a later stage. In two studies of the entire state of Illinois by McLafferty and Wang and by Wang and colleagues, spatial access to primary care was inversely associated with late-stage breast cancer diagnosis, but travel distance to mammography was not [139, 140]. In a study of New Jersey, Roche and colleagues found that geographic clusters of late-stage breast cancer were strongly correlated with area-level sociodemographic characteristics, but not correlated with the location of mammography facilities [141]. Studying all incident breast cancers diagnosed 2000–2001 in Virginia, more than 8000 cases, Schroen and colleagues found no association between travel distance to the nearest mammography facility and either tumor size of invasive cancers or the likelihood of *in situ* disease [142]. Among the nearly 6000 breast cancer cases diagnosed in New Hampshire from 1998 through 2004, Celaya and colleagues found no significant association between travel time to the nearest mammography facility and later stage at diagnosis [143]. Similarly, looking at more than 1000 breast cancer patients in one large integrated health care system in Washington State in the 1990s, Onega and colleagues found no significant relationship between travel time to the nearest radiology facility and stage at diagnosis [144]. Exploring different analytic methods, Goovaerts found clusters of late-stage breast cancer diagnoses in three counties in Southwestern Michigan, but no significant association between late-stage diagnosis and proximity to mammography facilities [145].

Three studies that took a national perspective on geographic access to mammography and stage at breast cancer diagnosis had findings similar to those of the aforementioned studies of single cities, states, and regions. Marchik and colleagues used data from the population-based Surveillance, Epidemiology and End Results (SEER) cancer registry program, which covered about 14% of the U.S. population during the period of analysis. Among breast cancer cases diagnosed in SEER areas in 2000, there was no significant relationship between the proportion of advanced-stage cancers (stages III and IV) and the number of mammography facilities per population or per land area [146]. There was a positive correlation between number of mammography facilities per population and the incidence of *in situ* cancers in both white and African-American women, but these associations were only significant when analysis was limited to women living in counties with at least 30,000 white or African-American women, respectively. Looking only at invasive breast cancers diagnosed 2004 through 2006 in 10 states, Henry and colleagues found no association between late-stage diagnosis and either travel time to diagnosing facility or to the nearest mammography facility [147]. Finally, using U.S. Cancer Statistics Registry data for almost one million breast cancers diagnosed 2004–2009 in 40 states, Mobley and colleagues found that while some area-level characteristics were associated with late-stage diagnosis, distance to the nearest mammography provider was not [148].

12.7   Mobile Mammography Facilities

In the late 1960s, Philip Strax, a radiologist and a principal investigator of the HIP screening mammography trial, became the first person to develop and successfully operate a self-contained mobile unit for screening mammography [149]. Many, if not most, of the studies reviewed above, particularly those using FDA data on certified mammography facilities, likely included both mobile and stationary facilities in their analyses, although most did not explicitly acknowledge or describe this. Few studies, if any, included the service locations of mobile facilities, that is, the geographic locations to which mobile units travel to provide mammograms.

While in theory mobile mammography should be a mechanism for improving geographic access to screening, very few U.S. studies have explicitly examined this effect. A study by Elkin and Swartz, mapping all FDA-certified mammography facilities in 2010, as well as the service locations visited by 97 mobile facilities, found that more than 85% of mobile facilities were in metropolitan areas, and half of all mobile service locations were within 10 miles of at least 10 stationary facilities [150]. Other studies suggest that mobile mammography may increase access for underserved populations, even if stationary facilities are geographically accessible. For example, among women living in West Virginia in the 2000s, those who were screened in a mobile mammography unit were younger (40–49 vs. 50 and older), had lower income, were more likely to be uninsured, and less likely to have seen an OB/GYN or any doctor in the prior year, and have lower perceived risk of breast cancer but greater knowledge about screening than their peers who were screened at a stationary facility serving a similar part of the state [151]. A study of women screened by a university cancer center's mobile and stationary facilities in 2014 in South Carolina also found that those who used the mobile unit were younger and less likely to have health insurance [152]. The same study found that more black, Hispanic, and single women were screened by the mobile unit. Thus, even when facilities serve similar geographic areas, mobile units may be reaching a systematically different segment of the screening-eligible population. Of concern, however, women using mobile mammography may be less likely to return for recommended additional imaging [152].

12.8   Human Resources for Mammography

All of the studies reviewed here focus on the number and location of mammography facilities, under the implicit assumption that women need access to mammography equipment in order to receive and benefit from screening mammograms. This is a reasonable assumption, but it ignores the human resources that are required for screening mammography, specifically the technologists who perform mammograms and the radiologists who interpret them. Several studies in the 2000s raised concerns about the supply of qualified mammographers. Among 575 breast imaging practices that responded to a survey in 2003–2004, 29% reported unfilled positions for radiologists who read mammograms, and 30% reported unfilled mammography technologist positions [153]. In a survey of New York and New Jersey radiology residents in 2007–2008, Baxi and colleagues found mixed attitudes and beliefs about breast imaging [154]. Most respondents agreed that mammography is an attractive subspecialty because there are few calls or emergencies (81%) and because it offers flexible work schedules (84%), and that the emergence of new technology (e.g., MRI, CT) makes breast imaging more interesting (88%). However, a majority of respondents also agreed that reading mammograms is stressful (76%), that the reimbursement rate for reading mammography is too low (71%), and that the risk of malpractice in mammography is high (97%). While recent estimates suggest that the U.S. is not facing a shortage of radiologists in general [155], it is not clear whether the supply of qualified mammographers is meeting current demand and whether it will in the future. A 2016 review of job postings on the American

College of Radiology's Career Center online portal found that of all jobs specifying a subspecialty area, breast imaging accounted for the greatest proportion, and of non-breast imaging jobs, about 30% explicitly indicated interest in candidates willing to perform breast imaging [156].

12.9 Challenges in Interpreting the Literature

Despite the sizable volume of scholarship devoted to understanding geographic access to mammography and its implications for use and outcomes, numerous aspects of this literature present challenges to its interpretation. The most notable are described below, with some recommendations for readers and investigators (Table 12.1).

12.9.1 Heterogeneous Data Sources and Cohort Definitions

The studies reviewed above use a variety of data sources to identify mammography utilization and presumed outcomes (stage at diagnosis). These sources vary widely in their purpose, methods of data collection, and scope and granularity of information, as well as in the populations they represent. For example, surveys like the BRFSS

Table 12.1 Challenges and recommendations to understand geospatial data

Challenge	Recommendations
Data sources and cohorts vary across studies; screening and diagnostic mammograms not always distinguished	Data sources, cohort inclusion and exclusion criteria should be clearly described
	Mammogram as predictor or endpoint should be clearly identified as screening or diagnostic
Measures of geographic access (distance, travel time, resource availability, resource coverage) and geographic boundaries vary across studies	Access measures and boundaries should be clearly described and chosen based on research question, availability of data, and potential application of findings
Analytic methods vary across studies; individual and contextual factors are often combined	Unit of analysis should be consistent with research question
	Multi-level models should be considered when both individual and contextual factors are included
	Potential sources of residual confounding should be identified
Lack of interdisciplinary training, collaboration, and publication impairs comprehension and usability of findings across different relevant audiences	Funding mechanisms should incentivize interdisciplinary collaboration
	Graduate courses in geography and epidemiology/health services research should be cross-listed and available to students across programs or departments

and California Health Interview Survey are designed explicitly to learn about health behaviors and risk factors, and collect self-reported information about the use mammography. Medicare claims, which are designed for billing, and health system records, which track clinical care and events, collect information about mammograms actually performed. Although the latter may more reliably identify use of mammography, as they are not subject to biases in recall and reporting, they may reflect limited or non-representative populations: Medicare does not generally cover women under age 65, and patients in one health care system may differ systematically from patients in other systems, even in the same geographic region. Additionally, as previously noted, some studies of geographic access and mammography utilization included women with a history of breast cancer, self-reported or otherwise, while others excluded these women, and some used an endpoint of mammogram for any reason, while others explicitly limited their endpoint to a record or report of mammography for screening.

Studies of mammography access and cancer stage at diagnosis have predominantly used cancer registry data. Registries, in particular the SEER registries, generally have high rates of case ascertainment and therefore capture the relevant population comprehensively. But other registries vary widely in the amount and detail of cancer information, with some registries collecting granular data on numerous extent-of-disease and tumor characteristics, and others collecting much less information and in much broader categories. While researchers are clearly leveraging the range and variety of data sources available, the heterogeneity in data sources and cohort definitions may impair our ability to compare findings across studies and over time. When interpreting results, readers should note carefully the sources of data and collection methods, the sample inclusion and exclusion criteria, and the definitions of study endpoints and key predictors. Investigators should take great care to describe their data sources and make explicit their cohort and variable definitions, allowing readers to understand both the population to which results are generalizable and the scope and specificity of the study endpoint and each predictor of interest.

12.9.2   Variable Measures of Geographic Access and Boundaries

The studies reviewed here use a variety of different measures to operationalize the concept of geographic access. In a recent review of studies that used multilevel modeling to examine contextual and cancer outcomes, Zahnd and McLafferty grouped these measures in several useful categories [157]. Container measures describe the supply of a resource relative to the population intended to use the resource, such as mammography facilities or machines per female population age 40 and older. Distance measures would include the travel distance (by actual road networks) or straight-line distance ("as the crow flies") from a woman's residence to the location of the nearest mammography facility. Travel time to the nearest mammography facility – by private vehicle or public transportation – might also be included in this category. Coverage measures are based on spatial filtering procedures, and include accessibility measures based on the 2SFCA. A fourth group, not used in the studies reviewed in this chapter, are measures based on federal designations of resource shortage areas. Among the first three categories, each reflects a different conceptual approach to defining geographic access. It is not obvious that any particular measure is preferable to another, and different measures may be more or less appropriate in different contexts or to answer different questions. In the case of the relationship between mammography resources (facilities, machines) and use of mammography or breast cancer stage at diagnosis, most studies employed a distance or container measure.

Measures of travel time and distance may most closely reflect the investigator's research question, but using these measures alone omits consideration of total supply and demand for resources within a given geographic area. A woman may live very close to the nearest mammography facility, but her access to mammography could be impaired if there are many other women within the area and no other facilities. Container measures incorporate both supply of and demand for a resource within a geographic area, but they assume that all people within the area have equal access to the resource, and that they do not seek care outside of the area. Coverage measures such as the 2SFCA can address resource supply and demand *and* consideration of distance, and may therefore be preferable to distance and container measures. Lian and colleagues compared nine different geographic access measures for studying the relationship between mammographic facilities and late-stage breast cancer diagnosis among breast cancers diagnosed in Missouri in 2002–2006 using state cancer registry data [158]. Of all measures examined, two of the 2SFCA-based measures were associated with odds of late-stage breast cancer diagnosis, controlling for individual demographic characteristics and neighborhood socioeconomic status. The three measures of travel distance and time were not associated with stage at diagnosis. Perhaps more importantly, there was little correlation between travel time or distance and the 2SFCA-based measures. These findings suggest that results may vary depending on the measure of geographic accessibility. Therefore, when possible, investigators should try to use measures that incorporate both travel barriers (time or distance) and competition for resources (supply and demand). As GIS and spatial analysis procedures become increasingly integrated in popular and commonly used statistical software (e.g., SAS), and interest in geography and health grows, use of more rigorous approaches such as the 2SFCA method may become more common in the health services research and oncology literature.

A related challenge to interpreting studies of geographic access to mammography is variation in geographic thresholds, boundaries, and units of analysis. For measures of travel time and distance, when the unit of analysis is the individual woman or patient, subjects are typically georeferenced to the centroid of their census tract or zip code of residence, or to their street address, if available. In these studies, researchers must decide whether to study distance or time as a continuous or categorical measure, and if the latter, what the thresholds for different categories should be. It is fairly well accepted that different types or levels of care should have different thresholds [159]. For example, emergency and outpatient primary care services should be closer than specialty services or inpatient hospital care to be considered accessible. However, it is not necessarily clear where preventive services such as cancer screening fall on a continuum of reasonable proximity. Although it is generally considered part of primary care, screening mammography is recommended no more than once per year for women at average risk, and less frequent use (e.g., biennial) is appropriate for and may be preferred by some women. Diagnostic mammography may not be considered primary care, and patients may have greater willingness to travel in the presence of disease signs or symptoms.

In the case of container measures of geographic access, the investigator must choose a geographic container. Zahnd and McLafferty, in their of review of studies addressing a range of outcomes across different cancer types using different measures of geographic access, found that census tract was the most common unit (44% of studies included), followed by county (35%) and zip code (11%), with fewer studies using census block, metropolitan statistical area, state, or designated health service area [157]. They note that the more common units may be used for practical reasons, as they are available in many administrative data sources, and because numerous population and area characteristics – including sociodemographic and economic measures based on U.S. Census data and health care market characteristics based on other sources – have been aggregated and reported at one or more of these levels. However, these units – which reflect census data collection units, governmental jurisdictions, and, in the case of zip codes, postal delivery routes – may not be inherently associated with or meaningful to the delivery of cancer screening services or the allocation of health care resources. They also vary widely across the country in terms of their land area, population size, or both, and their boundaries may change over time. The boundaries of designated health service areas, such as primary care service areas (PCSAs) and hospital referral regions, are based on observed patterns of health care utilization, with PCSAs potentially appropriate for analyses of screening mammography. But these were used in few if any of the studies reviewed here. Ultimately, the choice of boundaries for defining container measures of geographic access or as the unit of analysis should have both conceptual and practical rationales, considering the research question and implications of findings, as well as the availability of important predictors and covariates.

12.9.3 Variation in Analytic Methods

Research design and statistical analysis are as much art as science. Consequently, for most studies, the investigator faces numerous decisions about analytic and statistical methods. In studies of associations between geographic access to mammography and its use or outcomes, investigators have used a variety of analytic approaches. While each has advantages and disadvantages, the variation across studies may impair comparisons of results.

In most studies reviewed here, the individual woman or breast cancer patient was the unit of analysis. This is an appropriate and desirable choice for making inferences, to the degree that important information regarding predictors and covariates is available at the individual level. Studies that use a geographic region as the unit of analysis, for example, comparing county-level mammography availability with county-level estimates of screening, are inherently ecological, and therefore results of such studies should not be interpreted to reflect individual effects or associations. At the same time, analyses at the individual level are subject to threats to internal validity, notably selection bias. As these studies are all observational, women who live near and far from mammography facilities, those who live in areas with many vs. few mammography machines per population, may differ in ways other than simply these respects. Nearly all of the studies reviewed here used multivariable regression methods to adjust associations for differences in other individual- and area-level characteristics. But in the non-randomized setting, it is impossible to control for all observed and unobserved potential confounders, and residual confounding likely remains to varying degrees. At a minimum, investigators should identify potential sources of residual confounding and describe, qualitatively if not quantitatively, their possible impact on conclusions.

While most studies reviewed here used multivariable regression, few used multilevel analytic methods. As noted by several authors and echoed by Zahnd and McLafferty, multilevel analyses are appropriate when individuals are geographically nested and contextual effects are of interest as key predictors of the outcome or as covariates. Multilevel analysis allows consideration of both individual-level and area-level factors, without conflating the two. In studies that use only a single-level regression model, household income, for example, is commonly defined at the area level, because it is rarely available at the individual level. It may not be clear whether the investigator conceptually considers this an area-level characteristic (a contextual effect), or is using it as a proxy for the unavailable individual-level attribute. At a minimum, investigators should make these assumptions explicit, and when possible, use multi-level regression methods to appropriately estimate and control for important individual and area characteristics.

Many of the aforementioned methodologic challenges – to both producers and consumers of the literature on geographic access to mammography – could be better addressed by enhanced interdisciplinary collaboration among investigators. Despite increasing interest among health services researchers and epidemiologists in the role of geography, and among health geographers in cancer screening, the disciplines remain rather separate in terms of training, institutions, and journals. The most useful studies, wherever they are published, involve collaboration among investigators with relevant and complementary expertise, and translation of technical terminology to facilitate comprehension by readers from different disciplinary backgrounds. Funding mechanisms that explicitly call for such interdisciplinary teams would provide an incentive for more collaboration among health services researchers, geographers, and epidemiologists to produce high-quality studies with actionable findings.

12.10 Conclusions and Policy Implications

The body of literature addressing geographic access to mammography suggests that geographic access may be positively associated with utilization of mammography, in particular for screening. However, the size of the association is probably small, and other factors likely have a greater influence on uptake of screening mammography. In some locations over some periods of time, geographic access to mammography has been associated with later stage at breast cancer diagnosis, but evidence supporting this relationship is fairly limited.

One might ask whether these questions should be pursued in future research, given the substantial number of studies already addressing them. As previously described, the number and distribution of mammography resources have changed over time, as have recommendations for breast cancer screening. In addition, health insurance reforms and changes in health care markets may influence the financial accessibility and availability of cancer screening services, including mammography. Rural areas are of particular concern, where health care access in general may be compromised by physician shortages and hospital closures. Rates of early-stage breast cancer diagnosis are lower among rural women compared with their urban peers [160]. Future studies of geographic access and its influence on the use of screening mammography will help us monitor changes in population characteristics, health insurance, and health care services, and their effects on access to care. Careful consideration of methodologic challenges and decisions may improve the quality of this literature and facilitate more appropriate comparisons across different studies.

In the absence of centralized health care planning in the U.S., one might reasonably wonder how results of these studies can be used to improve public health. At a minimum, they can help us identify areas and individuals that are underserved by the current system and therefore at risk of missing potentially beneficial cancer screenings. In areas where geographic access is correlated with use of screening mammography, a decline in the number of mammography facilities could jeopardize access for women who should be screened. Public health officials and safety net providers can better target limited resources and programs to populations in those areas. If studies reveal an increase in need, advocates can use the information to lobby for increased funding for breast cancer screening, for example, through the CDC's National Breast and Cervical Cancer Early Detection Program, which helps low-income, uninsured, and underinsured women gain access to breast and cervical cancer screening and diagnostic services in all 50 states, the District of Columbia, 6 U.S. territories, and 13 American Indian/Alaska Native tribes or tribal organizations. And in areas where screening rates decline without a concomitant change in geographic access to mammography, public health officials can devote time and resources to identifying other possible factors, such as financial barriers.

Beyond mammography, continued research in this area may yield findings relevant to other cancer screening services and preventive health behaviors, potentially informing the development and implementation of interventions – at individual and population levels – to ensure that regardless of their geographic location, people have access to the health care services designed to prevent disease or detect it early.

References

1. Shapiro S, Strax P, Venet L. Periodic breast cancer screening in reducing mortality from breast cancer. JAMA. 1971;215(11):1777–85.
2. Shapiro S, Venet W, Strax P, Venet L, Roeser R. Ten- to fourteen-year effect of screening on breast cancer mortality. J Natl Cancer Inst. 1982;69(2):349–55.
3. Shapiro S, Venet W, Strax P, Venet L. Periodic screening for breast cancer: the health insurance plan project and its sequelae, 1963–1986. Baltimore: Johns Hopkins University Press; 1988.
4. Shapiro S. Evidence on screening for breast cancer from a randomized trial. Cancer. 1977;39(suppl 6):2772–82.
5. Andersson I, Aspegren K, Janzon L, Landberg T, Lindholm K, Linell F, et al. Mammographic screening and mortality from breast cancer: the Malmo mammographic screening trial. BMJ. 1988;297(6654):943–8.
6. Bjurstam N, Bjorneld L, Duffy SW, Smith TC, Cahlin E, Erikson O, et al. The gothenburg breast cancer screening trial: preliminary results on breast cancer mortality for women aged 39–49. J Natl Cancer Inst Monogr. 1997;(22):53–5.
7. Frisell J, Lidbrink E, Hellstrom L, Rutqvist LE. Followup after 11 years—update of mortality results in the Stockholm mammographic screening trial. Breast Cancer Res Treat. 1997;45(3):263–70.
8. Roberts MM, Alexander FE, Anderson TJ, Chetty U, Donnan PT, Forrest P, et al. Edinburgh trial of screening for breast cancer: mortality at seven years. Lancet. 1990;335(8684):241–6.
9. Tabar L, Fagerberg G, Duffy SW, Day NE. The Swedish two county trial of mammographic screening for breast cancer: recent results and calculation of benefit. J Epidemiol Community Health. 1989;43(2):107–14.
10. Begg CB. The mammography controversy. Oncologist. 2003;7:174–6.
11. Duffy SW. Interpretation of the breast screening trials: a commentary on the recent paper by Gotzsche and Olsen. Breast. 2001;10(3):209–12.
12. Freedman DA, Petitti DB, Robins JM. On the efficacy of screening for breast cancer. Int J Epidemiol. 2004;33(1):43–55.
13. Gotzsche PC, Olsen O. Is screening for breast cancer with mammography justifiable? Lancet. 2000;355(9198):129–34.
14. Olsen O, Gotzsche PC. Cochrane review on screening for breast cancer with mammography. Lancet. 2001;358(9290):1340–2.
15. Olsen O, Gotzsche PC. Screening for breast cancer with mammography. Cochrane Database Syst Rev. (2001, 4).: CD001877
16. Boyle P, Autier P, Bartelink H, Baselga J, Boffetta P, Burn J, et al. European code against cancer and scientific justification: third version (2003). Ann Oncol. 2003;14(7):973–1005.
17. Fletcher SW, Black WC, Harris R, Rimer BK, Shapiro S. Report of the international workshop on screening for breast cancer. J Natl Cancer Inst. 1993;85(20):1644–56.
18. Screening recommendations of the forum panel. J Gerontol. 1992; 47 Speec No: 5.
19. Dodd GD. American cancer society guidelines from the past to the present. Cancer. 1993;72:1429–32.
20. Perry S. Recommendations of the consensus development panel on breast cancer screening. Cancer Res. 1978;38(2):476–7.
21. U.S. Preventive Services Task Force. Guide to clinical services. Baltimore: Williams and Wilkins; 1996.
22. Nelson HD, Fu R, Cantor A, Pappas M, Daeges M, Humphrey L. Effectiveness of breast cancer screening: systematic review and meta-analysis to update the 2009 U.S. preventive services task force recommendation. Ann Intern Med. 2016;164(4):244–55.
23. Mandelblatt JS, Cronin KA, Bailey S, Berry DA, de Koning HJ, Draisma G, et al. Effects of mammography screening under different screening schedules: model estimates of potential benefits and harms. Ann Intern Med. 2009;151(10):738–47.

24. Davis WW, Parsons VL, Xie D, Schenker N, Town M, Raghunathan TE, et al. State-based estimates of mammography screening rates based on information from two health surveys. Public Health Rep. 2010;125(4):567–78.
25. Gonzales FA, Willis GB, Breen N, Yan T, Cronin KA, Taplin SH, et al. An exploration of changes in the measurement of mammography in the National Health Interview Survey. Cancer Epidemiol Biomarker Prev. 2017;26(11):1611–8.
26. Hiatt RA, Klabunde C, Breen N, Swan J, Ballard-Barbash R. Cancer screening practices from National Health Interview Surveys: past, present, and future. J Natl Cancer Inst. 2002;94(24):1837–46.
27. Swan J, Breen N, Graubard BI, McNeel TS, Blackman D, Tangka FK, et al. Data and trends in cancer screening in the United States: results from the 2005 National Health Interview Survey. Cancer. 2010;116(20):4872–81.
28. U.S. Preventive Services Task Force. Screening for breast cancer: U.S. preventive services task force recommendation statement. Ann Intern Med. 2009;151(10):716–26.
29. Siu AL, Force USPST. Screening for breast cancer: U.S. preventive services task force recommendation statement. Ann Intern Med. 2016;164(4):279–96.
30. American College of Obstetricians and Gynecologists. Breast cancer risk assessment and screening in average-risk women. ACOG Practice Bulletin. 2017(179).
31. Oeffinger KC, Fontham ET, Etzioni R, Herzig A, Michaelson JS, Shih YC, et al. Breast cancer screening for women at average risk: 2015 guideline update from the American cancer society. J Amer Med Assoc. 2015;314(15):1599–614.
32. Onega T, Haas JS, Bitton A, Brackett C, Weiss J, Goodrich M, et al. Alignment of breast cancer screening guidelines, accountability metrics, and practice patterns. Am J Manag Care. 2017;23(1):35–40.
33. Tabar L, Vitak B, Chen HH, Duffy SW, Yen MF, Chiang CF, et al. The Swedish two-county trial twenty years later. Updated mortality results and new insights from long-term follow-up. Radiol Clin North Am. 2000;38(4):625–51.
34. Jonsson H, Tornberg S, Nystrom L, Lenner P. Service screening with mammography of women aged 70–74 years in Sweden: effects on breast cancer mortality. Cancer Detect Prev. 2003;27:360–9.
35. Lenner P, Jonsson H. Excess mortality from breast cancer in relation to mammography screening in northern Sweden. J Med Screen. 1997;4(1):6–9.
36. van Dijck JA, Verbeek AL, Beex LV, Hendriks JH, Holland R, Mravunac M, et al. Breast-cancer mortality in a non-randomized trial on mammographic screening in women over age 65. Int J Cancer. 1997;70(2):164–8.
37. McCarthy EP, Burns RB, Freunds KM, Ash AS, Shwartz M, Marwill SL, et al. Mammography use, breast cancer stage at diagnosis, and survival among older women. J Am Geriatr Soc. 2000;48(10):1226–33.
38. Smith-Bindman R, Kerlikowske K, Gebretsadik T, Newman J. Is screening mammography effective in elderly women? Am J Med. 2000;108:112–9.
39. Solin LJ, Schultz DJ, Legoretta AP, Goodman RL. Downstaging of breast carcinomas in older women associated with mammographic screening. Breast J. 1999;5(2):94–100.
40. Kerlikowske K, Salzmann P, Phillips KA, Cauley JA, Cummings SR. Continuing screening mammography in women aged 70 to 79 years: impact on life expectancy and cost-effectiveness. JAMA. 1999;282(22):2156–63.
41. U.S. Preventive Services Task Force. Screening for breast cancer: recommendations and rationale. Ann Intern Med. 2002;137(5 Part 1):344–6.
42. Leitch AM, Dodd GD, Costanza M, Linver M, Pressman P, McGinnis L, et al. American cancer society guidelines for the early detection of breast cancer: update 1997. CA Cancer J Clin. 1997;47(3):150–3.
43. Sabogal F, Merrill SS, Packel L. Mammography rescreening among older California women. Health Care Financ Rev. 2001;22(4):63–75.
44. Blanchard K, Colbert JA, Puri D, Weissman J, Moy B, Kopans DB, et al. Mammographic screening: patterns of use and estimated impact on breast carcinoma survival. Cancer. 2004;101(3):495–507.

45. Blustein J. Medicare coverage, supplemental insurance, and the use of mammography by older women. New Engl J Med. 1995;332(17):1138–43.
46. Burns RB, McCarthy EP, Freund KM, Marwill SL, Shwartz M, Ash A, et al. Black women receive less mammography even with similar use of primary care. Ann Intern Med. 1996;125(3):173–82.
47. Gilliland FD, Rosenberg RD, Hunt WC, Stauber P, Key CR. Patterns of mammography use among Hispanic, American Indian, and non-hispanic white women in New Mexico, 1994–1997. Am J Epidemiol. 2000;152(5):432–7.
48. Lee JR, Vogel VG. Who uses screening mammography regularly? Cancer Epidemiol Biomarker Prev. 1995;4(8):901–6.
49. McCarthy EP, Burns RB, Coughlin SS, Freund KM, Rice J, Marwill SL, et al. Mammography use helps to explain differences in breast cancer stage at diagnosis between older black and white women. Ann Intern Med. 1998;128(9):729–36.
50. Preston JA, Scinto JD, Ni W, Wang Y, Galusha D, Schulz AF, et al. Mammography underutilization among older women in Connecticut. J Am Geriatr Soc. 1997;45(11):1310–4.
51. Rahman SM, Dignan MB, Shelton BJ. Factors influencing adherence to guidelines for screening mammography among women aged 40 years and older. Ethn Dis. 2003;13(4):477–84.
52. Swan J, Breen N, Coates RJ, Rimer BK, Lee NC. Progress in cancer screening practices in the United States: results from the 2000 National Health Interview Survey. Cancer. 2003;97(6):1528–40.
53. Facione NC. Breast cancer screening in relation to access to health services. Oncol Nurs Forum. 1999;26(4):689–96.
54. Kruse J, Phillips DM. Factors influencing women's decision to undergo mammography. Obstet Gynecol. 1987;70(5):744–8.
55. Phillips KA, Kerlikowske K, Baker LC, Chang SW, Brown ML. Factors associated with women's adherence to mammography screening guidelines. Health Serv Res. 1998;33(1):29–53.
56. Potvin L, Camirand J, Beland F. Patterns of health services utilization and mammography use among women aged 50–59 years in the Quebec Medicare system. Med Care. 1995;33(5):515–30.
57. Rakowski W, Breen N, Meissner H, Rimer BK, Vernon SW, Clark MA, et al. Prevalence and correlates of repeat mammography among women aged 55–79 in the Year 2000 National Health Interview Survey. Prev Med. 2004;39(1):1–10.
58. Schootman M, Jeffe DB, Reschke AH, Aft RL. Disparities related to socioeconomic status and access to medical care remain in the United States among women who never had a mammogram. Cancer Causes Control. 2003;14(5):419–25.
59. Taplin SH, Ichikawa L, Yood MU, Manos MM, Geiger AM, Weinmann S, et al. Reason for late-stage breast cancer: absence of screening or detection, or breakdown in follow-up? J Natl Cancer Inst. 2004;96(20):1518–27.
60. Urban N, Anderson GL, Peacock S. Mammography screening: how important is cost as a barrier to use? Am J Public Health. 1994;84(1):50–5.
61. Zapka JG, Hosmer D, Costanza ME, Harris DR, Stoddard A. Changes in mammography use: economic, need, and service factors. Am J Public Health. 1992;82(10):1345–51.
62. Bryant H, Mah Z. Breast cancer screening attitudes and behaviors of rural and urban women. Prev Med. 1992;21(4):405–18.
63. Adams EK, Florence CS, Thorpe KE, Becker ER, Joski PJ. Preventive care: female cancer screening, 1996–2000. Am J Prev Med. 2003;25(4):301–7.
64. Rao RS, Graubard BI, Breen N, Gastwirth JL. Understanding the factors underlying disparities in cancer screening rates using the Peters-Belson approach: results from the 1998 National Health Interview Survey. Med Care. 2004;42(8):789–800.
65. Taylor VM, Taplin SH, Urban N, White E, Peacock S. Repeat mammography use among women ages 50–75. Cancer Epidemiol Biomarker Prev. 1995;4(4):409–13.
66. Kelaher M, Stellman JM. The impact of medicare funding on the use of mammography among older women: implications for improving access to screening. Prev Med. 2000;31(6):658–64.

67. Makuc DM, Freid VM, Parsons PE. Health insurance and cancer screening among women. Hyattsville: National Center for Health Statistics; 1994. Contract No.: 254
68. Haggstrom DA, Phillips KA, Liang SY, Haas JS, Tye S, Kerlikowske K. Variation in screening mammography and Papanicolaou smear by primary care physician specialty and gatekeeper plan (United States). Cancer Causes Control. 2004;15(9):883–92.
69. Phillips KA, Haas JS, Liang SY, Baker LC, Tye S, Kerlikowske K, et al. Are gatekeeper requirements associated with cancer screening utilization? Health Serv Res. 2004;39(1):153–78.
70. Barr JK, Reisine S, Wang Y, Holmboe EF, Cohen KL, Van Hoof TJ, et al. Factors influencing mammography use among women in medicare managed care. Health Care Financ Rev. 2001;22(4):49–61.
71. Carney PA, Harwood BG, Weiss JE, Eliassen MS, Goodrich ME. Factors associated with interval adherence to mammography screening in a population-based sample of New Hampshire women. Cancer. 2002;95(2):219–27.
72. Finney Rutten LJ, Iannotti RJ. Health beliefs, salience of breast cancer family history, and involvement with breast cancer issues: adherence to annual mammography screening recommendations. Cancer Detect Prev. 2003;27(5):353–9.
73. Finney Rutten LJ, Nelson DE, Meissner HI. Examination of population-wide trends in barriers to cancer screening from a diffusion of innovation perspective (1987–2000). Prev Med. 2004;38(3):258–68.
74. Halabi S, Skinner CS, Samsa GP, Strigo TS, Crawford YS, Rimer BK. Factors associated with repeat mammography screening. J Fam Pract. 2000;49(12):1104–12.
75. Harper AP. Mammography utilization in the poor and medically underserved. Cancer. 1993;72(4 Suppl):1478–82.
76. Lerman C, Rimer B, Trock B, Balshem A, Engstrom PF. Factors associated with repeat adherence to breast cancer screening. Prev Med. 1990;19(3):279–90.
77. Lerman C, Daly M, Sands C, Balshem A, Lustbader E, Heggan T, et al. Mammography adherence and psychological distress among women at risk for breast cancer. J Natl Cancer Inst. 1993;85(13):1074–80.
78. Rimer BK, Trock B, Engstrom PF, Lerman C, King E. Why do some women get regular mammograms? Am J Prev Med. 1991;7(2):69–74.
79. Stein JA, Fox SA, Murata PJ. The influence of ethnicity, socioeconomic status, and psychological barriers on use of mammography. J Health Soc Behav. 1991;32(2):101–13.
80. Stein JA, Fox SA, Murata PJ, Morisky DE. Mammography usage and the health belief model. Health Educ Q. 1992;19(4):447–62.
81. Stomper PC, Gelman RS, Meyer JE, Gross GS. New England mammography survey: public misconceptions of breast cancer incidence. Breast Dis. 1990;3:1–7.
82. White E, Urban N, Taylor V. Mammography utilization, public health impact, and cost-effectiveness in the United States. Annu Rev Public Health. 1993;14:605–33.
83. Calvocoressi L, Kasl SV, Lee CH, Stolar M, Claus EB, Jones BA. A prospective study of perceived susceptibility to breast cancer and nonadherence to mammography screening guidelines in African American and white women ages 40–79 years. Cancer Epidemiol Biomarker Prev. 2004;13(12):2096–105.
84. Glanz K, Resch N, Lerman C, Rimer BK. Black-white differences in factors influencing mammography use among employed female health maintenance organization members. Ethn Health. 1996;1(3):207–20.
85. Jepson C, Kessler LG, Portnoy B, Gibbs T. Black-white differences in cancer prevention knowledge and behavior. Am J Public Health. 1991;81(4):501–4.
86. Messina CR, Lane DS, Glanz K, West DS, Taylor V, Frishman W, et al. Relationship of social support and social burden to repeated breast cancer screening in the women's health initiative. Health Psychol. 2004;23(6):582–94.
87. Vernon SW, Laville EA, Jackson GL. Participation in breast screening programs: a review. Soc Sci Med. 1990;30(10):1107–18.

88. Lane DS, Caplan LS, Grimson R. Trends in mammography use and their relation to physician and other factors. Cancer Detect Prev. 1996;20(4):332–41.
89. Zapka JG, Stoddard A, Maul L, Costanza ME. Interval adherence to mammography screening guidelines. Med Care. 1991;29(8):697–707.
90. Fox SA, Murata PJ, Stein JA. The impact of physician compliance on screening mammography for older women. Arch Intern Med. 1991;151(1):50–6.
91. Hawley ST, Earp JA, O'Malley M, Ricketts TC. The role of physician recommendation in women's mammography use: is it a 2-stage process? Med Care. 2000;38(4):392–403.
92. Howe HL. Repeat mammography among women over 50 years of age. Am J Prev Med. 1992;8(3):182–5.
93. Lurie N, Slater J, McGovern P, Ekstrum J, Quam L, Margolis K. Preventive care for women. Does the sex of the physician matter? N Engl J Med. 1993;329(7):478–82.
94. Roetzheim R, Fox SA, Leake B, Houn F. The influence of risk factors on breast carcinoma screening of medicare-insured older women. National Cancer Institute Breast Cancer Screening Consortium. Cancer. 1996;78(12):2526–34.
95. Stoddard AM, Rimer BK, Lane D, Fox SA, Lipkus I, Luckmann R, et al. Underusers of mammogram screening: stage of adoption in five U.S. subpopulations. The NCI Breast Cancer Screening Consortium. Prev Med. 1998;27(3):478–87.
96. Taplin SH, Urban N, Taylor VM, Savarino J. Conflicting national recommendations and the use of screening mammography: does the physician's recommendation matter? J Am Board Fam Pract. 1997;10(2):88–95.
97. Finison KS, Wellins CA, Wennberg DE, Lucas FL. Screening mammography rates by specialty of the usual care physician. Eff Clin Pract. 1999;2(3):120–5.
98. Burns RB, Freund KM, Ash A, Shwartz M, Antab L, Hall R. Who gets repeat screening mammography: the role of the physician. J Gen Intern Med. 1995;10(9):520–2.
99. Lurie N, Margolis KL, McGovern PG, Mink PJ, Slater JS. Why do patients of female physicians have higher rates of breast and cervical cancer screening? J Gen Intern Med. 1997;12(1):34–43.
100. Baker LC, Phillips KA, Haas JS, Liang SY, Sonneborn D. The effect of area HMO market share on cancer screening. Health Serv Res. 2004;39(6 Pt 1):1751–72.
101. Decker SL, Hempstead K. HMO penetration and quality of care: the case of breast cancer. J Health Care Financ. 1999;26(1):18–32.
102. Ferrante JM, Gonzalez EC, Pal N, Roetzheim RG. Effects of physician supply on early detection of breast cancer. J Am Board Fam Pract. 2000;13(6):408–14.
103. Mammography Quality Standards Act, Pub. L. No. 102–539, 106 Stat. 3547(1992).
104. Mammography Quality Standards Reauthorization Act of 1998, Pub. L. No. PL 105–248(1998).
105. Mammography Quality Standards Reauthorization Act of 2004, Pub. L. No. PL 108–365(2004).
106. U.S. General Accounting Office. Mammography services: initial impact of new federal law has been positive. Washington, DC: U.S. General Accounting Office; 1995. Report No.: GAO/HEHS-96-17
107. U.S. General Accounting Officee. FDA's mammography inspections: while some problems need attention, facility compliance is growing. Washington, DC: U.S. General Accounting Office; 1997. Report No.: GAO/HEHS-97-25
108. U.S. General Accounting Office. Mammography services: impact of federal legislation on quality, access and health outcomes. Washington, DC: U.S. General Accounting Office; 1997. Report No.: GAO/HEHS-98-11
109. U.S. General Accounting Office. Mammography quality standards act: X-ray quality improved, access unaffected, but impact on health outcomes unknown. Washington, DC: U.S. General Accounting Office; 1998. Report No.: GAO/T-HEHS-98-164
110. U.S. Government Accountability Office. Mammography: capacity generally exists to deliver services. Washington, DC: U.S. General Accounting Office; 2002. Report No.: GAO-02-532

111. Korn JE, Casey-Paal A, Lazovich D, Ball J, Slater JS. Impact of the mammography quality standards act on access in Minnesota. Public Health Rep. 1997;112(2):142–5.
112. Fischer R, Houn F, Van De Griek A, Tucker SA, Meyers D, Murphy M, et al. The impact of the mammography quality standards act on the availability of mammography facilities. Prev Med. 1998;27:697–701.
113. Khan-Gates JA, Ersek JL, Eberth JM, Adams SA, Pruitt SL. Geographic access to mammography and its relationship to breast cancer screening and stage at diagnosis: a systematic review. Womens Health Issues. 2015;25(5):482–93.
114. Engelman KK, Hawley DB, Gazaway R, Mosier MC, Ahluwalia JS, Ellerbeck EF. Impact of geographic barriers on the utilization of mammograms by older rural women. J Am Geriatr Soc. 2002;50(1):62–8.
115. Meersman SC, Breen N, Pickle LW, Meissner HI, Simon P. Access to mammography screening in a large urban population: a multi-level analysis. Cancer Causes Control. 2009;20(8):1469–82.
116. Jackson MC, Davis WW, Waldron W, McNeel TS, Pfeiffer R, Breen N. Impact of geography on mammography use in California. Cancer Causes Control. 2009;20(8):1339–53.
117. Mobley LR, Kuo TM, Clayton LJ, Evans WD. Mammography facilities are accessible, so why is utilization so low? Cancer Causes Control. 2009;20(6):1017–28.
118. Rahman S, Price JH, Dignan M, Rahman S, Lindquist PS, Jordan TR. Access to mammography facilities and detection of breast cancer by screening mammography: a GIS approach. Int J Cancer Prev. 2009;2(6):403–13.
119. Luo W, Wang F. Measures of spatial accessibility to health care in a GIS environment: synthesis and case study in the Chicago region. Environ Plann B Plann Des. 2003;30:865–84.
120. Elting LS, Cooksley CD, Bekele BN, Giordano SH, Shih YC, Lovell KK, et al. Mammography capacity impact on screening rates and breast cancer stage at diagnosis. Am J Prev Med. 2009;37(2):102–8.
121. Jewett PI, Gangnon RE, Elkin E, Hampton JM, Jacobs EA, Malecki K, et al. Geographic access to mammography facilities and frequency of mammography screening. Ann Epidemiol. 2018;28(2):65–71 e2.
122. Assessment of the Availability of Mammography Services: Final Report. Lexington: Eastern Research Groupm, Inc. Prepared for the Office of Policy, Planning, and Legislation, Food and Drug Administration; 2001.
123. Coughlin SS, Leadbetter S, Richards T, Sabatino SA. Contextual analysis of breast and cervical cancer screening and factors associated with health care access among United States women, 2002. Soc Sci Med. 2008;66(2):260–75.
124. Elkin EB, Ishill NM, Snow JG, Panageas KS, Bach PB, Liberman L, et al. Geographic access and the use of screening mammography. Med Care. 2010;. in press
125. Zenk SN, Tarlov E, Sun J. Spatial equity in facilities providing low- or no-fee screening mammography in Chicago neighborhoods. J Urban Health. 2006;83(2):195–210.
126. Peipins LA, Graham S, Young R, Lewis B, Foster S, Flanagan B, et al. Time and distance barriers to mammography facilities in the Atlanta metropolitan area. J Community Health. 2011;36(4):675–83.
127. Onega T, Hubbard R, Hill D, Lee CI, Haas JS, Carlos HA, et al. Geographic access to breast imaging for US women. J Am Coll Radiol. 2014;11(9):874–82.
128. Elkin EB, Atoria CL, Leoce N, Bach PB, Schrag D. Changes in the availability of screening mammography, 2000–2010. Cancer. 2013;119(21):3847–53.
129. Peipins LA, Miller J, Richards TB, Bobo JK, Liu T, White MC, et al. Characteristics of US counties with no mammography capacity. J Community Health. 2012;37(6):1239–48.
130. Alford-Teaster J, Lange JM, Hubbard RA, Lee CI, Haas JS, Shi X, et al. Is the closest facility the one actually used? An assessment of travel time estimation based on mammography facilities. Int J Health Geogr. 2016;15:8.
131. Onega T, Lee CI, Benkeser D, Alford-Teaster J, Haas JS, Tosteson AN, et al. Travel burden to breast MRI and utilization: are risk and sociodemographics related? J Am Coll Radiol. 2016;13(6):611–9.

132. Elkin EB, Paige Nobles J, Pinheiro LC, Atoria CL, Schrag D. Changes in access to screening mammography, 2008–2011. Cancer Causes Control. 2013;24(5):1057–9.
133. Mandelblatt J, Andrews H, Kao R, Wallace R, Kerner J. Impact of access and social context on breast cancer stage at diagnosis. J Health Care Poor Underserved. 1995;6(3):342–51.
134. Gumpertz ML, Pickle LW, Miller BA, Bell BS. Geographic patterns of advanced breast cancer in Los Angeles: associations with biological and sociodemographic factors (United States). Cancer Causes Control. 2006;17(3):325–339.
135. Huang B, Dignan M, Han D, Johnson O. Does distance matter? Distance to mammography facilities and stage at diagnosis of breast cancer in Kentucky. J Rural Health. 2009;25(4):366–71.
136. Dai D. Black residential segregation, disparities in spatial access to health care facilities, and late-stage breast cancer diagnosis in metropolitan Detroit. Health Place. 2010; 16(5):1038–52.
137. Onitilo AA, Liang H, Stankowski RV, Engel JM, Broton M, Doi SA, et al. Geographical and seasonal barriers to mammography services and breast cancer stage at diagnosis. Rural Remote Health. 2014;14(3):2738.
138. Tarlov E, Zenk SN, Campbell RT, Warnecke RB, Block R. Characteristics of mammography facility locations and stage of breast cancer at diagnosis in Chicago. J Urban Health. 2009;86(2):196–213.
139. McLafferty S, Wang F. Rural reversal? Rural-urban disparities in late-stage cancer risk in Illinois. Cancer. 2009;115(12):2755–64.
140. Wang F, Guo D, McLafferty S. Constructing geographic areas for cancer data analysis: a case study on late-stage breast cancer risk in illinois. Appl Geogr. 2012;35(1–2):1–11.
141. Roche LM, Skinner R, Weinstein RB. Use of a geographic information system to identify and characterize areas with high proportions of distant stage breast cancer. J Public Health Manag Pract. 2002;8(2):26–32.
142. Schroen AT, Lohr ME. Travel distance to mammography and the early detection of breast cancer. Breast J. 2009;15(2):216–7.
143. Celaya MO, Berke EM, Onega TL, Gui J, Riddle BL, Cherala SS, et al. Breast cancer stage at diagnosis and geographic access to mammography screening (New Hampshire, 1998–2004). Rural Remote Health. 2010;10(2):1361.
144. Onega T, Cook A, Kirlin B, Shi X, Alford-Teaster J, Tuzzio L, et al. The influence of travel time on breast cancer characteristics, receipt of primary therapy, and surveillance mammography. Breast Cancer Res Treat. 2011;129(1):269–75.
145. Goovaerts P. Visualizing and testing the impact of place on late-stage breast cancer incidence: a non-parametric geostatistical approach. Health Place. 2010;16(2):321–30.
146. Marchick J, Henson DE. Correlations between access to mammography and breast cancer stage at diagnosis. Cancer. 2005;103(8):1571–80.
147. Henry KA, Boscoe FP, Johnson CJ, Goldberg DW, Sherman R, Cockburn M. Breast cancer stage at diagnosis: is travel time important? J Community Health. 2011;36(6):933–42.
148. Mobley LR, Kuo TM, Scott L, Rutherford Y, Bose S. Modeling geospatial patterns of late-stage diagnosis of breast cancer in the US. Int J Environ Res Public Health. 2017;14(5)
149. Gold RH, Bassett LW, Widoff BE. Highlights from the history of mammography. RadioGraphics. 1990;10:1111–31.
150. Elkin EB, Atoria CL, editors. Mobile mammography facilities and access to breast cancer screening. Washington, DC: ESRI Health GIS Conference; 2011.
151. Vyas A, Madhavan S, Kelly K, Metzger A, Schreiman J, Remick S. Do Appalachian women attending a mobile mammography program differ from those visiting a stationary mammography facility? J Community Health. 2013;38(4):698–706.
152. Stanley E, Lewis MC, Irshad A, Ackerman S, Collins H, Pavic D, et al. Effectiveness of a mobile mammography program. AJR Am J Roentgenol. 2017;209(6):1426–9.
153. Farria DM, Schmidt ME, Monsees BS, Smith RA, Hildebolt C, Yoffie R, et al. Professional and economic factors affecting access to mammography: a crisis today, or tomorrow? Results from a national survey. Cancer. 2005;104(3):491–8.

154. Baxi SS, Snow JG, Liberman L, Elkin EB. The future of mammography: radiology residents' experiences, attitudes, and opinions. AJR Am J Roentgenol. 2010;194(6):1680–6.
155. Sharafinski ME Jr, Nussbaum D, Jha S. Supply/demand in radiology: a historical perspective and comparison to other labor markets. Acad Radiol. 2016;23(2):245–51.
156. Misono AS, Saini S, Prabhakar AM. Radiology jobs: uncovering hidden and not-so-hidden opportunities from the ACR jobs board. J Am Coll Radiol. 2016;13(4):471–6.
157. Zahnd WE, McLafferty SL. Contextual effects and cancer outcomes in the United States: a systematic review of characteristics in multilevel analyses. Ann Epidemiol. 2017;27(11):739–48.. e3
158. Lian M, Struthers J, Schootman M. Comparing GIS-based measures in access to mammography and their validity in predicting neighborhood risk of late-stage breast cancer. PloS one. 2012;7(8):e43000.
159. Cromley EK, McLafferty S. GIS and public health. New York: Guilford Press; 2002.
160. Zahnd WE, Fogleman AJ, Jenkins WD. Rural-urban disparities in stage of diagnosis among cancers with preventive opportunities. Am J Prev Med. 2018;54(5):688–98.

Chapter 13
Spatial and Contextual Analyses of Stage at Diagnosis

Francis P. Boscoe and Lindsey Hutchison

Abstract We assess national trends in breast cancer incidence stratified by stage at diagnosis that suggest only a limited benefit to screening mammography. We then use a novel application of the spatial scan statistic to measure spatial patterns in the breast cancer stage distribution within New York State that highlight substantial socioeconomic disparities between locales. Finally, we report stage-specific breast cancer incidence rates as a function of median household income. This last analysis indicates that the greatest difference in early-stage breast cancer rates are found between middle and upper income groups, contradicting conventional wisdom that lack of health care access among the poorer population is the main driver of socio-economic disparities. Overall, consideration of stage at diagnosis is indispensable to conducting population-based breast cancer surveillance, assessing the efficacy of screening, and identifying geographic and socioeconomic disparities.

Keywords Incidence · Mortality · Screening mammography · Spatial scan statistic · Socioeconomic status · New York state

13.1 Introduction

In this chapter we consider spatiotemporal patterns and trends in breast cancer inci-dence in the United States and New York State, stratified by stage at diagnosis. As we will show, there are stark demographic differences between those diagnosed at early and late stage. Early stage diagnosis is more common, has high survival rates, and is strongly associated with higher socioeconomic status. Late stage diagnosis is less common, has low survival, and is associated with lower socioeconomic status.

We make use of the SEER Historic Stage A staging system, which classifies tumors into one of four stages: in situ (no stromal invasion or penetration of the basement membrane of the tissue), local (infiltration past the basement membrane

F. P. Boscoe (✉) · L. Hutchison
New York State Department of Health, New York State Cancer Registry, Albany, NY, USA
e-mail: fboscoe@albany.edu

© Springer Nature Switzerland AG 2019   313
D. Berrigan, N. A. Berger (eds.), *Geospatial Approaches to Energy Balance and Breast Cancer*, Energy Balance and Cancer 15, https://doi.org/10.1007/978-3-030-18408-7_13

but confined to the organ of origin), regional (extension beyond the organ of origin), or distant (metastatic or systemic disease) [1]We use the term "early stage" to refer to the combination of in situ and local stage and "late stage" to refer to the combination of regional and distant stage. The SEER Historic Stage A staging system has the advantages of being simple, comparable over a long time span, and recorded for nearly all incident cancers. We considered using the more detailed AJCC staging system, but we chose SEER Historic Stage A because of its simplicity, familiarity, and wide use in geographical studies [2, 3].

The chapter is organized as follows. We begin by examining long-term breast cancer mortality and incidence trends in the United States. We next assess spatial patterns in the stage distribution of breast cancer, using high-quality data from the New York State Cancer Registry and a novel application of the spatial scan statistic. From this analysis, we produce a map identifying geographic locations with the most unusual stage distributions, which suggests the presence of socioeconomic and racial/ethnic disparities. We then investigate the relationship of median household income to stage-specific incidence rates, finding contrary to conventional wisdom, most of the observed variation in rates occurs at the upper part of the income spectrum.

In order to begin to understand the demographic differences in breast cancer patients diagnosed at early versus late stage, we shall first consider long-term trends in breast cancer mortality (the lower line in Fig. 13.1). As the figure shows, during

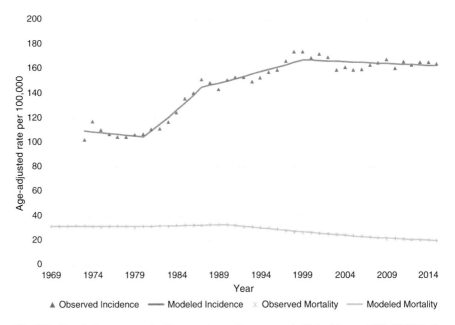

Fig. 13.1 Female breast cancer incidence and mortality rate trends, United States, 1969–2015 [4, 5]. The points represent measured values; the lines represent distinct trends within the data, as computed by SEER's Joinpoint software [6]. The number of distinct trends was limited to 4, otherwise the default settings within the software were used

the 1970s and 1980s, the rate remained essentially unchanged at 32–33 per 100,000. In 1990, it began a sharp drop of more than 2% per year, dropping below 30 in 1996 and below 25 in 2004. The downward trend eased slightly after 2007 but continued through 2015, the most recent data available at the time of writing, reaching an all-time low rate of 20 per 100,000. All told, the mortality rate dropped 39% in the quarter-century since 1990.

Death rates among women from all other causes also dropped during these years, but only by 15%. There are therefore many women alive today who would not be alive had the breast cancer mortality rates remained at their pre-1990 levels or had matched those of other diseases. This is a genuine success story, though one that is underappreciated, as the popular media often describe breast cancer as a growing epidemic [7]This perception is perhaps influenced by the steady incidence rates over this time period (the upper line in Fig. 13.1). The overall age-adjusted incidence rate of 165 in 2015 was nearly identical to the rate in 1997 (167) and higher than every year prior to 1997. The combination of level incidence, declining mortality, and a growing and aging population means that the number of breast cancer survivors is larger than it has ever been. While people are less likely to know someone who has died of breast cancer, they are more likely to know someone living with it, or to be living with it themselves. This "survivor's bias" contributes to the perception that breast cancer is a growing epidemic.

There are two primary ways that these incidence and mortality trends can be interpreted. One is to see both trends as largely a consequence of screening. In this interpretation, widespread adoption of routine mammography beginning in the 1980s has contributed to a steady high incidence rate even as it has reduced the death rate through earlier detection. The increases in rates of early stage disease are certainly consistent with a screening effect, particularly in situ which is asymptomatic and thus unlikely to be diagnosed in the absence of screening. A second interpretation is that the reduction in mortality can be seen as a consequence of improvements in chemotherapy, surgical methods, and other methods of treatment, while screening has merely served to inflate the incidence rate.

The truth likely falls somewhere in between [8], but just where has been a point of much contention. At one pole, Autier and Boniol in a lengthy position paper conclude that "the overwhelming evidence…is that improvements in patient management have played the preponderant role in the considerable reductions in breast cancer mortality…while the contribution of screening mammography itself has been marginal" [9, 10]. If early stage cancer rates increase while late stage cancer rates remain about the same, then it is more likely that the screening program is identifying tumors that would not have progressed further, and for which there was no treatment benefit. This phenomenon is known as overdiagnosis [11–13]. Using a conservative estimate that 1 in 8 breast cancer diagnoses is being overdiagnosed, one study estimated that 2–3 women will be treated unnecessarily for every woman who avoids a death from breast cancer through screening [14].

At the other extreme are studies which validate screening benefits for women beginning at age 40 or 50. For example, one recent simulation modeling study concluded that biennial mammography screening from age 50–74 reduces breast cancer

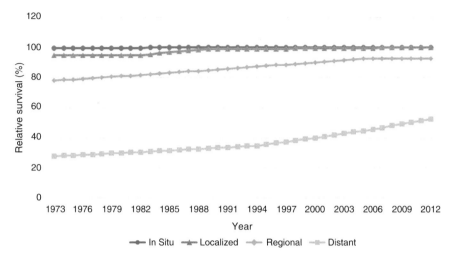

Fig. 13.2 3 year relative survival by stage, SEER 9, 1973–2012 [5]. The lines represent distinct trends within the data, as computed by SEER's Joinpoint software [6]

mortality by 24–32%, numbers that are in line with the earliest randomized trials which established the current breast cancer screening guidelines [15].

A well-established way to evaluate the efficacy of a screening mechanism is to evaluate the data by stage at diagnosis [16], which is the focus of this chapter. The earlier the stage at diagnosis, the more likely one is to survive the disease. This is seen in Fig. 13.2, which shows the 3 year relative survival by stage at diagnosis since 1973. For those diagnosed at early stage, the relative survival has been at 100% since 2009, meaning that those with cancer are no more likely to die than those without cancer. Indeed, the true value is over 100% – those with early stage breast cancer actually outlive their non-cancer peers, because they tend to be healthier in other respects – but the SEER∗Stat software used to generate this figure caps the value at 100%. More notable is the improvement in relative survival for late stage disease. This can only be attributable to improvements in treatment, not to screening – screening can only shift people to a higher line on the graph, it cannot change the shape of the line itself.

Incidence rates by stage at diagnosis are given in Fig. 13.3, and further clarify the picture. Over this 32 year period, in situ rates increased eightfold, local stage rates doubled, regional rates decreased modestly, and distant rates remained stable. If mammography was responsible for some of the downward trend in mortality, then we would also have expected to see a corresponding downward trend in late-stage disease. This is because an effective screening test works by identifying some cases of disease at an earlier, more treatable point. And yet distant rates did not change at all. As for regional stage rates, their decrease could at best account for only a modest share of the overall mortality reduction. Regional stage rates decreased from about 40 in 1990 to about 35 in 2014, a 12% drop at the same time overall mortality from breast cancer dropped by 39%. Regional breast cancer is also a relatively

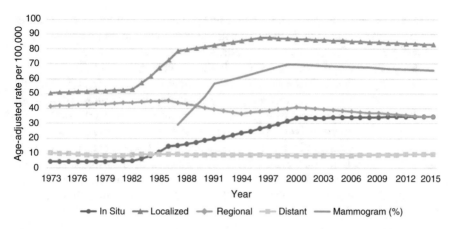

Fig. 13.3 Breast cancer rate vs. diagnosis year, by stage with unstaged rates being allocated to known stages as follows: 45% localized, 25% regional, and 30% distant. Joinpoint software [6] used in the same manner as Fig. 13.1. Lighter blue line indicates crude percent of women in the United States aged 40 and over having a mammogram within the past 2 years [17]

high-survival cancer, with relative survival in recent years of about 90%, so it is not the stage of origin for many of the cases that resulted in deaths. Regardless of any small impact on the regional-stage rate due to screening, it is difficult to argue in favor of a significant benefit of screening in the absence of any improvement in the distant-stage cancer rate.

One possible counterargument is that late stage disease would actually be increasing in the absence of screening, and screening has been effective in keeping it in check by maintaining the status quo. This has been tested by looking at trends among unscreened populations – either women under the age of 40 or places where screening had not yet been introduced. Breyer and Welch did the former in their 2012 paper [12], finding a 0.25% annual increase in late-stage disease among women under 40 and assuming this would also apply to women over 40. To be conservative, they also considered an annual increase twice as high (0.5%). These two assumptions resulted in overdiagnosis percentages of 31% and 26%, respectively, either of them arguing against the benefits of screening.

This analysis only extended to 2008, however. Advancing the timeline through 2015 reveals that late-stage breast cancer has been increasing more rapidly among women under 40 in recent years. Joinpoint analysis of data from 1976 (their starting year) through 2015 suggest an overall annual increase of 0.5% – matching their more conservative assumption – but consisting of no change from 1976–1996 and a 1.1% annual increase since. Specifically, between 1996 and 2015, the under-40 age-adjusted rate rose from about 6 per 100,000 to about 7.5 per 100,000. This suggests that their approach may have been insufficiently conservative and calls for a more formal reassessment of their methods.

In a related example, Lousdal et al. evaluated breast cancer rates before, during, and after the introduction of screening mammography in Norway among both the screening age and younger than screening age populations, and found that localized incidence rates more than doubled among the screening-age group and increased modestly among the younger group. Rates of advanced stage disease increased modestly regardless of age, suggesting a limited screening benefit [18].

Returning to Fig. 13.3, the early-stage trend lines do appear consistent with the wide adoption of screening mammography beginning in the 1980s. Both in situ and local stage cancer rates rose sharply throughout the 1980s and continued to increase steadily through the 1990s. Changes have been more modest in the 2000s, with in situ continuing to increase gradually and local stage decreasing modestly. Overall, the two lines track each other quite closely, with an absolute increase in rates since the early 1980s of about 30 per 100,000 in both instances. (The in situ rates experienced a much higher relative change, of course, since they began at such a lower level).

13.2   Spatial Patterns in Breast Cancer Incidence by Stage

We now turn our attention to the spatial patterns of stage at diagnosis, using data from New York State collected by the New York State Cancer Registry (NYSCR). The NYSCR is one of the oldest and largest cancer registries in North America, established in 1940 and population-based since 1976, with over three million tumors recorded since 1976 among New York State residents. It has achieved the highest level (gold) certification from the North American Association of Central Cancer Registries (NAACCR) every year since 2000.

We used a data set that comprises 200,074 tumors diagnosed among New York State resident women between 2006 and 2015. Because we took special effort to prepare this data set, and because of the geographical emphasis of the book, we describe the data set here in some detail, even while acknowledging that our analyses would have yielded essentially the same results if we had used the data as it existed at the time we were invited to contribute this chapter. The data set represents the total number of breast cancers diagnosed among the entire New York State population, excepting 595 tumors that were only diagnosed at death and had no clinical or staging information. (We located published obituaries for several of these patients which suggested that the cause of death was something other than breast cancer and that the cause of death was therefore miscoded on the death certificate, which further supports their exclusion).

Nearly all of these tumors (199,966; 99.95%) were geocoded to the census tract of residence at the time of diagnosis. Geocoding was performed using the AGGIE geocoder hosted at Texas A&M University (http://geoservices.tamu.edu/About/) or by clerical review by NYSCR staff. Of the 108 ungeocoded tumors, 8 had no address information whatsoever and were excluded from all spatial analyses. For the remaining 100 tumors, we imputed a census tract by randomly matching the tumor to one with the same ZIP code at diagnosis. Overall, we believe this data set to be among the most complete and accurate small-area geographic cancer data sets ever

Table 13.1 Female breast cancer stage distribution in NY data, diagnosis years 2006–2015. All tumors with unknown stage are known to be invasive, which means they are known not to be in situ

Stage	Count	Percent	Percent among invasive
In situ	48,536	24.3%	–
Local	96,360	48.2%	63.6%
Regional	42,177	21.1%	27.8%
Distant	8572	4.3%	5.7%
Unknown	4421	2.2%	2.9%

compiled and it should have applicability well beyond its use here. While it cannot be released publicly owing to confidentiality concerns, outside investigators may apply to the NYSCR to use it in formal research projects.

The stage distribution in the New York data are shown in Table 13.1, using the SEER Summary Stage 2000 staging system. Nearly half of all tumors were diagnosed at local stage, about one-quarter in situ, and one-fifth regional. Only about 4% of tumors were diagnosed at distant stage and for about 2% the stage was unknown. Since tumors with unknown stage are known to be invasive, and thus cannot be in situ, Table 13.1 also lists the stage distribution among invasive tumors.

Although the number of tumors with unknown stage is small, we were nevertheless concerned with any potential bias resulting from the data not being missing at random. In particular, there was a strong downward trend in missingness, with tumors in 2006 missing stage 50% more often than in 2015. There was also geographic structure among the cases with missing stage – the percent missing was closer to 1% in much of upstate New York, 4–5% in parts of New York City, and 7% in one rural county. Imputation of missing stage has become common practice in recent years to ameliorate these problems [19, 20], and so we followed this practice.

Imputation was performed by matching each case with missing stage information randomly to cases with known stage information [21], matched on age, tumor grade, census tract poverty rate, race/ethnicity, histology, and surgery type, with each of these variables classified broadly into 4–8 categories. Where there were fewer than five available match candidates, the matching criteria were relaxed by omitting variables in the reverse order listed, beginning with surgery type. 60% of the imputations were based on matching all six variables; 99% were based on matching four variables. A total of five imputed data sets were created, to ensure that the spatial analysis was not sensitive to the characteristics of a single imputation.

The distribution of the imputed stages was quite different than the distribution of known stages, with a disproportionately greater number of distant stage cases, as seen in Table 13.2. This means that unstaged cases tended to share more of the characteristics of tumors with distant stage.

We used the multinomial version of Kulldorff's spatial scan statistic [22] to evaluate geographic areas of unusual stage distribution across New York State in the 2006–2015 period, primarily using SaTScan software version 9.5. The multinomial

Table 13.2 Distribution of known versus imputed stages

Stage	Known	Imputed
Local	65.5%	45.7%
Regional	28.7%	24.0%
Distant	5.8%	30.3%

spatial scan statistic is able to identify unusual stage distributions involving high or low distributions of any stage alone or in combination. For example, the statistic is able to identify areas of unusually high distant stage, unusually low in situ stage, or unusually high local plus regional stage. We considered this an improvement over the more commonly used binary approach, such as considering in situ versus other stages, distant stage versus other stages, and so on. Indeed, we began with that approach but decided otherwise when the ensuing number of results, and their accompanying maps, became excessive and difficult to summarize. Our aim instead was to find a way to identify the locations of the most unusual stage distributions on a single map, drawn from the set of all possible stage distributions.

When we say "all possible", we are actually referring only to all possible distributions that are circular in shape. Specifically, there were approximately 4893[2]/2, or about 12 million, possible areas to consider, where 4893 is the number of census tracts in New York State and a possible area consists of each census tract and its nearest neighbors, where the number of neighbors ranges from zero to half of the state. While the areas are not literally circular, as the number of neighbors grows larger the shape more closely approaches a circle. We stop upon reaching half the state because by convention, unusual distributions covering more than half of the state are not considered unusual, because they represent the majority. By convention, clusters represent a minority of the population.

In general, SaTScan software produces a very large number of candidate areas with unusual stage distributions. Typically, the areas that are selected for depiction on a map are the non-overlapping areas with the highest log-likelihood ratios (LLR). The LLR is a measure of the likelihood that the data inside a circle are different than the data outside it. For the multinomial model, the equation is complex and we refer the reader to the paper by Jung et al. 2010 rather than reproduce it here [22]. A limitation of the LLR is that it tends to identify areas containing large numbers of cases but with only small differences in rates or proportions, often in the neighborhood of 5%. Given the complex multifactorial nature of cancer patterns and outcomes, such small differences are rarely of interest to medical or public health researchers even if they are statistically significant. Boscoe et al. proposed that the effect size, as measured by the relative risk, should also be considered in deciding which circles to report, and this innovation has been incorporated into the most recent release of SaTScan [23]. However, it applies only to the binary statistical models (specifically, the Poisson and Bernoulli models), not to the multinomial model. After some trial and error, we settled on the Gini coefficient as a reasonable analog to the relative risk suitable for use with the multinomial model. The ensuing analysis was conducted using SAS version 9.4 (SAS Institute, Cary, NC).

The Gini coefficient is used most often in economics to measure the wealth inequality of a nation, with values ranging from 0 (representing perfect equality, where all persons have equal wealth) to 1 (representing perfect inequality, where one person has all the wealth and the rest have nothing). Here we used the Gini coefficient to measure the stage inequality, where a value of 0 meant that the circular area under consideration matched the stage distribution of the state exactly, and a value of 1 meant that all the people were diagnosed at the same stage. Our goal was to restrict the reporting of areas to those which both exceeded a LLR threshold as well as a Gini threshold. The LLR threshold was obtained through Monte Carlo simulation. 999 random permutations of the data were generated assuming the cancer risk was uniform, after adjusting for age. We stored the highest LLR from each simulated data set, and used the 50th highest value among the stored values to represent the level that was reached by chance 5% of the time, corresponding to a p-value of 0.05.

Since, to our knowledge, we were the first researchers to apply a Gini coefficient to filter results from a SaTScan multinomial model result, there were no historical examples to help decide what was a suitable cutoff value. The global Gini coefficient for economic equality is often given at around 0.6, but levels of cancer stage inequality are much smaller than this. A higher Gini threshold results in fewer areas being selected for display, while a lower Gini threshold results in more areas being selected. Figure 13.4 shows the relationship in our dataset. We settled upon a threshold value of 0.13 which resulted in about 10% of the census tracts being defined as part of a cluster area, with 20 cluster areas overall. These areas are mapped in Fig. 13.5 and their stage distributions and some basic demographic characteristics are given in Table 13.3.

The disparities in stage distribution within New York State were quite dramatic. The percentage of in situ cases ranged from a low of 12.7% in the cluster in Livingston County (cluster 14) to a high of 34.5% in one of the Nassau County

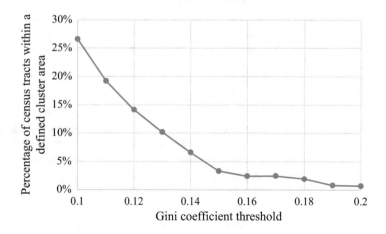

Fig. 13.4 Relationship between Gini coefficient threshold and cluster coverage

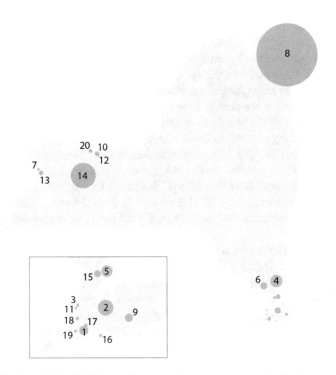

Fig. 13.5 Areas in New York State with unusual breast cancer stage distributions as determined by multinomial model in SaTScan. The stage distributions for each of the 20 areas are given in Table 13.3

clusters (cluster 9). Similarly, the local stage percentage ranges from 36.4 to 63.5, regional from 13.1 to 34.7, and distant from 0.8 to 12.2. The cluster locations and demographics suggest that the stage distributions reflect socioeconomic and racial/ ethnic disparities. The areas with unusually high early stage disease occupy some of the wealthiest places in the state, indeed the world, centered on locales such as the Upper East Side of Manhattan (clusters 3 and 11) and the affluent New York City suburbs of Scarsdale (cluster 15) and Great Neck (cluster 2). Conversely, areas with unusually high late stage disease are found in less-affluent areas such as inner-city Buffalo (cluster 7) and Rochester (clusters 10 and 12) and less prosperous neighborhoods in Brooklyn (clusters 1, 17, and 18). Notably, no cluster appears in the Bronx, which by many measures is the lowest-ranking county in the state socioeconomically. This points to an ethnic influence, as the Bronx is primarily Hispanic (specifically, Dominican and Puerto Rican) while the highlighted parts of Brooklyn are primarily black, both African-American and Afro-Caribbean.

A few of the clusters show patterns other than a straightforward early/late stage divide, such as the cluster in Clinton County in the northeastern corner of the state (number 8), which has an ordinary distribution of late stage disease but relatively few in situ cases. This particular cluster is unlikely to have been identified had the

Table 13.3 Areas with unusual stage distribution in New York State. See Fig. 13.5 for map. Percent White Non-Hispanic is from Table P9 of the 2010 Census

	County/NYC borough	In situ (%)	Local (%)	Regional (%)	Distant (%)	Percent white non-hispanic	Percent below poverty
1	Brooklyn	19.3	42.6	30.2	8.0	6.3	23.0
2	Nassau	34.0	47.4	16.3	2.3	74.9	4.6
3	Manhattan	34.3	47.2	15.4	3.2	84.7	6.7
4	Westchester	32.2	51.1	14.4	2.2	80.4	4.8
5	Westchester	30.6	54.6	13.1	1.7	57.6	5.3
6	Rockland	33.6	48.5	15.5	2.4	70.5	5.0
7	Erie	20.2	36.4	34.7	8.7	11.9	37.6
8	Clinton	13.0	59.5	23.2	4.2	93.9	12.1
9	Nassau	34.5	46.3	16.8	2.4	87.7	3.7
10	Monroe	14.2	52.5	26.1	7.2	27.9	37.7
11	Manhattan	34.4	47.7	14.4	3.5	74.4	6.7
12	Monroe	16.7	63.5	17.7	2.2	76.8	14.5
13	Erie	16.0	49.2	26.3	8.5	71.4	20.0
14	Livingston	12.7	54.0	28.5	4.8	78.1	14.2
15	Westchester	33.1	49.0	17.1	0.8	83.8	3.2
16	Queens	16.7	43.7	27.3	12.2	17.0	24.0
17	Brooklyn	19.2	42.6	33.4	4.7	1.2	36.2
18	Brooklyn	17.8	44.2	31.1	6.9	34.9	39.9
19	Brooklyn	17.2	44.7	29.0	9.2	67.6	34.2
20	Monroe	16.6	62.6	17.8	2.9	85.9	5.4

multinomial model not been used. We know from previous work with colorectal cancer [24] that certain facilities diagnose in situ disease conservatively; that is, they are more apt to classify ambiguous cases as free of disease. However, there is really no problem with ambiguity in the case of breast cancer, as the boundaries between nonreportable disease and in situ stage, and between in situ and local stage, are clearly drawn. The cause of this cluster therefore remains unknown.

A potential weakness of the multinomial SaTScan-based approach is that since it is based on proportions rather than rates, it does not reflect the true underlying risk of disease. For example, suppose more than 40% of the cases in a region were diagnosed at distant stage, a proportion many times above the state average. This would seem to be cause for grave concern, but suppose also that the overall incidence rate of cancer here was one-tenth the state average. The distant stage rate would be roughly equal to the state average, while the rates for the other stages would be exorbitantly low. The unusual stage distribution might still be of some concern here, but much less so than it would appear at first glance. We spent considerable effort trying to incorporate the underlying risk of disease into our analytical approach, but could not find a satisfactory solution. However, we know from having worked with cancer surveillance data for many years that something as extreme as in the example above is unlikely, and that the variation in the proportions far exceeds the variations in the underlying risk. Supporting this point, a purely rate-based approach was used in a separate New York State Department of Health project [25], and it showed quite limited geographic variation in breast cancer rates for the 2011–2015 period.

13.3 Income and Breast Cancer Incidence by Stage

We next consider more explicitly the relationship between income and stage distribution. To measure this, we assigned each case in the study to a median household income percentile value based on the 2010 census tract of residence at diagnosis, where the 100th percentile corresponded to the highest earners.[1] Because there are over 4800 tracts in New York, each percentile consisted of 48 or 49 tracts. Income data were obtained from American Community Survey Table S1903; we used the 2006–2010 version for cases diagnosed in those years and the 2011–2015 version for cases diagnosed in those years.

We then calculated incidence rates by stage for each income percentile (Fig. 13.6). The populations used in the rate calculations were single-year age and sex-specific estimates using iterative proportional fitting to reconcile the tract-level populations in the 2010 census with the county-level estimates published for other years [26]. The incidence rates were fit to a polynomial of order 3 to permit a nonlinear relationship. Figure 13.6 shows a strong positive relationship between income and the

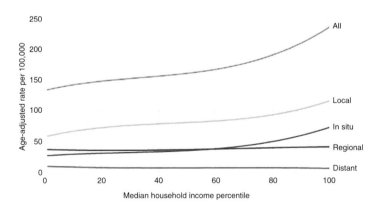

Fig. 13.6 Cancer rate vs. median household income percentile, by stage, New York State, 2006–2015

---

[1] Because median household income is based on a survey of households, 58 census tracts without households (primarily college campuses, prisons, and military bases) were excluded from this part of the analysis.

incidence rates of in situ and local stage breast cancer, no relationship for regional stage, and a weak negative relationship for distant stage. For in situ, the rates range from about 30 per 100,000 among the poorest to 80 per 100,000 among the most affluent, a 167% difference. Half of this variation occurs among the top 20% of the income range. That is, the range is the same among the top 20% of income (55–80) as for those in the bottom 80% (30–55). The coefficient of determination (r^2) for the fitted curve is 0.96, with no strong individual outliers. To the extent that the curve fails to fit the data, it does so at the highest incomes – the curve slightly under predicts the rates for percentiles 95 through 99 and greatly under predicts the top percentile. Individual data points are not shown for clarity, but we have made the raw data and the equations for the fitted curves available for download [27].

For local stage, the range is about 60 per 100,000 among the poorest to 115 per 100,000 among the most affluent, nearly a two-fold difference. As with in situ, the variation is skewed toward the upper range of income, with half of the range in the top 30% of income. The coefficient of determination for the fitted curve is 0.94, again with no unusual outliers. The curve underpredicted the rates for the top two percentiles.

For regional stage, there was little relationship by income, with the rate close to 40 per 100,000 at all income levels. For distant stage, there was a negative trend, with rates of about 10 per 100,000 among the poorest and 6.5 per 100,000 among the most affluent, a difference of 35%. Here, the variation was skewed toward the poor end of the range, with half of the variation found among the bottom 15%. There were a number of individual outliers in these data; for example, the rate for the 89th percentile was 10 and for the 14th percentile was 6.4, the reverse of what would have been expected. The coefficient of determination was 0.31, indicative of a weak trend.

These results suggest that wealthier people are more likely to get screened for breast cancer and that there are also additional risks more common to wealthier populations. There is solid evidence in the literature in support of both of these conclusions, though together they fail to explain all of the rate differences. Regarding screening, we had difficulty finding detailed data on screening rates by income level. The Centers for Disease Control's Behavioral Risk Factor Surveillance System is a telephone-based survey that asks questions about mammography utilization. In terms of income, it distinguishes only between those below and above household incomes of $25,000 and $50,000, corresponding to the 7th and 37th percentiles in the 2011–2015 period. In response to the question "Have you had a mammogram in the past 2 years?", the percentage of New York State women aged 50–74 years answering yes in 2016 was 76% among households below $25,000, 78% between $25,000 and less than $50,000, and 83% for those equal to or greater than $50,000 [28]. The numbers trend in the expected direction, but do not differ by much – regardless of income, it seems a solid majority of women are receiving mammograms at least biannually.

We also located an independent source of mammography data from the same year from the National Committee for Quality Assurance (NCQA) that was based on actual medical claims and stratified by insurer type [29]. In these data, just over 70% of women aged 50–74 years with a commercial or Medicare HMO or PPO had a screening mammogram within the past 2 years, versus about 59% among those with Medicaid HMO coverage. These numbers are quite a bit lower than the BRFSS figures, suggesting those values might be inflated. There is reason to believe that social desirability bias is present in the BRFSS survey; that is, that respondents are apt to report themselves as healthier and in greater compliance with health guidelines than is actually the case. Regardless, even a roughly 10% disparity in mammography utilization is not enough to account for a two-fold difference in cancer incidence by income. Moreover, the NCQA only distinguish between the poorest individuals (the Medicaid members) and the remainder of the population (those with other insurance). In New York State, that is roughly 25% of the population, but in most states, it is much lower than this.

Prior work has found that it is not only the utilization of mammography but the technical sophistication of the mammogram itself that varies by social class [30]. In the early 2000s, wealthier women in New York State were much more likely to be receiving digital mammograms than their less-affluent counterparts, though there was ample local variation. Today virtually all mammograms are digital, but the diffusion of innovation cycle is now being repeated with 3-dimensional tomography. In general, more advanced technologies are more sensitive and thus result in more positive diagnoses, though often at the cost of more false positives, though our previous work suggested the net effect is small.

Aside from health care utilization, the positive relationship between wealth and breast cancer incidence has mainly been explained in terms of lifetime exposure to estrogen [31–35]. In their exhaustive review article Klassen and Smith noted 9 risk factors for breast cancer: earlier age of menarche, later age at first birth or nulliparity, higher birth weight or leg length, greater postmenopausal body mass index and weight gain later in life, lower premenopausal body mass index, higher contraceptive use, lower physical activity, lower rate of breast feeding, and greater alcohol consumption [34]. Each of these translates directly to estrogen exposure or is a marker for one of the other risk factors with the exception of alcohol which could also influence breast cancer through nonhormonal pathways. All, with the exception of physical activity, carry greater risk for the more affluent. Unfortunately, none of these measures are collected by cancer registries and to independently measure them was beyond our capabilities. A recent study by Ryabov using data from the National Center for Health Statistics to relate fertility with income does seem to match the cancer data quite well, however [36]. The total fertility rate ranges from about 1 for the wealthiest counties to about 3 in the poorest counties, where 2.1 is the replacement level where the population would be stable in the absence of migration. These data are at the county level; using data at the census tract level would likely magnify the relationship further, since many counties are highly heterogeneous with regard to income.

Klassen and Smith argue that trading sources of estrogen exposure is perhaps not necessary, that income is indeed the relevant measure of concern. As they write:

Breast cancer research to date has primarily sought to explain the effect of social class on the essentially biological process of carcinogenesis by identifying more proximal individual behaviors and exposures that vary by social class. This is basically a compositional interpretation of class, assuming that social class is, in any given society, a marker for certain behaviors and exposures, each of which adds to a woman's composite profile for disease risk. This approach is clearly an important strategy for cancer control through risk reduction. However, although this behavioral approach has produced a great deal of information leading to both interventions and further research inquiries, the decomposition of social phenomena into composite lists of behaviors may fail to capture fundamental effects of social position, for two reasons. The first is that behaviors do not occur in random combination, but as mutually reinforcing patterns within socially regulated lifestyles. Thus we may test risk behavior combinations that are possible in statistical models but rare in most societies. Moreover, single behaviors or factors, such as body size, are not likely to have uniform impact, but are likely modified by social class and context. Finally, a more intellectually compelling reason to consider social class as a direct health effect on breast cancer is that it may inform our understanding not only of the relationship of social class to this one disease process, but to a wider range of health outcomes, and indeed the relationship of social inequality to health [34].

A recent analysis using data from Switzerland provides some useful context [33]. Despite having been conducted in another country and lacking some of the precision of the New York data set, the results were essentially identical to our own. Stage proportions between the most and least affluent areas varied to a similar degree. This is, as the authors wrote, "despite universal health insurance coverage, high health expenditures, the highest average household net financial wealth worldwide, and one of the highest life expectancies in the world" [33]. What is interesting is how the authors framed their interpretation of their results. Like other studies we have reviewed, the primary framing was in terms of the ways that the poor are different from the rest of the population: "possible reasons…might be related to differences in health care access, cancer awareness and/or other attitudes about cancer (e.g., cancer fatalism)". But our data suggest that the differences between the wealthy and the middle class are of even greater importance. It is hard to understand how a woman in the 60th percentile of income, in either the United States or in Switzerland, would have different access to screening services or would be less "aware" of breast cancer than a woman in the 90th percentile.

Yet similar gradients in health and socioeconomic status have been found in a wide range of studies. For example, Marmot cites findings in Sweden that people with Ph.Ds have lower mortality than those with master's degrees, and that the middle of the social hierarchy in England has seven fewer years of healthy life than the top [37]. He concludes this must relate to how relative position translates into subtle manifestations of social and psychosocial conditions. While higher relative position generally confers a health advantage, in the case of breast cancer it appears to confer a disadvantage, in the form of over diagnosis. We originally found the results in Fig. 13.6 to be counterintuitive and seemingly unexplainable, but after reading Marmot's work, we adopt his view that "the scientific challenge…is to understand why inequalities in health run from top to bottom of the social hierarchy" [37]. In the case of breast cancer incidence, cumulative estrogen exposure and screening frequency can explain some of the gradient, but much remains unexplained. In contrast to Klassen and Smith we do think it would be useful to pursue the decomposition of social phenomena into specific behaviors, in the hope that some of them may prove to be modifiable.

13.4 Summary

Female breast cancer is a substantial burden in New York State, the United States, and throughout the world. While the breast cancer mortality rate has been dropping in the United States since 1990, steady high incidence rates since the mid 1990s and an aging population mean that breast cancer has the appearance of a growing epidemic. The incidence and mortality trends are likely due to the influence of widespread adoption of routine mammography screening as well as improvements in breast cancer treatments. The increase in survival rates for late stage disease can only be explained by improved treatments. If mammography can be credited for the decreasing mortality rates, then late stage disease should be decreasing as well, however this is not the case and suggests at best a weak benefit of screening mammography.

A Gini coefficient was applied to the multinomial version of Kulldorff's spatial scan statistic and was used to evaluate geographic areas of unusual stage distribution of nearly 200,000 geocoded female breast cancer cases in New York State between 2006 and 2015. The disparities in stage distribution within New York State are pronounced, and the identified clusters are strongly suggestive of socioeconomic and racial/ethnic disparities with areas of unusually high early stage disease occupying some of the wealthiest places and areas with unusually high late stage disease being in poorer areas.

The strong positive relationship between wealth and breast cancer incidence has been widely documented, however the underlying causes of this phenomenon are still subject to debate. Here we have quantified the relationship in a particularly precise manner. Factors such as breast cancer screening utilization, lifetime exposure to estrogen, and alcohol consumption can explain much, but not all, of the difference in breast cancer incidence between social classes. However, it is difficult to pinpoint each exposure's role in the breast cancer disease process.

Each of these topics – incidence and survival rate trends, geographic patterns, and the relevance of socioeconomic status on breast cancer – are informed by stratifying the available surveillance data by stage at diagnosis. Future surveillance work of this type should further consider molecular subtypes. Breast cancer is not one disease but rather a common symptom of several diseases that can be distinguished, at least partially, by the estrogen receptor (ER), progesterone receptor (PR), and human growth factor-neu receptor (HER2) biomarkers. Central cancer registries do collect this information, though it has only recently been sufficiently complete for analytic use. The 2015 edition Annual Report to the Nation on the Status of Cancer reported these data by state [20], but application to small geographic areas has been limited thus far.

References

1. Young JL Jr, Roffers SD, LAG R, Fritz AG, Hurlbut AA, editors. SEER summary staging manual – 2000: codes and coding instructions. Bethesda: National Cancer Institute, NIH Pub. No. 01-4969; 2001.
2. Steele CB, Li J, Huang B, Weir HK. Prostate cancer survival in the United States by race and stage (2001–2009): findings from the CONCORD-2 study. Cancer. 2017;123(Suppl 24):5160–77.
3. Jim MA, Pinheiro PS, Carreira H, Espey DK, Wiggins CL, Weir HK. Stomach cancer survival in the United States by race and stage (2001-2009): findings from the CONCORD-2 study. Cancer. 2017;123(Suppl 24):4994–5013.
4. Surveillance, Epidemiology, and End Results (SEER) Program (www.seer.cancer.gov) SEER*Stat Database: Mortality – All COD, Aggregated With State, Total U.S. (1969-2015) <Katrina/Rita Population Adjustment>, National Cancer Institute, DCCPS, Surveillance Research Program, released December 2017. Underlying mortality data prov;ided by NCHS www.cdc.gov/nchs.
5. Surveillance, Epidemiology, and End Results (SEER) Program (www.seer.cancer.gov) SEER*Stat Database: Incidence - SEER 9 Regs Research Data, Nov 2017 Sub (1973–2015) <Katrina/Rita Population Adjustment> – Linked To County Attributes – Total U.S., 1969–2016 Counties, National Cancer Institute, DCCPS, Surveillance Research Program, released April 2018, based on the November 2017 submission.
6. Joinpoint Regression Program [computer program]. Version 4.6.0.0. Rockville, MD: National Cancer Institute; 2018.
7. Schneider AP II, Zainer CM, Kubat CK, Mullen NK, Windisch AK. The breast cancer epidemic: 10 facts. Linacre Q. 2014;81:244–77.
8. American Cancer Society. How common is breast cancer? https://www.cancer.org/cancer/breast-cancer/about/how-common-is-breast-cancer.html. Accessed 26 Mar 2018.
9. Autier P, Boniol M. Mammography screening: a major issue in medicine. Eur J Cancer. 2018;90:34–62.
10. Bleyer A, Baines C, Miller AB. Impact of screening mammography on breast cancer mortality. Int J Cancer. 2016;138(8):2003–12.
11. Nelson HD, et al. Screening for breast cancer: an update for the U.S. preventive services task force. Ann Intern Med. 2009;151(10):727–37.
12. Bleyer A, Welch HG. Effect of three decades of screening mammography on breast-cancer incidence. N Engl J Med. 2012;367:1998–2005.
13. Pace LE, Keating NL. A systematic assessment of benefits and risks to guide breast cancer screening decisions. JAMA. 2014;311(13):1327–35.
14. Siu, AL on behalf of the U.S. Preventive Services Task Force. Screening for breast cancer: U.S. preventive services task force recommendation statement. Ann Intern Med. 2016;164(4):279–96.
15. Mandelblatt JS, Stout NK, Schechter CB, van den Broek JJ, Miglioretti DL, Krapcho M, et al. Collaborative modeling of the benefits and harms associated with different U.S. breast cancer screening strategies. Ann Intern Med. 2016;164(4):215–25.
16. International Agency for Research on Cancer. Breast cancer screening. IARC Press: 2002.
17. Table 070. Use of mammography among women 40 years of age and over, by selected characteristics: United States, selected years 1987-2015. Atlanta: Centers for Disease Control and Prevention https://www.cdc.gov/nchs/hus/contents2016.htm#070.
18. Lousdal ML, Kristiansen IS, Moller B, Stouring H. Trends in breast cancer stage distribution before, during and after introduction of a screening programme in Norway. Eur J Pub Health. 2014;24(6):1017–22.
19. Eisemann N, Waldmann A, Katalinic A. Imputation of missing values of tumour stage in population-based cancer registration. BMC Med Res Methodol. 2011;11:129.

20. Kohler BA, Sherman RL, et al. Annual report to the nation on the status of cancer, 1975-2011, featuring incidence of breast cancer subtypes by race/ethnicity, poverty and state. JNCI. 2015;107(6):djv048.
21. Andridge RR, Little RJA. A review of hot deck imputation for survey non-response. Int Stat Rev. 2010;78(1):40–64.
22. Jung I, Kulldorff M, Richard OJ. A spatial scan statistic for multinomial data. Stat Med. 2010;29(18):1910–8. https://doi.org/10.1002/sim.3951.
23. Boscoe FP, McLaughlin CC, Schymura MJ, Kielb CL. Visualization of the spatial scan statistic using nested circles. Health Place. 2003;9(3):273–7.
24. Boscoe FP, Hutchison LM. Differential reporting of in situ colorectal cancer in New York State and the United States. J Registry Manag. 2018;45(1):33–6.
25. Boscoe FP, Talbot TO, Kulldorff M. Public domain small-area cancer incidence data for New York State, 2005–2009. Geospat Health. 2016;11(1):304.
26. Boscoe FP. Population estimates by census tract, New York State, by age and sex, 1990–2016. Online: https://figshare.com/articles/Population_Estimates_by_Census_Tract_New_York_State_by_Age_and_Sex_1990-2016_/6813029. 2018
27. Boscoe FP. Breast cancer rates by stage and household income percentile, New York State, 2006–2015. Online: https://figshare.com/articles/Breast_cancer_rates_by_stage_and_household_income_percentile_New_York_State_2006-2015/6815357. 2018.
28. New York State Department of Health. BRFSS Brief Number 1714: Breast Cancer Screening New York State Adult Women, 2016. https://www.health.ny.gov/statistics/brfss/reports/docs/1714_brfss_breast_cancer.pdf. Accessed 20 July 2018.
29. National Committee for Quality Assurance. State of health care quality: breast cancer screening. http://www.ncqa.org/report-cards/health-plans/state-of-health-care-quality/2017-table-of-contents/breast-cancer. Accessed 11 July 2018.
30. Boscoe FP, Zhang X. Visualizing the diffusion of digital mammography in New York State. Cancer Epidemiol Biomark Prev. 2017;26(4):490–4.
31. Akinyemiju TF. The association of early life socioeconomic position on breast cancer incidence and mortality: a systematic review. Int J Public Health. 2018;63(9):787–97.
32. Chen X. A temporal analysis of the association between breast cancer and socioeconomic and environmental factors. GeoJournal 2017; in press.
33. Feller A, Schmidlin K, Bordoni A, Bouchardy C, Bulliard J-L, Camey B, Konzelmann I, Maspoli M, Wanner M, Clough-Gorr KM. Socioeconomic and demographic disparities in breast cancer stage and presentation and survival: a Swiss population-based study. Int J Cancer. 2017;141(8):1529–39.
34. Klassen AC, Smith KC. The enduring and evolving relationship between social class and breast cancer burden: a review of the literature. Cancer Epidemiol. 2011;35:217–34.
35. Lyle G, Hendrie GA, Hendrie D. Understanding the effects of socioeconomic status along the breast cancer continuum in Australian women: a systematic review of evidence. Int J Equity Health. 2017;16:182.
36. Ryabov I. On the relationship between development and fertility: the case of the United States. Comp Popul Stud. 2015;40(4):465–88.
37. Marmot M. The health gap: the challenge of an unequal world: the argument. Int J Epidemiol. 2017;46(4):1312–8.

Chapter 14
Geographic Variation in Medical Neighborhoods for Breast Cancer Care: Diagnosis and Beyond

Jennifer Tsui, Michelle Doose, and Kevin A. Henry

Abstract The health care system in the United States (U.S.) is a fragmented system with little coordination between primary care and specialty care. Along the cancer care continuum, failures in the delivery of adequate processes of care, defined as the "types of care provided and the transitions between them," directly result in suboptimal care quality and outcomes for cancer patients. The Agency for Healthcare Research and Quality defines a "medical neighborhood" as the "patient-centered medical home (PCMH) and the constellation of other clinicians providing health care services to patients within it, along with communication and social service organizations and state and local public health agencies." The increasing health care consolidation in the U.S. over the past decade, including the acquisition of independent physician practices into hospital and other integrated systems, could have profound impact on the geography of medical neighborhoods for cancer patients and access to cancer care services across population subgroups and geographic areas. In this chapter, we describe emerging research in medical neighborhoods and cancer care delivery and recommendations for future geographic-based research to better inform ways to address breast cancer care and cancer disparities. We specifically identify emerging models of care that facilitate cancer care coordination and focus on geographic access and medical neighborhood factors required to meet the needs of medically underserved populations.

Keywords Breast cancer · Cancer care delivery · Medical neighborhoods · Geographic access to care · Health care redesign

J. Tsui (✉) · M. Doose
Department of Population Science, Rutgers Cancer Institute of New Jersey,
New Brunswick, NJ, USA

Rutgers, School of Public Health, Rutgers, The State University of New Jersey,
New Brunswick, NJ, USA
e-mail: jk1341@cinj.rutgers.edu

K. A. Henry
Department of Geography and Urban Studies, Temple University, Philadelphia, PA, USA

Fox Chase Cancer Center, Temple University, Philadelphia, PA, USA

© Springer Nature Switzerland AG 2019
D. Berrigan, N. A. Berger (eds.), *Geospatial Approaches to Energy Balance and Breast Cancer*, Energy Balance and Cancer 15, https://doi.org/10.1007/978-3-030-18408-7_14

14.1 Overview

The U.S. health care system is a fragmented system with little coordination between primary care and specialty care. Understanding the context of real-world cancer care delivery, both within oncology and primary care, and how these settings interact within the geospatial context for patients is critical to achieving high quality breast cancer care for all populations [1]. Taplin's framework for improving the quality of cancer care shows that there are many processes of care that proceed the diagnosis of breast cancer into treatment [2]. Along the cancer care continuum, failures in the delivery of adequate processes of care, defined as the "types of care provided and the transitions between them," directly results in suboptimal care quality and outcomes for cancer patients [3]. Although geospatial disparities in cancer incidence and mortality are well documented [4–12], less is understood about the geospatial context of breast cancer care transitions, from diagnosis to treatment and from treatment to survivorship care. Furthermore, the implementation of a geospatial perspective of "medical neighborhoods" for cancer care utilization has been limited, but is necessary in identifying strategies to improve breast cancer care from diagnosis and beyond [13].

The Agency for Healthcare Research and Quality (AHRQ) defines a "medical neighborhood" as the "patient-centered medical home (PCMH) and the constellation of other clinicians providing health care services to patients within it, along with communication and social service organizations and state and local public health agencies" [14]. It was first coined by Elliot Fisher in 2008 given that patients with chronic illness required specialty care outside the medical home [15]. The medical home model is an approach where primary care delivers comprehensive, coordinated and continuous health care for patients. However, it does not refer to a specific geographic place or location, but rather the care settings that serve these patients. The concept of medical neighborhoods focuses on centralized health care coordination through primary care providers "surrounded by specialty clinics, ancillary service providers, and hospitals" [16]. In addition to key providers in the neighborhood, interoperable electronic medical records to streamline referrals and tests/procedures as well as "collaborative care agreements" to delineate roles and expectations between the primary care physicians and specialists are necessary requisites for a functional medical neighborhood [17–20]. Recent health reforms to promote medical neighborhoods, including efforts such as Accountable Care Organizations (ACO) to provide financial incentives for accountability and shared care across providers within neighborhoods, are currently being adopted and evaluated across the country [14]. A depiction of the BlueCross BlueShield ACO and Medical Neighborhood is shown in Fig. 14.1. To date, most of the literature on medical neighborhoods has focused on improving the health of the general population as well as for certain medical conditions, such as diabetes, behavioral health, kidney disease, and children with complex care needs [21–24]. Geographic/spatial access to breast cancer care and the interaction among these "neighbors" to deliver high-quality care from treatment and beyond care have been underexplored.

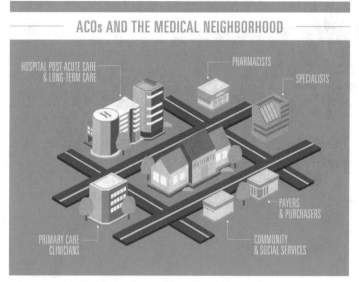

Source: https://www.bcbs.com/the-health-of-america/articles/bright-idea-how-accountable-care-organizations-are-changing

Fig. 14.1 ACOs and the medical neighborhood

Much of the research on geographic/spatial access to health care resources has focused on geographic variations in access to mammography facilities, source for treatment (e.g. surgery, radiation, etc.), and oncologists (Fig. 14.2). However, very limited research has focused on understanding and conceptualizing medical neighborhoods for cancer care delivery, particularly during a time of rapid health care reorganization and redesign efforts (e.g. PCMH, ACOs). The increasing health care consolidation in the U.S. over the past decade, including the acquisition of independent physician practices into hospital and other integrated systems, could have profound impact on the geography of medical neighborhoods for cancer patients [25–27]. For example, in community oncology settings, shifts from independent oncology practices to larger system affiliations have led to new referral patterns and underlying infrastructure that can affect primary care-oncology care relationships [28, 29]. In addition, new interventions to improve care delivery and care coordination, including patient navigation, telehealth, and nurse care management, could also impact the geography of medical neighborhoods [30]. From a disparities perspective, it is also unclear whether medical neighborhoods for cancer care manifest differently across population subgroups and within geographic areas. Our prior work, examining patterns of cancer care across diverse population subgroups in the New Jersey State Cancer Registry, indicates substantial differences in geospatial patterns of treatment by race/ethnicity, insurance type, and area-level factors [31]. In this chapter, we describe emerging research in this area and recommendations for future geographic-based research to better inform ways to address breast cancer care and cancer disparities.

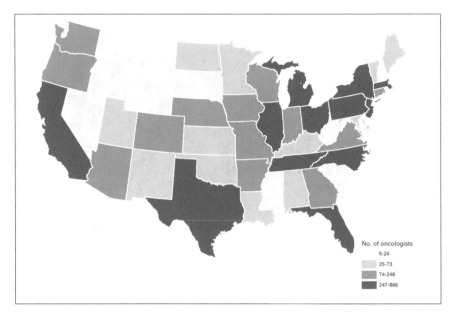

Fig. 14.2 Distribution of oncologists, 2016 ASCO oncology practice census, state of cancer care in American report. http://ascopubs.org/doi/10.1200/JOP.2016.020743

14.2 Current State of Cancer Care by Geographic Accessibility and Distribution

14.2.1 Regional Variations in Cancer Care

Geographic variations in breast cancer access, quality of care, and costs of care have been well-documented. Much of this work has focused on populations ages 65 years and older using Medicare data. One of the key sources to map and summarize how medical resources are distributed and used in the U.S. is the Dartmouth Atlas Project; this project summarizes how medical resources, including breast cancer screening and oncology services, are utilized and distributed in the U.S [32, 33]. While the Dartmouth Atlas has been instrumental in documenting geographic variations in medical resources, services, and costs across the U.S., it does not directly focus on how geographic access and travel burden (e.g. travel distance or time) to services can result in delays in diagnosis, influence the choice of treatment, and ultimately impact outcomes.

In the last decade, there has been an increased emphasis on how geographic access to medical services can influence the utilization of health services and outcomes [34, 35]. Geographic accessibility is an important enabling factor, which can facilitate or inhibit the use of health services. Geographic accessibility specifically describes the relationship between the availability of services (supply), the number of people needing a service (demand), the spatial variation of services from one place to another, and the spatial interaction between health services and the population [36, 37]. Sufficient geographic access to health care services can be realized through the addition of more physicians, specialists or services, and optimizing access to health care by adding more where gaps in geographic access exist [38–40]. However, gaps in geographic access remain in some areas due to market failures resulting from hospital and clinic closures as well as failures to retain and attract physicians and specialists (e.g. rural areas) [41–44]. Gaps in geographic access have also resulted from limited physician participation in the Medicaid program. Physician hesitancy to accept Medicaid patients has been attributed to low reimbursement rates, extra administrative burden of processing claims, and delays in reimbursement [45–47]. The need for increased physician participation in Medicaid is even more important following Medicaid eligibility expansion in several states under the Affordable Care Act [47]. However, a recent study by Neprash and colleagues reported most physicians either maintained or only slightly increased their Medicaid participation and increased participation was driven by physicians in expansions states only [48].

Poor geographic access to services resulting in long travel times from a patient's residence to their provider can be a key factor that can influence access to diagnosis and treatment services for cancer as well as delays in diagnosis and the types of treatment received [35]. The requirement of repeated visits for diagnosis, treatment, and follow-up of cancer further magnifies the importance of travel distance/time that currently must also be managed by the patient. Studies examining geographic access to services are generally conceptualized around the idea that a deficit or maldistribution of supply and/or populations or poor geographic access (e.g. long travel distances or time to health services, lower density of serviced per area, higher capacity) can result in barriers to conveniently accessing services and possible geographic disparities in health service utilization rates, treatments received, and poorer outcomes. A review study by Ambroggi et al. focused on cancer care and geographic access, found that increasing travel requirements for patients is associated with more advanced disease at diagnosis, inappropriate treatment, a worse prognosis, and a worse quality of life [35].

While long travel distances/times to access care is often conceptualized as a barrier to access care, distance and time might be perceived differently for people with varying resources (e.g. car ownership, access to public transit, income, social support, and time availability), and for people who have experiences living in different geographic contexts [49]. A study by Buzza and colleagues found that among rural veterans in eight Midwestern states a number of patient factors compounded long travel times to care including health status, functional impairment, travel cost, and work or family obligations [50]. They also found that perceptions of travel distance to care were seen differently based on the type of care required. For example, Veterans perceived the same travel distance as more burdensome when seeking care for basic services (e.g. laboratory), when compared with specialty care (e.g. cardiology). Other studies have also found that the relationships between travel distance/time on use of health services can differ across race/ethnic communities. For example, a study by Koizumi and colleagues found some racial/ethnic groups to be less likely to travel further for mental health services compared to other groups [51]. At the same time, other work suggests that some groups rely on services within their own ethnic communities that are often linguistically and culturally more concordant with racial/ethnic minority patients, and thus may be willing to travel further in distance or time to reach providers in community enclaves [52–55]. Regardless of how distance/time is overcome to access care, researchers should move beyond simply operationalizing travel distance/time as a concept that is linearly associated with geographic access. More research is needed on how distance/time as a barrier to breast cancer care, specifically, is perceived by patients, and how barriers to care resulting from travel distance/time are mediated by patient factors and geographic context [50].

In the context of the medical neighborhood for cancer care, it is unclear whether patients are more likely to seek clinicians in close proximity to their place or residence or located in other communities that are further away, based on one's employment location, access to racial/ethnic or language concordance, or preference for specific providers due to other reasons (e.g. reputation of oncologists, car ownership, poverty, financial or time resources). It is also unclear what role proximity to care plays in patient referral patterns. The literature on medical neighborhoods is very focused on the efficient coordination between providers and the group of clinicians providing health care services to patients within the neighborhood, along with community and social service organizations. However, there is little in the literature about how geographic or perceived distance to these services fits in or how geographic barriers to care will impact prevention and care opportunities in medical neighborhoods.

14.2.2 Surgery

Studies have shown that primary therapy after breast cancer diagnosis is influenced by travel distance or time to these services. Vora et al. found that patients located in surgical deserts (counties with fewer than six surgeons per 100,000 population) were much less likely to receive breast reconstruction surgery after adjusting for median household income, insurance, race, age, and type of comorbidity [56]. Other related measures of geographic access, including density of specialists per area and the types of facilities available, also showed important relationships between treatments received and outcomes. Albornoz et al. found that treatment centers with the highest volume of cases were located in metropolitan areas and those centers with the highest treatment volume were less likely to have surgery-related complications than those centers with a lower treatment volume [57]. However, a recent study by Keating et al., which examined patterns of care for breast cancer patients in four major U.S. cities, observed that Black women with breast cancer were less likely to receive care at high-quality hospitals (i.e. hospitals with greater volume of surgery) and more likely to receive care at hospitals with a higher proportion of Black patients after accounting for distance and other hospital characteristics [58]. Similar findings were found for Hispanic and Asian women. Despite being in close proximity to higher volume/high quality hospitals, minority patients may receive care at lower volume hospitals due to language or cultural concordance or due to actual or perceived discrimination in high volume hospital settings. Another reason may be that minority women were more likely to select their surgeon based on their doctor's referral compared with White women who were more likely to select their surgeon based on their reputation [59].

14.2.3 Radiation Therapy

A majority of studies have found that early-stage breast cancer patients who lived further away from radiation therapy facilities were more likely to receive a mastectomy instead of breast conserving surgery followed by radiation therapy [35, 60–64]. Time to initiating therapy has also been shown to be influenced by travel time/distance to services. Wheeler et al. found that the structural and organizational characteristics of the health system including distance to these organizations explained some of the racial/ethnic disparities in initiating radiation therapy [65]. Greater travel distance to radiation therapy was associated with late initiation of therapy and private/for-profit facilities had timelier initiation to treatment compared to government-owned or National Cancer Institute-designed centers. A study by Celeya et al. noted that New Hampshire women with early-stage breast cancer living more than 20 miles from a radiation treatment facility are not only less likely to have breast conserving surgery (BCS), but if they do so, they are significantly less likely to receive post-operative radiation that would reduce their risk of recurrence [61]. They also found that winter season also influenced treatment. In the winter season the proportion of women electing BCS, whom forgo radiation, is higher than the summer season, which is likely related to the difficulty of traveling during winter. Studies completed in New Mexico and Florida also found a lower likelihood of radiation after BCS with increasing travel distance to the nearest radiation therapy facility [62, 63].

A study by Lin et al. found that women with early stage-breast cancer in South Dakota, one of the most rural states in the U.S., who had to travel over 90 min to a radiation therapy facility were about 1.5 times more likely to receive a mastectomy, with increasing rates for travel times over 120 min [66]. In New Jersey, the most urbanized state in the U.S., Goyal et al. found that breast cancer patients residing >9.2 miles compared with ≤9.2 miles from radiation facility were 44% more likely to receive mastectomy than BCS and patients requiring >19 min compared with ≤19 min of travel time were 36% more likely to receive mastectomy than BCS [67]. Including data from 30% of the U.S. population (10 states), Boscoe and colleagues found a generally increasing likelihood of mastectomy with increasing distance to nearest radiation therapy and a monotonically increasing likelihood of mastectomy with increasing distance to surgical facility [60]. While Boscoe et al. hypothesized that women living far from treatment and radiation would be more likely to choose mastectomy, they also noted that some women were by-passing local options and traveling further to care where they would receive mastectomy. It was noted that this could be due to the multifaceted characteristics of this group, including patients who elect to travel long distances to seek the best (or perceived best) care, those whose prior medical histories call for more specialized care, those who were referred from smaller to larger cancer centers for any number of reasons, and perhaps even those whose insurance coverage dictated longer travel.

14.2.4   Survivorship Care

It is estimated that 1.7 million new cancer cases will be diagnosed in 2018 and the number of cancer survivors in the U.S. will reach over 18 million by 2020 [68, 69]. Professional cancer organizations have issued clinical practice guidelines for long-term follow-up of cancer patients [70–74]. Several recent reports and guidelines have been updated to recommend the systematic delivery of cancer survivorship care in conjunction with primary care [75–78]. While several care transitions initiatives have been implemented or piloted by AHRQ or Centers for Medicare and Medicaid Services (CMS) to improve transitions between acute hospitalizations and long-term care or back to primary care [79, 80], few strategies have been developed to focus on improving the transition from active cancer treatment to long-term survivorship care. Recent studies have shown implementation of cancer survivorship care is limited in primary care settings [81]. Other models of cancer survivorship care are often extension models in oncology settings [82, 83]. Most of these models implemented are extensions of oncologic care but vary widely in approach and scope of care based on the context where they are operationalized [82, 84]. Few studies to date have examined geographic influences on access to survivorship care given the limited implementation of survivorship care overall.

Current studies focused on geographic access to breast cancer care and cancer care as whole are limited by the availability of data. While SEER-Medicare data has provided data to answer many questions about breast cancer outcomes, this data resource is limited to population 65 and older who account for 43.2% of new breast cancer cases [85]. For example, a study found that the per capita rate of oncologists in an area had a negative relationship with the proportion of patients over 65 who were receiving chemotherapy [86], but it is unclear if this relationship is consistent for younger populations with cancer. As indicated in the literature review above, cancer registry data can be used in certain situations to examine geographic access (e.g. place of diagnosis), but it is currently unclear if all cancer registries collected information about where treatments occurred and whether the data quality are consistent across registries. In several of the studies using registry data to examine use of radiation after surgery travel time to the 'nearest' radiation facility was used rather than travel time to the actual radiation facility because these data were missing from the cancer registry data. Some registries capture information about treatments performed and what organization submitted the treatment information, but with an increasing number of partnered and affiliate hospitals, it is not always clear where the patient was actually treated. To properly study the utilization of health services and document and address any gaps in access in medical neighborhoods, new procedures and methods of data collection are needed to accurately capture this information.

14.3   Coordination of Oncology Services Across the Cancer Care Continuum: Geographic Availability, Co-Location, & Integrated Systems

14.3.1   Care Coordination

Over the course of treatment, breast cancer patients may transition their care from chemotherapy, surgery, and radiation while going back and forth from primary care to address the cancer diagnosis, side-effects from treatment, and disease management of comorbidities, and other non-cancer care [87]. Medical and patient advocacy organizations have long been advocating for better care coordination between medical providers and across health systems, which has garnered new attention since the passing of the Affordable Care Act [88]. However, the implementation and evaluation of care coordination initiatives to improve delivery of care, reduce overuse, and improve cancer outcomes are lacking, especially in the context of the medical neighborhood [1]. A major impediment to understanding whether current care coordination efforts are effective is the lack of consensus in the definition of care coordination roles and activities from the patient, provider, and healthcare system perspectives. For example, in the context of coordinating care for cancer survivors, work by our study team in PCMH settings has revealed provider-reported lack of clarity in the respective roles and responsibilities of PCPs and oncologists during transition points in the cancer care continuum [89]. Primary care providers caring for cancer survivors also report a lack of guidance on appropriate follow-up care plans for cancer survivors. National guidelines on cancer survivorship care indicate that long-term systematic care should take place within primary care settings as the number of cancer survivors continues to increase [72, 76, 90, 91]. However, recent studies, including those by our study team, have shown implementation of systematic survivorship care is extremely limited within primary care [92–95].

The National Quality Forum (NQF) in 2007 defined care coordination as the "function that helps ensure that the patient's needs and preferences for health services and information sharing across people, functions, and sites are met over time" [96]. AHRQ developed a working definition of care coordination: *"Care coordination is the deliberate organization of patient care activities between two or more participants (including the patient) involved in a patient's care to facilitate the appropriate delivery of health care services. Organizing care involves the marshalling of personnel and other resources needed to carry out all required patient care activities, and is often managed by the exchange of information among participants responsible for different aspects of care.*" One care coordination measure defined by AHRQ to date is specific for breast cancer patients (i.e. quality of patient and practice management among hospital surgery centers) [97]. Commonly known care coordination mechanisms and activities are not traditionally geographically bound: patients sharing medical records with providers (e.g., treatment summary, survivorship care plan), active communication between providers (i.e., faxed discharged summary), and care coordination by a designated person (e.g., care coordinator/navigator). New emerging models of care delivery with promise to facilitate care coordination, including co-location of providers in the same physical location and integrated patient-centered care within a single healthcare system, are increasingly reliant on geographic boundaries [98–100].

14.3.2   Co-Location

Few studies to date have examined the influence of co-location of cancer care services with primary care or other specialty providers on breast cancer outcomes. Elrashidi et al. systematic review and meta-analysis of 22 studies on the co-location of specialty care (i.e. behavioral health, diabetes, cardiology, geriatrics, nephrology, and infectious disease) with primary care found an association with increased patient satisfaction, primary care provider satisfaction, outpatient visits, and reduced wait for appointments [101]. It is has been hypothesized that if multispecialty cancer care (and non-cancer care) is delivered within the same location or practice, that "providers will improve communication, collaboration, and coordination."[101, 102] Co-location may increase collaboration between providers who may have an increased opportunity to see each other and each other's patient notes within the same electronic health record system. Additionally, it may remove barriers to care such as travel time and appointment wait times if patients are able to schedule their visits concurrently. Co-location of staff can also facilitate team-based care such as multidisciplinary cancer conferences/tumor boards [81, 94, 103]. The fragmented delivery of breast cancer care across the cancer care continuum remains a major impediment for high-quality cancer care; however, measures of fragmentation and co-location and its associated mechanisms that influence cancer care outcomes remains poor [104, 105].

14.3.3   Integrated Delivery Systems

Factors associated with breast cancer awareness and knowledge [106], adherence to adjuvant endocrine therapy [107, 108], chemotherapy-related adverse events [109], disparities in utilization of breast cancer treatment [110], and incidence and survival [111, 112] have been examined within integrated single health care systems. Integrated health systems consist of delivery settings where all health services from primary to specialty care are part of the same organization and located in the same practice. The expectations are that interoperable electronic medical records are available for all participating care team members to coordinate care and avoid duplication of medical services. Since 1999 the National Institutes for Health funds the Cancer Research Network (CRN) research programs to study integrated health delivery systems across the cancer care continuum [113, 114]. Today there are 8 non-profit health care systems and 4 sites that comprise CRN. One breast cancer screening study among 7 CRN health care systems found that late stage breast cancer diagnosis compared with early stage was associated with no prior mammography or clinical breast exam [115]. However, not all cancer care will be integrated into single health care systems. As a result, research is needed to examine the delivery of oncology services via inter-organizational care coordination/collaboration within a patient's medical neighborhood; that is the sharing of cancer care between independent health care systems [116].

14.4 Emerging Models to Facilitate Care Coordination: Implications for Geospatial Access and Medical Neighborhoods for Breast Cancer Care

The significant and ongoing shift in health care organization and delivery over the past several years is likely having a direct impact on the structure of medical neighborhoods for breast cancer care. These emerging models of delivery, organization and payment, include the overall increase in health care consolidation (both vertical and horizontal), the implementation of patient-centered medical homes and accountable care organizations, and the introduction of oncology care models and multispecialty care teams. We describe each of these emerging models below and their potential, or emerging evidence, impact on breast cancer care to date.

14.4.1 Consolidation of Oncology Practices

Over the last decade, there has been rapid health care delivery consolidation in the U.S., including the acquisition of independent physician practices into hospital and other integrated systems, which can have profound effects in primary care delivery and management for cancer patients [25–27]. Based on the American Society of Clinical Oncology (ASCO) State of Oncology Practice in America report for 2018, trends in consolidation for oncology practices have continued in recent years, with a 9.4% decreased in the number of oncology practices overall from 2013 to 2017 and a 25% increase in the size of oncology practices from 2016–2017 [117]. In the same report, approximately 34% of oncology practices indicated some change in organizational structure over the past year as well. In community oncology settings, shifts from independent oncology practices to larger system affiliations has led to new referral patterns and underlying infrastructure that can affect primary care-oncology care relationships [29, 118]. Our recent study on existing primary care-oncology relationships within varying settings found that nearly all primary care practices observed with existing formal primary care-oncology relationships were embedded within healthcare systems and that these formal relationships noted ease of communication and transfer of patient information, timely referrals, and direct access to oncologists [119]. In contrast, practices with informal relationships in our study noted the benefits of having close engagement with specific oncologists. There is limited evidence on whether formal primary care-oncology relationships impact long-term outcomes for cancer patients more positively compared to informal relationships, but ongoing monitoring of whether the increasing number of system/hospital owned practices may provide additional infrastructure for primary care to establish more feasible, formal relationships with oncologists is needed.

14.4.2   Patient-Centered Medical Homes

Newly emerging research for improved care coordination has also stemmed from the Chronic Care Model and new models of health care delivery, including Patient-Centered Medical Home (PCMHs) and Accountable Care Organizations (ACOs) [120, 121]. These new models focus on reshaping the health system environment by organizing the delivery and coordination of patient care activities and holding system and providers accountable to the health care outcomes of their patients [122, 123]. For example, the PCMH, first introduced in 2007, is a widely touted model designed to enhance quality and safety in primary care practices [124–126]. The PCMH model integrates best practices in access, prevention, chronic disease management, care coordination, and patient responsiveness using innovative health technology to improve communication through patient portals and other tools [127–131]. Core attributes of the PCMH include serving as the first contact for access to care and providing more proactive and effective coordination and integration of care. The relationship between PCMHs, and other innovative primary care settings, with oncology providers has been understudied. The few studies that have examined PCMH enrollment among breast cancer patients have found higher outpatient care utilization and costs among a single state Medicaid program, better follow-up mammography among breast cancer survivors, and fewer inpatient visits for chemotherapy-related adverse events [132–134].

14.4.3 Accountable Care Organizations

The Medicare Shared Savings Program Accountable Care Organization (ACO) was enacted into law as part of the Patient Protection and Affordable Care Act in March 2010 [31]. Other ACOs and ACO-like organizations have since been formed by Medicaid and private commercial insurance entities. As of August 2012, 55% of the U.S. population resided in a hospital service area (HSA) served by at least one of 227 ACOs, which varied by payer: 21% Medicare, 13% private, and 3% Medicaid [135]. ACOs were less likely to be located in high-poverty, rural regions, and in the South region of the U.S [135]. As of 2018, there are 550 Medicare ACOs and 12 states with Medicaid ACOs with 10 additional states pursing ACO formation (Fig. 14.3) [136–138].

The research on ACOs impact on breast cancer screening is emerging, yet findings are mixed. Several studies reported no significant increases in screening mammography at ACOs [139–142]. Another study reported a statistically significant (albeit small) increase in screenings while another study found a statistically significant reduction in screening mammograms for women greater than 75 years [139, 143]. A natural extension of ACO is the formation of medical neighborhoods to address the health of communities by linking providers, hospital systems, and

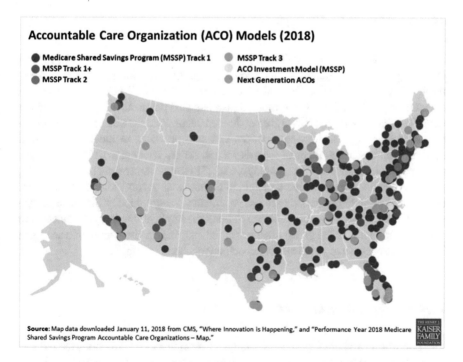

Accountable Care Organization (ACO) Models (2018)

● Medicare Shared Savings Program (MSSP) Track 1   ● MSSP Track 3
● MSSP Track 1+   ○ ACO Investment Model (MSSP)
● MSSP Track 2   ● Next Generation ACOs

Source: Map data downloaded January 11, 2018 from CMS, "Where Innovation is Happening," and "Performance Year 2018 Medicare Shared Savings Program Accountable Care Organizations – Map."

Fig. 14.3 Accountable care organization models in 2018, Kaiser family foundation, https://www.kff.org/aco-map-nooutline_1-11-18

social services [144]. Given the well documented delays or forgoing of necessary cancer care, medical neighborhoods may be able to address the additional socio-economic and other non-clinical needs of cancer patients [145, 146]. Research on breast cancer care within ACOs is currently missing from the literature as oncology practice grapples with the changing health care delivery landscape [147].

14.4.4   Community Oncology Medical Home (COME HOME)

In 2012, the Center for Medicare & Medicaid Innovation (CMMI) funded Innovative Oncology Business Solutions to launch their patient-centered oncology medical home at seven community practices within the U.S [148]. The main goal of COME HOME is to "improve health outcomes, enhance patient care experiences and significantly reduce costs of care by keeping patients out of the emergency department and hospital as much as possible" [149]. One study found that COME HOME had reduced hospitalizations and health care spending in comparison to matched practices [150].

14.4.5   Oncology Care Model

In 2016 the CMMI created the Oncology Care Model (OCM), a 5 year model to "test innovative payment strategies that promote high-quality and high-value cancer" through "care coordination fee and episode-based payments" [151, 152]. The first chemotherapy claim triggers a 6 month episode-based payment for nearly all cancer types for which additional 6 month episodes can occur. Practice transformation activities at eligible physician group practices and solo practices include: (1) enhanced services (i.e., electronic medical records access, patient navigation), (2) use of certified electronic health record technology, and (3) quality improvement. As of 2018, there are 184 participating practices and 13 commercial payers along with Medicare (Fig. 14.4) [152]. While OCMs are not specifically geographically bound (although payments are adjusted for geographic variation), the implications for tying cancer care coordination to physician group practices could also change the geographic access to breast cancer care (e.g. inpatient versus outpatient chemotherapy).

14.4.6   Team-Based Care

The definition of shared care, also known as team-based or collaborative care, is where the oncologists (e.g., medical, surgical, and/or radiation oncologists), primary care physician, and other specialists (e.g., endocrinologist, cardiologists) jointly participate in patient's care [153–155]. The concept of shared care is not new. Since the 1980s, shared care of diabetes care between primary care physicians

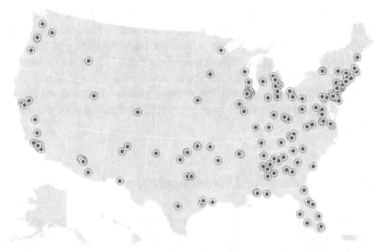

Source: Centers for Medicare & Medicaid Services

Fig. 14.4 Oncology care models, centers for medicare & medicaid services, https://innovation.cms.gov/initiatives/Oncology-Care

and hospital specialists was of much debate [156]. Limited studies, including randomized controlled trials, demonstrated that shared care improved care coordination, patient outcomes (e.g., morbidity, mortality), and for cancer, improved symptom management, treatment initiation, and adherence [156–162]. Recent studies evaluating primary care physicians involvement during cancer care demonstrated that Medicare breast cancer patients who reported greater primary care interaction had lower all-cause and cancer-specific mortality [163]. However, there is no literature on the type of provider involved and the type of comorbidity care delivered by that provider during breast cancer treatment [164].

Due to the rising number of cancer patients, especially among the aging population with complex health needs, and the increased complexity of cancer care with the advent of precision medicine, the U.S. health care system is in a state of crisis to deliver high-quality, coordinated cancer care to every patient [88, 165–167]. New studies are needed to capture processes of care, mechanisms, and activities of breast cancer care across the cancer continuum and within the context of a medical neighborhood. Emerging new models, including those described above, of cancer care are timely for this call to research.

14.5   Meeting the Cancer Care Needs of the Medically Underserved

Geospatial disparities in cancer incidence and mortality are well documented [4–11, 168]. Limited research has been conducted to understand geospatial boundaries for cancer care among low-income, racial/ethnic minority, and other vulnerable populations, both in rural and urban areas. While several studies to date have examined the relationship between geographic availability or access (e.g. travel distance) to cancer care services, there is a limited understanding of the multilevel factors that impact where cancer care is actually utilized [33, 64, 169]. As mentioned earlier, several of these studies also focus largely on elderly, Medicare-insured populations rather than a non-elderly, diverse population-based cancer cohorts, suggesting a need to better understand geographic boundaries for cancer care for disparity populations.

14.5.1 Cancer Care for Urban Populations

Factors related to urbanicity, or urban area characteristics, for example, can affect not only direct geographic/physical access to care but also humanistic elements, such as perceived lack of high quality care or perceptions on proximity to care within an individual's immediate neighborhood [170–172]. Local level determinants, including regulation of health care delivery services and insurance coverage, can also impact access to cancer care services [173]. Galea et al. also suggest focusing on the role of urban living conditions that help illuminate the complexities of life in urban settings and the interaction of service systems, social environment, the urban physical environment, and demographics of urban residents [173].

With a projected workforce shortage of oncologists by 2020, there is a real concern for the lack of timely access to cancer care due to the current geographic maldistribution of oncologists [174]. An important, yet underexplored area is the geographic access to oncologists within safety-net systems who serve a predominantly Medicaid insured and uninsured population. More research is needed to focus on referral patterns and delays in access to specialists for vulnerable patients in urban settings, where geographic availability of cancer care services is high but accessibility may be limited due to other patient, health care, and structural factors. Additionally, the oncology workforce struggles to racially/ethnically represent the U.S. population they serve [175]. Overall, 9% of physicians identified as African American/Black, Hispanic/Latino, or American Indian/Alaska Native [176]. African Americans (4%) and Hispanics (5%) have the lowest participation rates in hematology/oncology fellowships [175]. At the same time, minority physicians (African Americans, Latinos, and Pacific Islanders) are more likely to practice in medically underserved areas compared with non-Hispanic White physicians [177]. Given that safety-net hospitals and clinics are more likely to serve minority populations, there is a real problem of racial/ethnic (and linguistic) provider-patient concordance. Unfortunately, limited studies are available to determine whether racial/ethnic and linguistic concordance between the patient and provider are associated with improved cancer outcomes [178, 179].

14.5.2   Cancer Care for Rural Populations

It is estimated that rural residents, including those in rural Appalachia, experience higher rates of late-stage diagnosis and mortality from breast cancer compared to women in urban areas [180, 181]. However, in the 2017 State of Cancer Care in America report, only 1 oncologist per 100,000 rural residents compared to 5 oncologists per 100,000 urban residents were reported across the U.S [175]. In addition, residents in rural communities have higher proportions of poverty, lower educational attainment, and experience more co-morbidities. Rural areas also have lower geographic access to oncologists (Fig. 14.2), fewer treatment facilities for radiation and cancer clinical trials, and face increased travel burden to accessing cancer care services [182, 183]. In recent years, a rising interest and implementation of ehealth and telemedicine for oncology has developed both in the U.S. and abroad [184–191]. While empirical evidence of telemedicine on cancer outcomes is still incomplete, many have suggested that telemedicine can improve access to cancer-related specialist in low access areas, increase communication between multidisciplinary teams, reduce travel burden for patients in rural areas, and reduce overall disparities for breast cancer [192–195].

14.6   Summary and Areas for Future Research

While several studies have examined the relationship between geographic availability or access (e.g. travel distance) to cancer care services, there is a limited understanding of the multilevel factors that impact where cancer care is actually utilized [33, 64, 169]. Furthermore, geospatial analyses on cancer care spending and surgical outcomes have employed geographies such as those defined by the Dartmouth Atlas of Health Care based on Medicare data, which may be limited for non-Medicare, minority populations, and other subgroups in urban areas [32, 33, 169]. Cancer prevention and control research should continue to leverage and expand on existing data sources, such as cancer registries, to understand geospatial aspects of cancer care delivery and identify multilevel strategies to improve care quality and outcomes. An understanding of urban environments and the urban population context can help to better define and inform the role medical neighborhoods play in cancer care for disadvantaged groups.

As discussed above, several emerging models for care coordination and cancer care delivery are promising to potentially improve care for breast cancer patients in both rural and urban environments where care is currently limited. However, future research is needed to better understand how geography impacts breast cancer care from treatment and beyond. First, the accuracy and quality of facility information reported to cancer registries should be explored further. The utility of cancer registry data for treatment location could be better examined, presenting an opportunity to improve on the quality of the information that is currently being collected routinely by registries. Datasets that provide information of patterns and locations of care throughout the care continuum from diagnosis and beyond and from multiple payer sources is also required to better understand the cancer experiences of non-Medicare patients. Second, more comprehensive data, including mixed methods designs that incorporate qualitative information from patients, are needed to understand how geography impacts accessibility and choice of breast cancer treatment locations across population subgroups. Qualitative interview data on the impact of a breast cancer diagnosis and follow-up care processes with employment, financial burden, and other social and health care needs will help to inform the current understanding of how medical neighborhoods, and more specifically cancer care neighborhoods, are defined by different communities.

Conflict of Interest None of the authors have any potential conflicts of interest to disclose.

References

1. Parry C, Kent EE, Forsythe LP, Alfano CM, Rowland JH. Can't see the forest for the care plan: a call to revisit the context of care planning. J Clin Oncol. 2013;31:2651–3.
2. Taplin SH, Anhang Price R, Edwards HM, et al. Introduction: understanding and influencing multilevel factors across the cancer care continuum. J Natl Cancer Inst Monogr. 2012;2012:2–10.
3. Zapka JG, Taplin SH, Solberg LI, Manos MM. A framework for improving the quality of cancer care. Cancer Epidemiol Biomark Prev. 2003;12:4.
4. Roche LM, Niu X, Henry KA. Invasive cervical cancer incidence disparities in New Jersey—a spatial analysis in a high incidence state. J Health Care Poor Underserved. 2015;26:1173–85.
5. Henry KA, Sherman R, Farber S, Cockburn M, Goldberg DW, Stroup AM. The joint effects of census tract poverty and geographic access on late-stage breast cancer diagnosis in 10 US States. Health Place. 2013;21:110–21.
6. Boscoe FP, Johnson CJ, Sherman RL, Stinchcomb DG, Lin G, Henry KA. The relationship between area poverty rate and site-specific cancer incidence in the United States. Cancer. 2014;120:2191–8.
7. Roche LM, Niu X, Stroup AM, Henry KA. Disparities in female breast cancer stage at diagnosis in New Jersey: a spatial-temporal analysis. J Public Health Manag Pract. 2017;23:477–86.
8. Henry KA, Sherman RL, McDonald K, et al. Associations of census-tract poverty with sub-site-specific colorectal cancer incidence rates and stage of disease at diagnosis in the United States. J Cancer Epidemiol. 2014;2014:823484.
9. Harper S, Lynch J, Meersman SC, Breen N, Davis WW, Reichman MC. Trends in area-socioeconomic and race-ethnic disparities in breast cancer incidence, stage at diagnosis, screening, mortality, and survival among women ages 50 years and over (1987–2005). Cancer Epidemiol Biomark Prev. 2009;18:121–31.
10. Pardo-Crespo MR, Narla NP, Williams AR, et al. Comparison of individual-level versus area-level socioeconomic measures in assessing health outcomes of children in Olmsted County, Minnesota. J Epidemiol Community Health. 2013;67:305.
11. Hu S, Sherman R, Arheart K, Kirsner RS. Predictors of neighborhood risk for late-stage melanoma: addressing disparities through spatial analysis and area-based measures. J Invest Dermatol. 2014;134:937–45.

12. Towne SD Jr. Socioeconomic, geospatial, and geopolitical disparities in access to health care in the US 2011–2015. Int J Environ Res Public Health. 2017;14

13. Pham HH. Good neighbors: how will the patient-centered medical home relate to the rest of the health-care delivery system? J Gen Intern Med. 2010;25:630–4.

14. Taylor EF, Lake T, Nysenbaum J, Peterson G, Meyers D. Coordinating care in the medical neighborhood: critical components and available mechanism. In: Mathematica policy research. Rockville: Agency for Healthcare Resaerch and Quality; 2011.

15. Fisher ES. Building a medical neighborhood for the medical home. N Engl J Med. 2008;359:1202–5.

16. Huang X, Rosenthal MB. Transforming specialty practice—the patient-centered medical neighborhood. N Engl J Med. 2014;370:1376–9.

17. Feuerstein JD, Sheppard V, Cheifetz AS, Ariyabuddhiphongs K. How to develop the medical neighborhood. J Med Syst. 2016;40:196.

18. Kirschner N, Greenlee M. The patient-centered medical home neighbor: the interface of the patient-centered medical home with specialty/subspecialty practices. A position paper of the American college of Physicians. Philadelphia 2010.

19. Greenberg JO, Barnett ML, Spinks MA, Dudley JC, Frolkis JP. The "medical neighborhood": integrating primary and specialty care for ambulatory patients. JAMA Intern Med. 2014;174:454–7.

20. Spatz C, Bricker P, Gabbay R. The patient-centered medical neighborhood: transformation of specialty care. Am J Med Qual. 2014;29:344–9.

21. Bojadzievski T, Gabbay RA. Patient-centered medical home and diabetes. Diabetes Care. 2011;34:1047–53.

22. Smith ZG, McNicoll L, Clark TL, et al. Medical neighborhood model for the care of chronic kidney disease patients. Am J Nephrol. 2016;44:308–15.

23. The Working Party Group on Integrated Behavioral H, Baird M, Blount A, et al. Joint principles: integrating behavioral health care into the patient-centered medical home. Ann Fam Med. 2014;12:183–5.

24. Nielsen M, Olayiwola J, Grundy P, Grumbach K. The patient-center medical home's impact on cost & quality: an annual update of the evidence, 2012–2013. Washington, D.C.: Patient-Centered Primary Care Collaborative; 2014.

25. Christianson JB, Carlin CS, Warrick LH. The dynamics of community health care consolidation: acquisition of physician practices. Milbank Q. 2014;92:542–67.

26. Carlin CS, Feldman R, Dowd B. The impact of hospital acquisition of physician practices on referral patterns. Health Econ. 2016;25:439–54.

27. Essary AC, Green EP, Gans DN. Compensation and production in family medicine by practice ownership. Health Serv Res Manag Epidemiol. 2016;3: 2333392815624111.

28. Bach PB. Limits on Medicare's ability to control rising spending on cancer drugs. N Engl J Med. 2009;360:626–33.

29. Conti RM. Expanding the scope of the national practice oncology benchmark would be a critical source for understanding outpatient oncology practice costs and profits in a time of change. J Oncol Pract. 2015;11:e95–7.

30. Gorin SS, Haggstrom D, Han PKJ, Fairfield KM, Krebs P, Clauser SB. Cancer care coordination: a systematic review and meta-analysis of over 30 years of empirical studies. Ann Behav Med. 2017;51:532–46.

31. Tsui J, McGee-Avila JK, Henry KA, et al. Factors associated with geospatial patterns of cancer care among diverse, urban populations in New Jersey: a new perspective on medical neighborhoods for oncology care. Under Review. 2018.

32. The Henry J. Kaiser family foundation. Summary of the affordable care act. Available from URL: https: //www.kff.org/health-reform/fact-sheet/summary-of-the-affordable-care-act/ Accessed 29 June 2018.

33. Keating NL, Kouri EM, He Y, Freedman RA, Volya R, Zaslavsky AM. Location isn't everything: proximity, hospital characteristics, choice of hospital, and disparities for breast cancer surgery patients. Health Serv Res. 2016;51:1561–83.

34. Schroeder MC, Chapman CG, Nattinger MC, et al. Variation in geographic access to chemotherapy by definitions of providers and service locations: a population-based observational study. BMC Health Serv Res. 2016;16:274.
35. Ambroggi M, Biasini C, Del Giovane C, Fornari F, Cavanna L. Distance as a barrier to cancer diagnosis and treatment: review of the literature. Oncologist. 2015;20:1378–85.
36. Guagliardo MF. Spatial accessibility of primary care: concepts, methods and challenges. Int J Health Geogr. 2004;3:3.
37. Henry KA, McDonald K. Geographic Access to Health Services. In: Boscoe FP, editor. Geographic Health Data: Fundamental Techniques for Analysis. Wallingford: CABI International Press; 2013.
38. Wang F. Measurement, optimization, and impact of health care accessibility: a methodological review. Ann Assoc Am Geogr. 2012;102:1104–12.
39. Decker SL. No association found between the medicaid primary care fee bump and physician-reported participation in medicaid. Health Aff. 2018;37:1092–8.
40. Long SK. Physicians may need more than higher reimbursements to expand medicaid participation: findings from Washington State. Health Aff. 2013;32:1560–7.
41. Kamerow DB. Is the national health service corps the answer? (for placing family doctors in underserved areas). J Am Board Fam Med. 2018;31:499–500.
42. Renner DM, Westfall JM, Wilroy LA, Ginde AA. The influence of loan repayment on rural healthcare provider recruitment and retention in Colorado. Rural Remote Health. 2010;10:1605.
43. Ricci S, Tergas AI, Long Roche K, et al. Geographic disparities in the distribution of the U.S. gynecologic oncology workforce: a society of gynecologic oncology study. Gynecol Oncol Rep. 2017;22:100–4.
44. United States Government Accountability Office. Rural hospital closures: number and characteristics of affected hospitals and contributing factors, 2018.
45. Decker SL. In 2011 nearly one-third of physicians said they would not accept new Medicaid patients, but rising fees may help. Health Aff (Millwood). 2012;31:1673–9.
46. Gottlieb JD, Shapiro AH, Dunn A. The complexity of billing and paying for physician care. Health Aff (Millwood). 2018;37:619–26.
47. Long SK. Physicians may need more than higher reimbursements to expand Medicaid participation: findings from Washington State. Health Aff (Millwood). 2013;32:1560–7.
48. Neprash HT, Zink A, Gray J, Hempstead K. Physicians' participation in medicaid increased only slightly following expansion. Health Aff. 2018;37:1087–91.
49. Nemet GF, Bailey AJ. Distance and health care utilization among the rural elderly. Soc Sci Med. 2000;50:1197–208.
50. Buzza C, Ono SS, Turvey C, et al. Distance is relative: unpacking a principal barrier in rural healthcare. J Gen Intern Med. 2011;26(Suppl 2):648–54.
51. Koizumi N, Rothbard AB, Kuno E. Distance matters in choice of mental health program: policy implications for reducing racial disparities in public mental health care. Adm Policy Ment Health. 2009;36:424–31.
52. Mobley LR, Kuo T-MM, Andrews L. How sensitive are multilevel regression findings to defined area of context?: a case study of mammography use in California. Med Care Res Rev. 2008;65:315–37.
53. Gany FM, Herrera AP, Avallone M, Changrani J. Attitudes, knowledge, and health-seeking behaviors of five immigrant minority communities in the prevention and screening of cancer: a focus group approach. Ethn Health. 2006;11:19–39.
54. Ngo-Metzger Q, Sorkin DH, Phillips RS, et al. Providing high-quality care for limited English proficient patients: the importance of language concordance and interpreter use. J Gen Intern Med. 2007;22(Suppl 2):324–30.
55. Yang JS, Kagawa-Singer M. Increasing access to care for cultural and linguistic minorities: ethnicity-specific health care organizations and infrastructure. J Health Care Poor Underserved. 2007;18:532–49.

56. Vora H, Chung A, Lewis A, et al. Reconstruction among patients undergoing mastectomy: the effect of surgical deserts. J Surg Res. 2018;223:237–42.
57. Albornoz CR, Cordeiro PG, Hishon L, et al. A nationwide analysis of the relationship between hospital volume and outcome for autologous breast reconstruction. Plast Reconstr Surg. 2013;132:192e–200e.
58. Keating NL, Kouri E, He Y, Weeks JC, Winer EP. Racial differences in definitive breast cancer therapy in older women: are they explained by the hospitals where patients undergo surgery? Med Care. 2009;47:765–73.
59. Freedman RA, Kouri EM, West DW, Keating NL. Racial/ethnic differences in patients' selection of surgeons and hospitals for breast cancer surgery. JAMA Oncol. 2015;1:222–30.
60. Boscoe FP, Johnson CJ, Henry KA, et al. Geographic proximity to treatment for early stage breast cancer and likelihood of mastectomy. Breast. 2011;20:324–8.
61. Celaya MO, Rees JR, Gibson JJ, Riddle BL, Greenberg ER. Travel distance and season of diagnosis affect treatment choices for women with early-stage breast cancer in a predominantly rural population (United States). Cancer Causes Control. 2006;17:851–6.
62. Voti L, Richardson Lisa C, Reis Isildinha M, Fleming Lora E, MacKinnon J, Coebergh Jan Willem W. Treatment of local breast carcinoma in Florida. Cancer. 2005;106:201–7.
63. Athas WF, Adams-Cameron M, Hunt WC, Amir-Fazli A, Key CR. Travel distance to radiation therapy and receipt of radiotherapy following breast-conserving surgery. J Natl Cancer Inst. 2000;92:269–71.
64. Onega T, Duell EJ, Shi X, Wang D, Demidenko E, Goodman D. Geographic access to cancer care in the U.S. Cancer. 2008;112:909–18.
65. Wheeler SB, Carpenter WR, Peppercorn J, Schenck AP, Weinberger M, Biddle AK. Structural/organizational characteristics of health services partly explain racial variation in timeliness of radiation therapy among elderly breast cancer patients. Breast Cancer Res Treat. 2012;133:333–45.
66. Lin Y, Wimberly MC, Da Rosa P, Hoover J, Athas WF. Geographic access to radiation therapy facilities and disparities of early-stage breast cancer treatment. Geospat Health. 2018;13:622.
67. Goyal S, Chandwani S, Haffty BG, Demissie K. Effect of travel distance and time to radiotherapy on likelihood of receiving mastectomy. Ann Surg Oncol. 2015;22:1095–101.
68. Society AC. Cancer facts & figures. Atlanta: American Cancer Society; 2018.
69. American Cancer Society. Cancer treatment & survivorship facts & figures 2016–2017. Atlanta: American Cancer Society; 2016.
70. Khatcheressian JL, Hurley P, Bantug E, et al. Breast cancer follow-up and management after primary treatment: American society of clinical oncology clinical practice guideline update. J Clin Oncol. 2013;31:961–5.
71. Meyerhardt JA, Mangu PB, Flynn PJ, et al. Follow-up care, surveillance protocol, and secondary prevention measures for survivors of colorectal cancer: American society of clinical oncology clinical practice guideline endorsement. J Clin Oncol. 2013;31:4465–70.
72. Mohler JL. The 2010 NCCN clinical practice guidelines in oncology on prostate cancer. J Natl Compr Canc Netw. 2010;8:145.
73. American Society of Clinical Oncology. Guidelines, tools, & resources. Available from URL: https://www.asco.org/practice-guidelines/quality-guidelines/guidelines Accessed 29 June 2018.
74. National Comprehensive Cancer Network. NCCN guidelines. Available from URL: https://www.nccn.org/professionals/physician_gls/f_guidelines.asp Accessed 29 June 2018.
75. Cohen EE, LaMonte SJ, Erb NL, et al. American cancer society head and neck cancer survivorship care guideline. CA Cancer J Clin. 2016;66:203–39.
76. El-Shami K, Oeffinger KC, Erb NL, et al. American cancer society colorectal cancer survivorship care guidelines. CA Cancer J Clin. 2015;65:428–55.
77. Runowicz CD, Leach CR, Henry NL, et al. American cancer society/American society of clinical oncology breast cancer survivorship care guideline. J Clin Oncol. 2016;34:611–35.
78. Skolarus TA, Wolf AM, Erb NL, et al. American cancer society prostate cancer survivorship care guidelines. CA Cancer J Clin. 2014;64:225–49.

79. Dy SM, Ashok M, Wines RC, Rojas Smith L. A framework to guide implementation research for care transitions interventions. J Healthc Qual. 2015;37:41–54.
80. Kim CS, Flanders SA. Transitions of care. Ann Intern Med. 2013;158
81. Rubinstein EB, Miller WL, Hudson SV, et al. Cancer survivorship care in advanced primary care practices: a qualitative study of challenges and opportunities. JAMA Intern Med. 2017;177:1726–32.
82. Halpern MT, Viswanathan M, Evans TS, Birken SA, Basch E, Mayer DK. Models of cancer survivorship care: overview and summary of current evidence. J Oncol Pract. 2015;11:e19–27.
83. Howell D, Hack TF, Oliver TK, et al. Models of care for post-treatment follow-up of adult cancer survivors: a systematic review and quality appraisal of the evidence. J Cancer Surviv. 2012;6:359–71.
84. Campbell MK, Tessaro I, Gellin M, et al. Adult cancer survivorship care: experiences from the LIVESTRONG centers of excellence network. J Cancer Surviv. 2011;5:271–82.
85. National Cancer Institute. Cancer stat facts: female breast cancer. Available from URL: https://seer.cancer.gov/statfacts/html/breast.html Accessed 17 Oct 2018.
86. Chandak A, Nayar P, Lin G. Rural-urban disparities in access to breast cancer screening: a spatial clustering analysis. J Rural Health. 2018;35(2):229–35.
87. Sussman J, Baldwin LM. The interface of primary and oncology specialty care: from diagnosis through primary treatment. J Natl Cancer Inst Monogr. 2010;2010:18–24.
88. Medicine Io. In: Levit L, Balogh E, Nass S, Ganz PA, editors. Delivering high-quality cancer care: charting a new course for a system in Crisis. Washington, DC: National Academies Press; 2013.
89. Tsui J, Howard J, O'Malley, et al. The relationship between patient centered medical homes and oncology practices: implications for improving transitions in care. Under Review. 2018.
90. Desch CE, Benson AB III, Smith TJ, et al. Recommended colorectal cancer surveillance guidelines by the American society of clinical oncology. J Clin Oncol. 1999;17:1312.
91. Ligibel JA, Denlinger CS. New NCCN guidelines for survivorship care. J Natl Compr Canc Netw. 2013;11:640–4.
92. Nekhlyudov L, O'Malley DM, Hudson SV. Integrating primary care providers in the care of cancer survivors: gaps in evidence and future opportunities. Lancet Oncol. 2017;18:e30–8.
93. Oeffinger KC, Argenbright KE, Levitt GA, et al. Models of cancer survivorship health care: moving forward. Am Soc Clin Oncol Educ Book. 2014;34:205–13.
94. O'Malley D, Hudson SV, Nekhlyudov L, et al. J Cancer Surviv. 2017;11:13. https://doi.org/10.1007/s11764-016-0555-2.
95. Rubinstein E, Miller WL, Hudson SV, et al. Cancer survivorship care in advanced primary care practices: a qualitative study of challenges and ppportunities. JAMA Intern Med. 2017;177(12):1726–32.
96. National Quality Forum (NQF). Preferred practices and performance measures for measuring and reporting care coordination: a consensus report. Washington, DC: National Quality Forum; 2010.
97. Katz SJ, Morrow M, Hawley ST, et al. Coordinating cancer care: patient and practice management processes among surgeons who treat breast cancer. Med Care. 2010;48:45–51.
98. National Institute of Mental Health. Integrated Care. Available from URL: https://www.nimh.nih.gov/health/topics/integrated-care/index.shtml Accessed 25 June 2018.
99. Weaver SJ, Che XX, Petersen LA, Hysong SJ. Unpacking care coordination through a multiteam system lens: a conceptual framework and systematic review. Med Care. 2018;56:247–59.
100. Drury M, Yudkin P, Harcourt J, et al. Patients with cancer holding their own records: a randomised controlled trial. Br J Gen Pract. 2000;50:105–10.
101. Elrashidi MY, Mohammed K, Bora PR, et al. Co-located specialty care within primary care practice settings: a systematic review and meta-analysis. Healthcare. 2018;6:52–66.
102. Gesme DH, Wiseman M. Expanding practice to provide integrated cancer care. J Oncol Pract. 2010;6:325–7.

103. Gagliardi AR, Honein-AbouHaidar G, Stuart-McEwan T, et al. How do the characteristics of breast cancer diagnostic assessment programmes influence service delivery: a mixed methods study. Eur J Cancer Care (Engl). 2018;27:e12727.
104. Spinks T, Ganz PA, Sledge GW Jr, et al. Delivering high-quality cancer care: the critical role of quality measurement. Healthc (Amst). 2014;2:53–62.
105. Ponce N, Glenn B, Shimkhada R, Scheitler AJ, Ko M. Addressing barriers to breast cancer care in California. The 2016–2017 landscape for policy change. Los Angeles: UCLA Center for Health Policy Research; 2018.
106. Kwan ML, Shen L, Munneke JR, et al. Patient awareness and knowledge of breast cancer-related lymphedema in a large, integrated health care delivery system. Breast Cancer Res Treat. 2012;135:591–602.
107. Kroenke CH, Hershman DL, Gomez SL, et al. Personal and clinical social support and adherence to adjuvant endocrine therapy among hormone receptor-positive breast cancer patients in an integrated health care system. Breast Cancer Res Treat. 2018;170(3):623–31.
108. Kwan ML, Roh JM, Laurent CA, et al. Patterns and reasons for switching classes of hormonal therapy among women with early-stage breast cancer. Cancer Causes Control. 2017;28:557–62.
109. Rashid N, Koh HA, Baca HC, et al. Clinical impact of chemotherapy-related adverse events in patients with metastatic breast cancer in an integrated health care system. J Manag Care Spec Pharm. 2015;21:863–71.
110. Kurian AW, Lichtensztajn DY, Keegan THM, et al. Patterns and predictors of breast cancer chemotherapy use in Kaiser Permanente Northern California, 2004–2007. Breast Cancer Res Treat. 2013;137:247–60.
111. Keegan TH, Kurian AW, Gali K, et al. Racial/ethnic and socioeconomic differences in short-term breast cancer survival among women in an integrated health system. Am J Public Health. 2015;105:938–46.
112. Roseland ME, Pressler ME, Lamerato LE, et al. Racial differences in breast cancer survival in a large urban integrated health system. Cancer. 2015;121:3668–75.
113. Wagner EH, Greene SM, Hart G, et al. Building a research consortium of large health systems: the cancer research network. JNCI Monographs. 2005;2005:3–11.
114. Geiger Ann M, Buist Diana SM, Greene Sarah M, Altschuler A, Field Terry S. Survivorship research based in integrated healthcare delivery systems. Cancer. 2008;112:2617–26.
115. Taplin SH, Ichikawa L, Yood MU, et al. Reason for late-stage breast cancer: absence of screening or detection, or breakdown in follow-up? JNCI. 2004;96:1518–27.
116. Gagliardi AR, Dobrow MJ, Wright FC. How can we improve cancer care? A review of interprofessional collaboration models and their use in clinical management. Surg Oncol. 2011;20:146–54.
117. Polite BN, Seid JE, Levit LA, et al. A new look at the state of cancer care in America. J Oncol Pract. 2018;14(7):397–9.
118. Bach PB. Limits on Medicare's ability to control rising spending on cancer drugs. N Engl J Med. 2009;360(6)
119. Tsui J, Howard J, Miller WL, et al. Opportunities for improving cancer care management through primary care-oncology relationships. Under Review. 2018.
120. Meyers D, Peikes D, Genevro J, et al. The roles of patient-centered medical homes and accountable care organizations in coordinating patient care. Rockville: Agency for Healthcare Research and Quality; 2010.
121. American Society of Clinical Oncology. The state of cancer care in America, 2016: a report by the American society of clinical oncology. J Oncol Pract. 2016;12:339–83.
122. Brantley-Sieders DM, Fan KH, Deming-Halverson SL, Shyr Y, Cook RS. Local breast cancer spatial patterning: a tool for community health resource allocation to address local disparities in breast cancer mortality. PLoS One. 2012;7:e45238.
123. Rosenthal TC. The medical home: growing evidence to support a new approach to primary care. J Am Board Fam Med. 2008;21:427–40.

124. Adaji A, Melin GJ, Campbell RL, Lohse CM, Westphal JJ, Katzelnick DJ. Patient-centered medical home membership is associated with decreased hospital admissions for emergency department behavioral health patients. Popul Health Manag. 2017;21(3):172–9.
125. Crabtree BF, Nutting PA, Miller WL, Stange KC, Stewart EE, Jaen CR. Summary of the National Demonstration Project and recommendations for the patient-centered medical home. Ann Fam Med. 2010;8(Suppl 1).: S80–90; S92
126. Kilo CM, Wasson JH. Practice redesign and the patient-centered medical home: history, promises, and challenges. Health Aff (Millwood). 2010;29:773–8.
127. Bodenheimer T, Wagner EH, Grumbach K. Improving primary care for patients with chronic illness. JAMA. 2002;288:1909–14.
128. Grumbach K, Bodenheimer T. A primary care home for Americans: putting the house in order. JAMA. 2002;288:889–93.
129. Arrow K, Auerbach A, Bertko J, et al. Toward a 21st-century health care system: recommendations for health care reform. Ann Intern Med. 2009;150:493–5.
130. Berenson RA, Hammons T, Gans DN, et al. A house is not a home: keeping patients at the center of practice redesign. Health Aff. 2008;27:1219–30.
131. Davis K, Schoenbaum SC, Audet AM. A 2020 vision of patient-centered primary care. J Gen Intern Med. 2005;20:953–7.
132. Kohler RE, Goyal RK, Lich KH, Domino ME, Wheeler SB. Association between medical home enrollment and health care utilization and costs among breast cancer patients in a state Medicaid program. Cancer. 2015;121:3975–81.
133. Wheeler SB, Kohler RE, Goyal RK, et al. Is medical home enrollment associated with receipt of guideline-concordant follow-up care among low-income breast cancer survivors? Med Care. 2013;51:494–502.
134. Goyal RK, Wheeler SB, Kohler RE, et al. Health care utilization from chemotherapy-related adverse events among low-income breast cancer patients: effect of enrollment in a medical home program. N C Med J. 2014;75:231–8.
135. Lewis VA, Colla CH, Carluzzo KL, Kler SE, Fisher ES. Accountable care organizations in the United States: market and demographic factors associated with formation. Health Serv Res. 2013;48:1840–58.
136. Barnes AJ, Unruh L, Chukmaitov A, van Ginneken E. Health reform monitor: accountable care organizations in the USA: types, developments and challenges. Health Policy. 2014;118:1–7.
137. Center for Health Care Strategies I. Medicaid accountable care organizations: state update. Available from URL: https://www.chcs.org/resource/medicaid-accountable-care-organizations-state-update/ Accessed 2 May 2018.
138. The Henry J. Kaiser Family Foundation. 8 FAQs: medicare ACO models. Available from URL: https://www.kff.org/faqs-medicare-accountable-care-organization-aco-models/ Accessed 19 June 2018.
139. Resnick MJ, Graves AJ, Thapa S, et al. Medicare accountable care organization enrollment and appropriateness of cancer screening. JAMA Intern Med. 2018;178:648–54.
140. Narayan AK, Harvey SC, Durand DJ. Impact of medicare shared savings program accountable care organizations at screening mammography: a retrospective cohort study. Radiology. 2017;282:437–42.
141. Pope G, Kautter J, Leung M, Trisolini M, Adamache W, Smith K. Financial and quality impacts of the medicare physician group practice demonstration. Medicare Medicaid Res Rev. 2014;4: mmrr2014–2004-2003-a2001
142. Lewis VA, Colla CH, Carluzzo KL, Kler SE, Fisher ES. Accountable care organizations in the United States: market and demographic factors associated with formation. Health Serv Res. 2013;48:1840–58.
143. Song Z, Safran DG, Landon BE, et al. Health care spending and quality in year 1 of the alternative quality contract. N Engl J Med. 2011;365:909–18.
144. Tipirneni R, Vickery KD, Ehlinger EP. Accountable communities for health: moving from providing accountable care to creating health. Ann Fam Med. 2015;13:367–9.

145. Ko NY, Battaglia TA, Gupta-Lawrence R, et al. Burden of socio-legal concerns among vulnerable patients seeking cancer care services at an urban safety-net hospital: a cross-sectional survey. BMC Health Serv Res. 2016;16:196.
146. Weaver KE, Rowland JH, Bellizzi KM, Aziz NM. Forgoing medical care because of cost: assessing disparities in healthcare access among cancer survivors living in the United States. Cancer. 2010;116:3493–504.
147. Mehta AJ, Macklis RM. Overview of accountable care organizations for oncology specialists. J Oncol Pract. 2013;9:216–21.
148. Waters TM, Webster JA, Stevens LA, et al. Community oncology medical homes: physician-driven change to improve patient care and reduce costs. J Oncol Pract. 2015;11:462–7.
149. Innovative Oncology Business Solutions I. Come home program. Available from URL: http://www.comehomeprogram.com/ Accessed 26 June 2018.
150. Colligan EM, Ewald E, Keating NL, et al. Two innovative cancer care programs have potential to reduce utilization and spending. Med Care. 2017;55:873–8.
151. Kline RM, Muldoon LD, Schumacher HK, et al. Design challenges of an episode-based payment model in oncology: the centers for medicare & medicaid services oncology care model. J Oncol Pract. 2017;13:e632–45.
152. Centers for Medicare and Medicaid Services. Oncology care model. Available from URL: https://innovation.cms.gov/initiatives/oncology-care/ Accessed 26 June 2018.
153. Sada Y, Street RL, Singh H, Shada R, Naik AD. Primary care and communication in shared cancer care: a qualitative study. Am J Manag Care. 2011;17:259–65.
154. O'Toole E, Step MM, Engelhardt K, Lewis S, Rose JH. The role of primary care physicians in advanced cancer care: perspectives of older patients and their oncologists. J Am Geriatr Soc. 2009;57(Suppl 2):S265–8.
155. Oeffinger KC, McCabe MS. Models for delivering survivorship care. J Clin Oncol. 2006;24:5117–24.
156. Greenhalgh PM. Shared care for diabetes. A systematic review. Occas Pap R Coll Gen Pract. 1994;67:i–viii, 1–35.
157. Hickman M, Drummond N, Grimshaw J. A taxonomy of shared care for chronic disease. J Public Health Med. 1994;16:447–54.
158. Taplin SH, Weaver S, Salas E, et al. Reviewing cancer care team effectiveness. J Oncol Pract. 2015;11:239–46.
159. Bosch M, Faber MJ, Cruijsberg J, et al. Review article: effectiveness of patient care teams and the role of clinical expertise and coordination: a literature review. Med Care Res Rev. 2009;66:5s–35s.
160. Griffin S. Diabetes care in general practice: meta-analysis of randomised control trials. BMJ. 1998;317:390–6.
161. Shojania KG, Ranji SR, McDonald KM, et al. Effects of quality improvement strategies for type 2 diabetes on glycemic control: a meta-regression analysis. JAMA. 2006;296:427–40.
162. Walsh JME, McDonald KM, Shojania KG, et al. Quality improvement strategies for hypertension management: a systematic review. Med Care. 2006;44:646–57.
163. Roetzheim RG, Ferrante JM, Lee JH, et al. Influence of primary care on breast cancer outcomes among Medicare beneficiaries. Ann Fam Med. 2012;10:401–11.
164. Doose M, McGee-Avila J, Stroup AM, et al. Shared care during breast and colorectal cancer treatment: is it associated with patient-reported care quality? Under review. 2018.
165. Weir HK, Thompson TD, Soman A, Moller B, Leadbetter S. The past, present, and future of cancer incidence in the United States: 1975 through 2020. Cancer. 2015; 121:1827–37.
166. Nekhlyudov L, Levit L, Hurria A, Ganz PA. Patient-centered, evidence-based, and cost-conscious cancer care across the continuum: translating the institute of medicine report into clinical practice. CA Cancer J Clin. 2014;64:408–21.
167. Institute of Medicine. Crossing the quality chasm: a new health system for the 21st century. Washington, DC: National Academies Press; 2001.

168. Singh GK, Miller BA, Hankey BF, Edwards BK. Persistent area socioeconomic disparities in U.S. incidence of cervical cancer, mortality, stage, and survival, 1975–2000. Cancer. 2004;101:1051–7.

169. Keating NL, Landrum MB, Lamont EB, Bozeman SR, McNeil BJ. Area-level variations in cancer care and outcomes. Med Care. 2012;50:366–73.

170. Hasse JE, Lathrop RG. Land resource impact indicators of urban sprawl. Applied Geogr. 2003;23:159–75.

171. Fan Y, Song Y. Is sprawl associated with a widening urban-suburban mortality gap? J Urban Health. 2009;86:708–28.

172. Vlahov D, Galea S. Urbanization, urbanicity, and health. J Urban Health. 2002;79:S1–s12.

173. Galea S, Freudenberg N, Vlahov D. Cities and population health. Soc Sci Med. 2005;60: 1017–33.

174. Erikson C, Salsberg E, Forte G, Bruinooge S, Goldstein M. Future supply and demand for oncologists: challenges to assuring access to oncology services. J Oncol Pract. 2007;3:79–86.

175. American Society of Clinical Oncology. The state of cancer care in America, 2017: a report by the American society of clinical oncology. J Oncol Pract. 2017;13:e353–94.

176. Association of American Medical Colleges. Diversity in the physician workforce: facts & figures 2014. Available from URL:. http://aamcdiversityfactsandfigures.org/section-ii-current-status-of-us-physician-workforce/ Accessed 29 June 2018.

177. Walker KO, Moreno G, Grumbach K. The association among specialty, race, ethnicity, and practice location among California physicians in diverse specialties. J Natl Med Assoc. 2012;104:46–52.

178. Meghani SH, Brooks JM, Gipson-Jones T, Waite R, Whitfield-Harris L, Deatrick JA. Patient–provider race-concordance: does it matter in improving minority patients' health outcomes? Ethn Health. 2009;14:107–30.

179. Malhotra J, Rotter D, Tsui J, Llanos AAM, Balasubramanian BA, Demissie K. Impact of patient-provider race, ethnicity, and gender concordance on cancer screening: findings from medical expenditure panel survey. Cancer Epidemiol Biomark Prev. 2017;26:1804–11.

180. Yao N, Alcala HE, Anderson R, Balkrishnan R. Cancer disparities in rural appalachia: incidence, early detection, and survivorship. J Rural Health. 2017;33:375–81.

181. Meilleur A, Subramanian SV, Plascak JJ, Fisher JL, Paskett ED, Lamont EB. Rural residence and cancer outcomes in the US: issues and challenges. Cancer Epidemiol Biomark Prev. 2013;22 https://doi.org/10.1158/1055-9965.EPI-1113-0404.

182. American Society of Clinical Oncology. Key trends in tracking supply of and demand for oncologists. Available from URL: https://www.asco.org/sites/new-www.asco.org/files/content-files/research-and-progress/documents/2015-cancer-care-in-america-report.pdf Accessed 28 June 2018.

183. Charlton M, Schlichting J, Chioreso C, Ward M, Vikas P. Challenges of rural cancer care in the United States. Oncology (Williston Park). 2015;29:633–40.

184. Santomauro M, Stroup SP. Improving urologic cancer care through telemedicine. Expert Rev Anticancer Ther. 2013;13:773–5.

185. Sabesan S, Larkins S, Evans R, et al. Telemedicine for rural cancer care in North Queensland: bringing cancer care home. Aust J Rural Health. 2012;20:259–64.

186. Ricke J, Bartelink H. Telemedicine and its impact on cancer management. Eur J Cancer. 2000;36:826–33.

187. McDonald E, Lamb A, Grillo B, Lucas L, Miesfeldt S. Acceptability of telemedicine and other cancer genetic counseling models of service delivery in geographically remote settings. J Genet Couns. 2014;23:221–8.

188. Kvedar J, Heinzelmann PJ, Jacques G. Cancer diagnosis and telemedicine: a case study from Cambodia. Ann Oncol. 2006;17(Suppl 8):viii 37–42.

189. Dorrian C, Ferguson J, Ah-See K, et al. Head and neck cancer assessment by flexible endoscopy and telemedicine. J Telemed Telecare. 2009;15:118–21.

190. Davison AG, Eraut CD, Haque AS, et al. Telemedicine for multidisciplinary lung cancer meetings. J Telemed Telecare. 2004;10:140–3.

191. Coelho JJ, Arnold A, Nayler J, Tischkowitz M, MacKay J. An assessment of the efficacy of cancer genetic counselling using real-time videoconferencing technology (telemedicine) compared to face-to-face consultations. Eur J Cancer. 2005;41:2257–61.
192. Freeman LW, White R, Ratcliff CG, et al. A randomized trial comparing live and telemedicine deliveries of an imagery-based behavioral intervention for breast cancer survivors: reducing symptoms and barriers to care. Psychooncology. 2015;24:910–8.
193. Kunkler IH, Fielding RG, Brebner J, et al. A comprehensive approach for evaluating telemedicine-delivered multidisciplinary breast cancer meetings in southern Scotland. J Telemed Telecare. 2005;11(Suppl 1):71–3.
194. Kunkler IH, Prescott RJ, Lee RJ, et al. TELEMAM: a cluster randomised trial to assess the use of telemedicine in multi-disciplinary breast cancer decision making. Eur J Cancer. 2007;43:2506–14.
195. Pruthi S, Stange KJ, Malagrino GD Jr, Chawla KS, LaRusso NF, Kaur JS. Successful implementation of a telemedicine-based counseling program for high-risk patients with breast cancer. Mayo Clin Proc. 2013;88:68–73.

Part IV
Cross-Cutting Topics

Chapter 15
Persistent Racial Disparities in Breast Cancer Mortality Between Black and White Women: What is the Role for Structural Racism?

Kirsten M. M. Beyer, Staci Young, and Amin Bemanian

Abstract Wide racial disparities in breast cancer mortality persist in the United States, providing troubling evidence that not all populations are benefitting equally from advances in cancer control.

However, the size of the racial disparity in breast cancer mortality varies geographically across the US, suggesting that disparities are not inevitable and may be related to characteristics of places. In this chapter, we examine structural racism in housing, including racial residential segregation, as a possible explanation for variation in the size of racial breast cancer disparities. In the sections to follow, we (1) provide an overview of structural racism and the ways in which it has manifested itself through housing discrimination in the United States, (2) review the literature linking institutional racism and racial segregation to breast cancer disparities, (3) provide a conceptual framework to theorize causal pathways linking institutional racism to breast cancer disparities, and (4) operationalize the framework by describing several metrics of housing discrimination and racial segregation and discussing their application to breast cancer survival.

We conclude with a focus on moving toward solutions to reduce disparities.

Keywords Breast cancer mortality · Structural racism · Housing discrimination · Segregation · African-American · Health disparities

K. M. M. Beyer (✉)
Institute for Health & Equity, Division of Epidemiology, Medical College of Wisconsin, Milwaukee, WI, USA
e-mail: kbeyer@mcw.edu

S. Young
Center for Healthy Communities and Research, Department of Family and Community Medicine, Medical College of Wisconsin, Milwaukee, WI, USA
e-mail: syoung@mcw.edu

A. Bemanian
Institute for Health & Equity, Medical College of Wisconsin, Milwaukee, WI, USA
e-mail: abemanian@mcw.edu

© Springer Nature Switzerland AG 2019
D. Berrigan, N. A. Berger (eds.), *Geospatial Approaches to Energy Balance and Breast Cancer*, Energy Balance and Cancer 15, https://doi.org/10.1007/978-3-030-18408-7_15

15.1 Breast Cancer Disparities in the United States: A Place-Based Phenomenon?

15.1.1 Breast Cancer Mortality Disparities Between Black and White Women

Wide racial disparities in breast cancer mortality (and survival) persist in the United States [1, 2], and may be growing [3, 4], providing troubling evidence that not all populations are benefitting equally from advances in cancer control that have transformed overall expectations for survival after breast cancer diagnosis across the country. These gaps exist despite the availability of early detection and treatment therapies known to lengthen survival among diverse population groups. Blacks/African Americans have the shortest survival among all racial groups for most cancers [5].

Notably, the gap between Black and White mortality rates has not always been present; as shown in Fig. 15.1 and reported in recent literature, mortality rates for Black and White women were approximately equal in the early 1980s; however, by 2012, there was a 42% higher death rate in Black women [6, 7]. Further, while breast cancer incidence had long been an example of a "reverse disparity," with incidence rates higher among White women than Black women, incidence rates at the national level converged in 2012, putting Black and White women nationally at approximately equal risk for incident breast cancer, although regional differences remain [7].

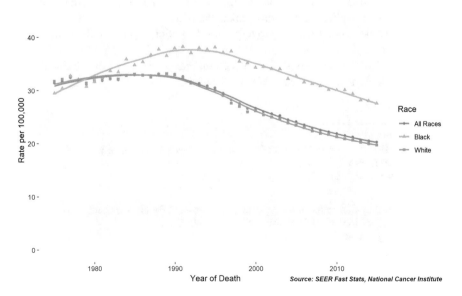

Fig. 15.1 Age-Adjusted US Mortality of Female Breast Cancer, By Race (1975-2015)

Individual and health care factors do not fully explain breast cancer survival disparities. Although Black women are more likely than Whites to be diagnosed at later stages of cancer progression [8], the 5 year breast cancer survival rate is disproportionately lower for Blacks than it is for Whites when considered by diagnosis stage [5]. Tumor biology, particularly higher prevalence of early onset ER negative and triple negative tumors in Black women, is considered a strong contributor to survival disparities [9–11]; however, disparities persist even after taking into account these factors [12, 13]. It is well known that there are differences in treatment offered to individuals by race for many health conditions [14], including longer time to adjuvant chemotherapy among Black and Hispanic breast cancer patients [15]. Some have suggested that equal access to health care can explain away differences in cancer survival [16, 17], while other studies have indicated this is not the case [2, 18–23]. Socio-economic status (SES), while an important predictor of cancer survival, has been shown to be insufficient to erase racial disparities [2]. Thus, the question remains – what are the root causes of the Black to White disparity in breast cancer mortality, and how can we close the gap?

15.1.2 Geographical Variation in the Magnitude of Breast Cancer Mortality Disparities

Importantly, recent studies have indicated that the size of the racial disparity in breast cancer mortality between Black and White women varies geographically across the United States [4, 7, 24, 25]. As illustrated in Fig. 15.2, calculations of Black to White mortality rate ratios using data from CDC wonder reveal no observable state-level disparity between Black and White women in Minnesota and Massachusetts, but a mortality rate ratio of over 1.60 in Mississippi, Louisiana, and Wisconsin [26]. This geographical variation suggests that disparities are not inevitable and may be related to the characteristics of places.

Most importantly, the reasons for this variation have not been explained. Determining the causes of this variation could lead to new strategies to reduce gaps, as new knowledge about successful programs or policies could be translated from places where gaps are small to reduce disparities in places where gaps are large.

In the next sections, we examine structural racism in housing, including racial residential segregation, as a possible explanation for variation in the size of racial breast cancer disparities. First, we provide a brief foundational overview of structural racism and the ways in which it has historically manifested itself through housing discrimination in the United States, including the ways in which these phenomena have differentially affected American cities and regions. We then review the literature that examines relationships between structural racism in housing, segregation, and racial breast cancer disparities. We then outline a conceptual framework to guide research examining structural racism and breast cancer disparities.

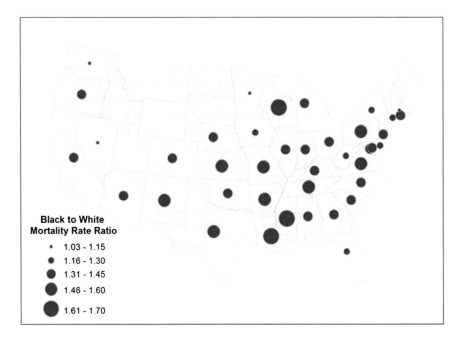

Black to White Mortality Rate Ratio

- 1.03 - 1.15
- 1.16 - 1.30
- 1.31 - 1.45
- 1.46 - 1.60
- 1.61 - 1.70

Fig. 15.2 Geographical variation in breast cancer mortality rate ratios by US State, 2010–2014

Finally, we operationalize the framework by describing several metrics of housing discrimination and racial segregation and discuss their application to breast cancer survival.

15.2 Structural Racism, Housing Discrimination, and Segregation in the United States

15.2.1 Defining Racism: Structural, Institutional, Interpersonal

We define racism following Williams and Mohammed [27] and others [28, 29] as "an organized system premised on the categorization and ranking of social groups into races, that devalues, disempowers and differentially allocates desirable societal opportunities and resources to racial groups regarded as inferior." A racialized social system means that racial phenomena have a structure in any given society, and racism operates within social relations among individuals from different races [29]. Researchers such as Harrell (2000) have articulated that racism occurs on multiple levels – cultural, institutional, and interpersonal – and it is expressed via implicit and explicit communication [30]. Racism can occur through cultural messaging (e.g. advertisements depicting ethnic minorities in stereotypic-conforming ways), and "institutional policies that restrict access to opportunities or resources" [31].

The concept of institutional racism has been applied to numerous sectors, including the medical/health care system. Health and medicine are seen as social institutions that reflect the larger norms, values and stratification systems of a given society [32]. Patterns of racism are legitimized through criteria and standards that exist in the medical complex that effectively discriminate against a racial group. Racism is thus manifested through "history, ideology, community relations, research, education and the professions and differential treatment [32]. Discriminatory acts can be in the form of *de jure* (mandated by law) or *de facto* (without any legal basis but sanctioned by practice). This can be perpetrated and reinforced by multiple agents, yet it is the state that "can enforce, enable, or condone discrimination, or alternatively it can outlaw discrimination and seek to redress its effects" [33]. Sociological research has focused on racial residential segregation as "a primary institutional mechanism of racism and fundamental cause of racial disparities in health" [34].

15.2.2 Racial Segregation and Housing Discrimination in the United States

Racial residential segregation in the United States began in earnest after the end of the Reconstruction era. Southern states created explicit segregationist laws during the Jim Crow period (1877–1950), and these policies led to the Great Migration of African-Americans from the South to the Northeast, Midwest, and West [35]. The Great Migration resulted in major demographic shifts for cities outside of the South. From 1910 to 1930, Black populations in Milwaukee and Chicago grew by 665% and 430% respectively; this resulted in growing racial tensions between the new Black residents and the existing White residents [36]. With little money and seeking social support, new Black migrants tended to live with family and friends who had arrived in northern cities earlier [35, 37], thus concentrating the Black populations of these cities in specific geographic areas within the cities. Neighborhoods undergoing demographic change began to experience "tipping," a phenomenon where small changes in a minority population would trigger an exodus by the existing majority residents [36, 38]. These migration patterns helped lead to the development of predominately Black neighborhoods in these cities [36, 39].

While northern cities did not have the full extent of Jim Crow laws, a combination of local and federal policies actively encouraged housing discrimination and residential segregation. Locally, restrictive racial housing covenants were used by landlords, homeowners, and subdivisions to prevent the sale or lease of property to minorities [35, 40]. In order to enforce these deeds and lease contracts, landlords and neighbors would use state and federal law enforcement agencies to sue or evict people found in violation of these covenants [40].

Federal policy during this period had a major impact on the development of racially segregated metropolitan areas across the country. Federal policy developed during the New Deal to promote home ownership included the creation of an entity known as the Home Owners' Loan Corporation (HOLC). The HOLC purchased mortgages and then reissued them with low down payments and interest rates, so more families would be able to actually own their homes [40]. However, the HOLC focused its efforts on neighborhoods which it considered financially stable, and asked local realtors to audit neighborhoods across the United States. The auditors promoted existing patterns of segregation by giving predominately minority neighborhoods low desirability grades and effectively reducing the likelihood of lending in those areas [40]. Maps created for numerous cities across the country illustrate these "low grade" neighborhoods using the color red (Fig. 15.3). This became the formal practice of "redlining," whereby areas of cities were systematically identified as too risky to receive home loans and were thus targeted for disinvestment. Over time, this practice resulted in less housing and economic development in minority neighborhoods, while homeownership and wealth increased in White neighborhoods.

Creation of the interstate highway system promoted suburbanization, encouraging further "White Flight" and the demolition of existing Black neighborhoods to make way for the construction of the new highways [35, 36, 39, 41].

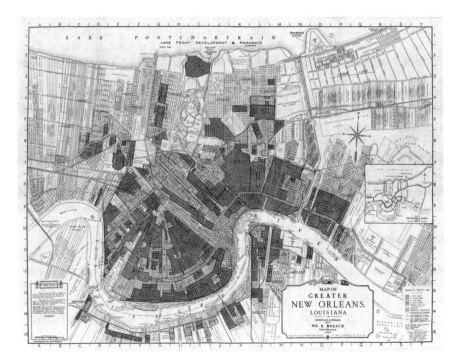

Fig. 15.3 HOLC Map for New Orleans, LA, 1939

After intense pressure from the Civil Rights Movement in the 1960s, the federal government passed several key pieces of legislation to rectify the wrongs of the Jim Crow Era. Among these laws was the Fair Housing Act (Title VIII of the Civil Rights Act), which banned discrimination in sale or rent of a property on the basis of race, color, religion, sex, or national origin. In order to help enforce Title VIII regulations, Congress passed the Home Mortgage Disclosure Act (HMDA) in 1975, with the purpose of increasing transparency in mortgage lending practices [42].

However, the effect of these policies on undoing the entrenched segregation in America's cities is controversial. Denton's analysis of thirty major metropolitan areas' segregation measures found little change from 1970 to 1990, but she argues that these policy changes may have prevented further segregation [43]. Over the past two decades there has been a steady but slow decrease in Black segregation, but many metropolitan areas continue to be characterized by significant racial residential segregation [44, 45]. Furthermore, enforcement of anti-discrimination statutes remains imperfect. Studies show the persistence of racial steering, where realtors and landlords present prospective residents with different housing options based on their race [46, 47]. The persistence of housing discrimination and racial segregation are part of the social environment within which health disparities, including in breast cancer, develop.

15.3 Housing Discrimination and Segregation as Underlying Causes of Breast Cancer Disparities

15.3.1 Housing Discrimination and Segregation as Fundamental Causes of Disparity

Housing discrimination and resultant patterns of racial segregation are significant and pervasive, and result in completely different distributions of neighborhood quality, disfavoring racial and ethnic minorities. Hypothesized pathways linking segregation to breast cancer survival include spatial access to quality health care, exposure to stressors, and local health behavioral norms [48, 49]. For instance, for-profit health systems may forgo the opening of clinics in lower income neighborhoods of metropolitan areas, given the expectation of little financial gain; grocery stores that stock fresh fruits and vegetables and potential employers may be among other entities unlikely to open establishments in lower income areas, furthering the socioeconomic decline of the neighborhoods. Lack of economic investment can lead, in turn, to the siting of hazardous facilities, increased crime, land vacancy, and lack of public amenities that support healthy nutrition, physical activity and social engagement, with implications for health disparities. However, despite the plausibility of the influence of segregation on breast cancer mortality and survival disparities, and widespread agreement that segregation is an important and possibly fundamental cause of health disparities [50, 51], few studies have examined these relationships, and both study approaches and results have been mixed [49, 52–55]. While the focus of this chapter is on Black to White disparities, studies have also examined relationships for other racial and ethnic groups [53, 56].

15.3.2   Relationships Across Places: Metropolitan Area Level Segregation and the Magnitude of Breast Cancer Mortality Disparities

Racism and racial residential segregation are widely considered to contribute to health disparities and may partially explain geographical variation in the size of breast cancer disparities observed across the country. Whitman et al. (2012) reported that segregation is one of two important correlates of the magnitude of the breast cancer mortality rate ratio between Black and White women in the United States, at the city-level [24]. Across metropolitan statistical areas (MSAs) in Georgia, Russell (2012) found that the largest breast cancer mortality disparities were found in highly segregated MSAs – similar to the finding by Whitman and others [55]. Examining the impact of MSA level segregation at the individual level, Russell (2012) further found that, for Black women, higher MSA level segregation was a predictor of increased breast cancer mortality, but the same was not found for all-cause mortality [55].

15.3.3   Place-Specific Relationships: Are Relationships Between Segregation, Discrimination and Disparity Uniform Across Places?

A number of studies have found that a higher proportion Black neighborhood composition is associated with poorer outcomes for Black women. Schootman et al. (2009) found that the percentage of the census tract population Black was – in combination with tumor grade and diagnosis stage – able to explain why Black women were more likely to develop breast cancer metastases than White women [49]. Pruitt (2015) found that the Black location quotient (see Table 15.1 for explanation of segregation measures) for a census tract – measuring the proportion of Black population in the tract compared to the proportion for the MSA overall – was associated with greater all-cause mortality after breast cancer diagnosis, but an association observed in unadjusted analyses for breast-cancer specific mortality was attenuated in fully adjusted models [53].

However, this has not been a uniform finding. Warner et al. (2010) found that Black women in tracts with a higher Black population experienced lower mortality [54], a finding that could suggest a protective effect via social support, similar to the notion of "ethnic enclaves." While Haas et al. (2008) found an association between

Table 15.1 Summary of several common measures of segregation previously used in the literature for studying relationship between health outcomes and segregation

Example measures of segregation	
Regional measures	Describes the level of segregation for large areas (e.g. MSAs, counties) by aggregating demographics of the subunits within the region
Dissimilarity [57]	Percent of the population of a racial group in the region that would have to move so that the group is evenly distributed across the region (i.e. all census tracts or ZCTAs within an MSA have an equal percentage of group X)
Isolation [57]	Probability of a random interaction between people living in the same subunit (e.g. ZCTA, census tract) will be between two people of the same race
Exposure [57]	Probability of a random interaction between people living in the same subunit (e.g. ZCTA, census tract) will be between two people of different races
Local measures	Describes the level of segregation experienced by people living within a specific geographic area (typically ZCTA, census tract) which can be normalized against the overall level of segregation in a larger geographic region
Racial composition or percent race	Proportion of people within a geographic area who are a specific race
Location quotient (LQ) [58]	Percent race within a subunit normalized against percent race of the region
Index of concentration at the extremes (ICE) [59, 60]	Difference between percent of subunit belonging in an "advantaged" class (e.g. racial majority group, high SES) and percent belonging in a "disadvantaged" class (e.g. racial minority group, low SES)
Local exposure/ Isolation (LEx/Is) [61]	Local extension of exposure and isolation indices described above. Likelihood of a random interaction between people of different races (exposure) or the same race (isolation) within a subunit normalized against the hypothetical likelihood of the interaction if there was zero dissimilarity in the region

Black census tract level isolation and inadequate breast cancer care, they did not find a relationship between Black isolation and breast cancer mortality among older women [62]. For White women, Russell (2012) found that increasing census tract percent Black was associated with higher all-cause mortality in Georgia [55]. Warner and Gomez (2010) found a similar relationship in California, with higher Black composition associated with greater risk for both all-cause and breast-cancer-specific mortality among White women [54].

Beyond breast cancer, some studies have indicated the potential importance of segregation and housing discrimination for other cancer sites. Hayanga (2013) found that segregation (dissimilarity) at the county level was associated with higher lung cancer mortality [63], and Chae (2013) found an association between a measure of area racism derived from internet searches and Black cancer mortality [64]. Additionally, recent studies have also highlighted the potential importance of historical policies and migration patterns on the observation of current day breast cancer disparities. In two studies incorporating a measure of Jim Crow states,

Krieger et al. identify potential relationships between birth in a Jim Crow state and breast cancer tumor type [65, 66]. Specifically, when studying changes in estrogen-receptor (ER) status, they found the greatest changes among Black women born in Jim Crow states (versus non-Jim Crow states) [65]. Furthermore, the authors emphasize the importance of historical and societal context when examining these racial and ethnic inequities among breast cancer patients.

15.4 A Conceptual Framework: Structural Racism and Breast Cancer Disparities

15.4.1 A Conceptual Framework

We propose a conceptual framework to guide research at the intersection of racism, segregation, and breast cancer disparities. This framework (Fig. 15.4) is adapted from the framework for the study of racism and health by Williams and Mohammed (2013) [27] to focus specifically on breast cancer survival (and mortality) disparities. The framework is conceptualized to have five distinct and causally related elements. The first element, *fundamental determinants of health*, emphasizes that determinants

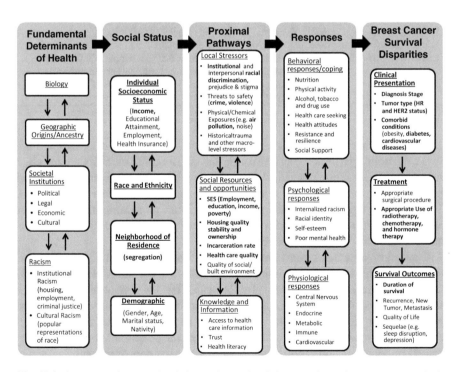

Fig. 15.4 Conceptual framework relating racism and racial segregation to breast cancer survival

of health and related disparities include not only biology, geographic origins, and the influence of societal institutions, but also racism at multiple levels.

The second element, *social status*, is influenced by these fundamental determinants. Social status is presented as groups or categories within which an individual can fall (e.g. race, socioeconomic status) that have health consequences. It is important to understand this element of the conceptual model focuses on the socially constructed aspects of these categories. For example, race is associated with specific biological genetic variations, but distinguishing explicit racial categories was developed to create a social hierarchy of cultures [67, 68]. Similarly, gender and the social conception of age is viewed distinct from biological sex and the physical aging process. These determinants can interact with each other. For example, the relationship between segregation and cancer survival can be dependent on the patient's race [54, 69]. Studies of racial breast cancer disparities often find conflicting evidence of whether disparities are driven by individual race, neighborhood segregation, socioeconomic status, or by specific interactions between these categories [53, 54, 61]. Statistical approaches such as multilevel multivariate analysis can help with separating the confounding effects of these determinants, but selection of a well specified model can be challenging.

The third element, *proximal pathways*, identifies the mechanisms that link fundamental health determinants and social categories to disparate breast cancer outcomes. These pathways include [1] different exposure to stressors (e.g. crime), [2] different access to social resources and opportunities (e.g. employment) and [3] different access to knowledge and information (e.g. cancer risk factor messages). These proximal pathways can vary with different social status categories. Collins and Williams (1999) reviewed evidence that racially segregated neighborhoods suffer from poorer health due to a combination of increased exposure to direct stressors (e.g. communicable diseases, environmental toxins) and decreased access to healthcare and social support resources [70]. One example of a proximal pathway in breast cancer outcomes can be access to screening services. Mobley et al. (2016) found that Black and American Indian female Medicaid patients were less likely to receive mammograms, while Hispanic and Asian/Pacific Islander patients were more likely to receive them, relative to Non-Hispanic White women [71]. Additionally, their study suggested that patients living in counties with higher Black and Asian isolation scores (see Table 15.1) were less likely to receive mammograms, while patients living in counties with higher Hispanic isolation scores were more likely to receive them [71]. By studying these proximal pathways it is possible to develop interventions to affect breast cancer outcomes.

The fourth element, human *responses* to these exposures, are categorized as [1] behavioral (e.g. poor nutrition) [2], psychological (e.g. poor mental health), and [3] physiological (e.g. inflammation). Behavioral responses such as alcohol and substance abuse can develop as a coping mechanism against societal stressors such as systematic racism [70, 72, 73]. Additionally, individuals living in segregated and economically deprived neighborhoods may develop poorer dietary and exercise habits due to limitations in their physical and social environments (e.g. lower quality grocery stores, less safe space for physical activity) [70, 74, 75]. Social stresses such as systematic racism have been postulated to affect physiologic response primarily through a mechanism known as allostatic load. Stress is believed to affect the body through the hypothalamic-pituitary-adrenal axis, which leads to changes in blood pressure, heart rate, and metabolism [76]. This allostatic stress may lead to changes in immune function and therefore have implications in cancer susceptibility and treatment [77, 78]. Brody et al. (2014) investigated the relationship between allostatic load and perceived discrimination in African-American adolescents, and found that discrimination was a significant predictor for increased allostatic load in adolescents who lacked strong emotional support networks [79]. There is additional evidence that discrimination affects brain structure in certain regions such as the prefrontal cortex and anterior cingulate cortex, which may lead to poorer mental health outcomes [76]. A meta-analysis of 134 articles by Pascoe et al. (2009) found that poorer mental health, stress response, and health behaviors were all significantly associated with increased perceived discrimination [80].

Ultimately, together, these exposures and responses produce different clinical presentations of breast cancer at diagnosis, including comorbid conditions, tumor type, and diagnosis stage. These factors influence length and quality of survival as well as breast cancer survival disparities. However, these factors do not cease to be relevant after clinical presentation. For example, access to health care matters not only for early diagnosis, but also in ensuring early, adequate, and ongoing treatment, and poor mental health post-diagnosis has been linked to poor survival.

15.4.2   Operationalizing the Framework

Racial residential segregation is an important and explicitly spatial mechanism by which social categories of people (e.g. by race) are disempowered, devalued, and differentially allocated resources. It also manifests itself through discriminatory housing practices. A number of approaches have been taken to derive measures of racial segregation – the spatial distribution of individuals by race over a given region. More recently, additional work has begun to focus more on the processes by which segregation takes hold – particularly by measuring the degree of bias in housing policies and practices [47, 81, 82].

We recently built upon our previous innovations in disease mapping [83–88] and innovations in the published literature [89] to develop two new metrics of housing discrimination [90]. In contrast to most previous measures of segregation, these new metrics capture an element of the *process* by which patterns of segregation arise and persist, and incorporate the *spatial relationships* among small area geographies, recognizing and leveraging spatial dependence to enhance estimation. To create these metrics, we undertook a novel use of adaptive spatial filtering (ASF) [83]; a grid of estimation points is placed across the study area, and for each grid point, a circular filter expands, based on a specified threshold, to obtain data from multiple locations until it can calculate a stable rate. We extended this method beyond rate calculations to incorporate statistical modeling and develop two measures of housing discrimination using the Home Mortgage Disclosure Act (HMDA) database [81]. The Racial Bias Index is estimated as the odds of denial of a mortgage for a Black applicant relative to a White applicant. The Redlining Index is estimated as the odds of denial of a mortgage in the local area, as compared to the study area as a whole.

In addition to these two housing discrimination measures, our group has also developed a new segregation metric, the Localized Exposure/Isolation index (LEx/Is) [91], that localizes the well-known measures of isolation and exposure (see Table 15.1) [92]. Preliminary analyses indicate that LEx/Is performs as well or better than other local metrics. Work is underway to extend the LEx/Is metrics to incorporate transportation patterns/networks.

We have examined relationships between our new indices (Racial bias, Redlining, and LEx/Is) and breast cancer survival in the Milwaukee-Waukesha-West Allis, WI MSA. Survival analyses revealed the Racial Bias Index to be significantly associated with poorer survival among Black women diagnosed with breast cancer; 81 related work has found similar relationships in colorectal cancer survival [93]. Using LEx/Is, we found that neighborhood Hispanic isolation was associated with poorer survival for women of all races in the Milwaukee MSA [91]. When the analysis was stratified by race, Hispanic isolation was no longer significantly associated with breast cancer survival in any particular race, but Black isolation was associated with increased breast cancer survival among Black women. These two findings suggest that Black women living in predominately White neighborhoods (low Black isolation, high Racial Bias Index) actually have worse survival outcomes than their counterparts who live in predominately Black neighborhoods, despite neighborhoods with high Black isolation tending to have higher levels of poverty [90, 91]. These results contribute to an overall literature on housing discrimination, segregation and breast cancer disparities that reveals complex and place dependent relationships; more work is needed to move this work toward policy and intervention.

15.5   Conclusions: Toward Solutions

Growing racial disparities in breast cancer mortality and survival are especially concerning and indicate the importance of examining the root causes and persistence of these disparities, in spite of early detection and treatment therapies. As individual and health care factors do not fully explain these disparities, it is critical for researchers to examine institutional and structural conditions that influence health outcomes. Racism and residential segregation are such examples of these conditions. In this chapter we outline the history of segregation in the United States as a multitude of local and federal policies that encouraged housing segregation and advanced racial inequalities in the living environment. The implications of this are realized in geographical variations of breast cancer disparities.

The conceptual framework presented in this chapter linking segregation to breast cancer survival is a useful tool to not only identify root causes but also potential solutions. Our work aligns with that of other researchers across multiple disciplines including public health, sociology, and epidemiology that point the way to efforts grounded in community engagement and critical discourse about institutional and structural racism [94–96]. Community engagement includes building and nurturing ongoing relationships among residents, advisory boards, researchers, and policymakers that are truly invested in health equity. Incorporating this process into scientific research agendas and policymaking is essential to improving health outcomes.

In aggregate, studies indicate that policy changes targeting housing discrimination, segregation and their adverse effects could result in decreased breast cancer survival disparities. However, more work is urgently needed to examine differences among places and population groups. Pathways by which segregation influences breast cancer survival disparities are not well understood, and this gap in knowledge prevents the strategic targeting of policies and interventions. Interventions require detailed, evidence-based recommendations in order to make a meaningful impact on disparities.

Ultimately, efforts to improve breast cancer outcomes, and health overall, should include the critical examination of policies implemented by societal institutions (i.e. political, legal, economic, cultural) and the myriad of ways in which racism affects health. Ongoing research to study how organizational and structural interventions lead to changes in health outcomes is particularly relevant and should be supported. This is especially critical as demographic changes continue across racialized societies and ongoing progress is necessary to dismantle the effects of racism.

References

1. Ward E, Jemal A, Cokkinides V, et al. Cancer disparities by race/ethnicity and socioeconomic status. CA Cancer J Clin [Internet] 2004;54(2):78–93. Available from: http://www.ncbi.nlm.nih.gov/entrez/query.fcgi?cmd=Retrieve&db=PubMed&dopt=Citation&list_uids=15061598.
2. Newman LA, Mason J, Cote D, et al. African-American ethnicity, socioeconomic status, and breast cancer survival. Cancer. 2002;94(11):2844–54.
3. Orsi JM, Margellos-Anast H, Whitman S. Black-White health disparities in the United States and Chicago: a 15-year progress analysis. Am J Public Health. 2010;100(2):349–56.
4. Hunt BR, Whitman S, Hurlbert MS. Increasing black: white disparities in breast cancer mortality in the 50 largest cities in the United States. Cancer Epidemiol. 2014;38(2):118–23.
5. DeSantis C, Naishadham D, Jemal A. Cancer statistics for African Americans. CA Cancer J Clin. 2013;63(3):151–66.
6. Ghafoor A, Jemal A, Ward E, Cokkinides V, Smith R, Thun M. Trends in breast cancer by race and ethnicity. CA Cancer J Clin. 2003;53(6):342–55.
7. Desantis CE, Fedewa SA, Sauer AG, Kramer JL, Smith RA, Jemal A. Breast cancer statistics, 2015: convergence of incidence rates between black and white women. CA Cancer J Clin. 2016;66(1):31–42.
8. Iqbal J, Ginsburg O, Rochon PA, Sun P, Narod SA. Differences in breast cancer stage at diagnosis and cancer-specific survival by race and ethnicity in the United States. JAMA. 2015;313(2):165–73.

9. Stead LA, Lash TL, Sobieraj JE, et al. Triple-negative breast cancers are increased in black women regardless of age or body mass index. Breast Cancer Res. 2009;11(2):R18.
10. Bauer KR, Brown M, Cress RD, Parise CA, Caggiano V. Descriptive analysis of estrogen receptor (ER)-negative, progesterone receptor (PR)-negative, and HER2-negative invasive breast cancer, the so-called triple-negative phenotype. Cancer. 2007;109(9):1721–8.
11. Lund MJ, Trivers KF, Porter PL, et al. Race and triple negative threats to breast cancer survival: a population-based study in Atlanta, GA. Breast Cancer Res Treat. 2009;113(2):357–70.
12. Wallace TA, Martin DN, Ambs S. Interactions among genes, tumor biology and the environment in cancer health disparities: examining the evidence on a national and global scale. Carcinogenesis. 2011;32(8):1107–21.
13. Menashe I, Anderson WF, Jatoi I, Rosenberg PS. Underlying causes of the black-white racial disparity in breast cancer mortality: a population-based analysis. J Natl Cancer Inst. 2009;101(14):993–1000.
14. Nelson A. Unequal treatment: confronting racial and ethnic disparities in health care. J Natl Med Assoc. 2002;94(8):666.
15. Vandergrift JL, Niland JC, Theriault RL, et al. Time to adjuvant chemotherapy for breast cancer in national comprehensive cancer network institutions. J Natl Cancer Inst. 2013;105(2):104–12.
16. Komenaka IK, Martinez ME, Pennington RE Jr, et al. Race and ethnicity and breast cancer outcomes in an under insured population. J Natl Cancer Inst. 2010;102(15):1178–87.
17. Bach PB, Schrag D, Brawley OW, Galaznik A, Yakren S, Begg CB. Survival of blacks and whites after a cancer diagnosis. JAMA. 2002;287(16):2106–13.
18. Du XL, Lin CC, Johnson NJ, Altekruse S. Effects of individual-level socioeconomic factors on racial disparities in cancer treatment and survival. Cancer. 2011;117(14):3242–51.
19. Albain KS, Unger JM, Crowley JJ, Coltman CA Jr, Hershman DL. Racial disparities in cancer survival among randomized clinical trials patients of the Southwest oncology group. J Natl Cancer Inst. 2009;101(14):984–92.
20. Alexander DD, Waterbor J, Hughes T, Funkhouser E, Grizzle W, Manne U. African-American and Caucasian disparities in colorectal cancer mortality and survival by data source: an epidemiologic review. Cancer Biomark. 2007;3(6):301–13.
21. Newman LA, Griffith KA, Jatoi I, Simon MS, Crowe JP, Colditz GA. Meta-analysis of survival in African American and white American patients with breast cancer: ethnicity compared with socioeconomic status. J Clin Oncol. 2006;24(9):1342–9.
22. Wojcik BE, Spinks MK, Optenberg SA. Breast carcinoma survival analysis for African American and white women in an equal-access health care system. Cancer. 1998;82(7):1310–8.
23. Jatoi I, Becher H, Leake CR. Widening disparity in survival between white and African-American patients with breast carcinoma treated in the US department of defense healthcare system. Cancer. 2003;98(5):894–9.
24. Whitman S, Orsi J, Hurlbert M. The racial disparity in breast cancer mortality in the 25 largest cities in the United States. Cancer Epidemiol. 2012;36(2):e147–51.
25. Freund KM. The racial disparity in breast cancer mortality in the 25 largest cities in the United States. Cancer Epidemiol. 2012;36(5):497.
26. Centers for Disease Control and Prevention. United States cancer statistics: public information data [Internet]. 2016; 2016 December 20. Available from: https://wonder.cdc.gov/cancer. HTML
27. Williams DR, Mohammed SA. Racism and health I: pathways and scientific evidence. Am Behav Sci. 2013;57(8) https://doi.org/10.1177/0002764213487340.
28. Williams DR, Chung A-M. Racism and health. Closing gap Improv heal minor elders new Millenn; 2004. p. 69–80.
29. Bonilla-Silva E. Rethinking racism: toward a structural interpretation. Am Sociol Rev. 1997;62:465–80.
30. Harrell SP. A multidimensional conceptualization of racism-related stress: implications for the well-being of people of color. Am J Orthopsychiatry. 2000;70(1):42–57.
31. Brondolo E, Gallo LC, Myers HF. Race, racism and health: disparities, mechanisms, and interventions. J Behav Med. 2009;32(1):1–8.

32. King G. Institutional racism and the medical/health complex: a conceptual analysis. Ethn Dis. 1996;6(1–2):30–46.
33. Krieger N, Berkman LF. Discrimination and health. In: Social epidemiology; 2000. p. 36–75.. Available from: https://books.google.es/books?hl=es&lr=&id=ReTRAwAAQBAJ&oi=fnd&p g=PA63&ots=TPHeZ1EK1F&sig=e4PYzESbuhfj6mCA19aNU_G1eMs&redir_esc=y#v=on epage&q&f=false.
34. Williams DR, Sternthal M. Understanding racial-ethnic disparities in health. J Health Soc Behav 2010;51(1 suppl): S15–S27. Available from: http://hsb.sagepub.com/content/51/1_ suppl/S15.abstract%5Cnhttp://hsb.sagepub.com/content /51/1_suppl/S15.full%5Cnhttp://hsb. sagepub.com/content/51/1_suppl/S15.full.pdf
35. Tolnay SE. The African American "great migration" and beyond. Annu Rev Sociol. 2003;29(1):209–32.
36. Gurda J. The making of Milwaukee. Milwaukee: Milwaukee County Historical Society; 2006.
37. White KJC, Crowder K, Tolnay SE, Adelman RM. Race, gender, and marriage: destination selection during the great migration. Demography. 2005;42(2):215–41.
38. Schelling TC. Dynamic models of segregation. J Math Sociol. 1971;1(2):143–86.
39. Price-Spratlen T, Guest AM. Race and population change: a longitudinal look at cleveland neighborhoods. Sociol Forum. 2002;17(1):105–36.
40. Rothstein R. The color of law. New York: Liveright; 2017.
41. Connerly CE. From racial zoning to community empowerment -The interstate highway system and the African American community in Birmingham, Alabama. J Plan Educ Res. 2002;22(2):99–114.
42. McCoy PA. The home mortgage disclosure act: a synopsis and recent legislative history. J R Estate Res. 2007;29(4):381–97.
43. Denton NA. Half empty or half full: segregation and segregated neighborhoods 30 years after the fair housing act. City. 1999;4(3):107–22.
44. Frey WH. Census shows modest declines in black-white segregation. Washington, DC: Brookings; 2015.
45. Frey WH. Analysis of 1990, 2000, and 2010 census decennial census tract data. Brookings Institution University Michigan Social Science Data Analysis 2010;
46. Yinger J. Measuring racial discrimination with fair housing audits: caught in the act. Am Econ Rev. 1986;76(5):881–93.
47. Hanson A, Hawley Z, Taylor A. Subtle discrimination in the rental housing market: evidence from e-mail correspondence with landlords. J Hous Econ. 2011;20(4):276–84.
48. Russell E, Kramer MR, Cooper HLF, Thompson WW, Arriola KRJ. Residential racial composition, spatial access to care, and breast cancer mortality among women in Georgia. J Urban Heal. 2011;88(6):1117–29.
49. Schootman M, Jeffe DB, Gillanders WE, Aft R. Racial disparities in the development of breast cancer metastases among older women. Cancer. 2009;115(4):731–40.
50. Williams DR, Collins C. Racial residential segregation: a fundamental cause of racial disparities in health. Public Health Rep. 2001;116(5):404–16.
51. Collins CA, Williams DR. Segregation and mortality: the deadly effects of racism?. Sociol Forum, 14(3) Springer; 1999. p. 495–523.
52. Schootman M, Jeffe DB, Lian M, Gillanders WE, Aft R. The role of poverty rate and racial distribution in the geographic clustering of breast cancer survival among older women: a geographic and multilevel analysis. Am J Epidemiol. 2009;169(5):554–61.
53. Pruitt SL, Lee SJC, Tiro JA, Xuan L, Ruiz JM, Inrig S. Residential racial segregation and mortality among black, white, and Hispanic urban breast cancer patients in Texas, 1995–2009. Cancer. 2015;121:1845–55.
54. Warner ET, Gomez SL. Impact of neighborhood racial composition and metropolitan residential segregation on disparities in breast cancer stage at diagnosis and survival between black and white women in California. J Community Health. 2010;35(4):398–408.
55. Russell EF, Kramer MR, Cooper HLF, Gabram-Mendola S, Senior-Crosby D, Arriola KRJ. Metropolitan area racial residential segregation, neighborhood racial composition, and breast cancer mortality. Cancer Causes Control. 2012;23(9):1519–27.

56. Keegan THM, Quach T, Shema S, Glaser SL, Gomez SL. The influence of nativity and neighborhoods on breast cancer stage at diagnosis and survival among California Hispanic women. BMC Cancer. 2010;10(1):1.
57. Massey DS, Denton NA. The dimensions of residential segregation. Soc Forces. 1988;67(2):281–315.
58. Sudano JJ, Perzynski A, Wong DW, Colabianchi N, Litaker D. Neighborhood racial residential segregation and changes in health or death among older adults. Health Place. 2013;19:80–8.
59. Krieger N, Singh N, Waterman PD. Metrics for monitoring cancer inequities: residential segregation, the index of concentration at the extremes (ICE), and breast cancer estrogen receptor status (USA, 1992–2012). Cancer Causes Control. 2016;27(9):1139–51.
60. Massey DS. The prodigal paradigm returns: ecology comes back to sociology. In: Booth A, Crouter AC, editors. Does it take a village? Community effects on children, adolescents, and families. Mahwah: Lawrence Erlbaum; 2001. p. 41–8.
61. Bemanian A, Beyer KMM. Measures matter: the local exposure/isolation (LEx/is) metrics and relationships between local-level segregation and breast cancer survival. Cancer Epidemiol Biomarker Prev. 2017;26(4):516–24.
62. Haas JS, Earle CC, Orav JE, et al. Racial segregation and disparities in breast cancer care and mortality. Cancer. 2008;113(8):2166–72.
63. Hayanga AJ, Zeliadt SB, Backhus LM. Residential segregation and lung cancer mortality in the United States. JAMA Surg. 2013;148(1):37–42.
64. Chae DH, Clouston S, Hatzenbuehler ML, et al. Association between an internet-based measure of area racism and black mortality. PLoS One. 2015;10(4):e0122963.
65. Krieger N, Jahn JL, Waterman PD, Chen JT. Breast cancer estrogen receptor status according to biological generation: US black and white women born 1915–1979. Am J Epidemiol. 2018;187(5):960–70.
66. Krieger N, Jahn JL, Waterman PD. Jim crow and estrogen-receptor-negative breast cancer: US- born black and white non-hispanic women, 1992–2012. Cancer Causes Control. 2017;28(1):49–59.
67. Smedley A, Smedley BD. Race as biology is fiction, racism as a social problem is real: anthropological and historical perspectives on the social construction of race. Am Psychol. 2005;60(1):16–26.
68. Jorde L, Wooding S. Genetic variation, classification and "race". Nat Genet. 2004;36(11): 28–33.
69. Bemanian A, Beyer KMM. Exploration of the spatial distribution of liver cancer mortality in Wisconsin. In: International medical geography symposium. France: Angers. p. 2017.
70. Collins CA, Williams DR. Segregation and mortality: the deadly effects of racism? Sociol Forum. 14(3) Springer; 1999. p. 495–523.
71. Mobley LR, Subramanian S, Tangka FK, et al. Breast cancer screening among women with medicaid, 2006–2008: a multilevel analysis. J Racial Ethn Heal Disparities. 2016:2006–8.
72. Caetano R, Clark CL, Tam T. Alcohol consumption among racial/ethnic minorities: theory and research. Alcohol Health Res World. 1998;22(4):233–41.
73. Zapolski TCB, Pedersen SL, McCarthy DM, Smith GT. Less drinking, yet more problems: understanding African American drinking and related problems. Psychol Bull. 2014;140(1):188–223.
74. Schulz AJ, Williams DR, Israel BA, Lempert LB. Racial and spatial relations as fundamental determinants of health in Detroit. Milbank Q. 2002;80(4):677–707.
75. Morland K, Wing S, Diez Roux A, Poole C. Neighborhood characteristics associated with the location of food stores and food service places. Am J Prev Med. 2002;22(1):23–9.
76. Berger M, Sarnyai Z. "More than skin deep": "stress neurobiology and mental health consequences of racial discrimination". Stress. 2015;18(1):1–10.
77. Doyle DM, Molix L. Minority stress and inflammatory mediators: covering moderates associations between perceived discrimination and salivary interleukin-6 in gay men. J Behav Med. 2016;39(5):782–92.
78. McEwen BS. Protective and damaging effects of stress mediators. N Engl J Med. 1998;338(3):171–9.

79. Brody GH, Lei MK, Chae DH, Yu T, Kogan SM, Beach SRH. Perceived discrimination among African American adolescents and allostatic load: a longitudinal analysis with buffering effects. Child Dev. 2014;85(3):989–1002.

80. Pascoe EA, Smart Richman L. Perceived discrimination and health: a meta-analytic review. Psychol Bull. 2009;135(4):531–54.

81. Beyer KMM, Zhou Y, Matthews K, Bemanian A, Laud PW, Nattinger AB. New spatially continuous indices of redlining and racial bias in mortgage lending: links to survival after breast cancer diagnosis and implications for health disparities research. Heal Place 2016;40:34–43. Available from: https://doi.org/10.1016/j.healthplace.2016.04.014

82. Mendez DD, Hogan VK, Culhane JF. Stress during pregnancy: the role of institutional racism. Stress Heal. 2013;29(4):266–74.

83. Beyer KMM, Tiwari C, Rushton G. Five essential properties of disease maps. Ann Assoc Am Geogr [Internet] 2012 [cited 2014 Aug 29];102(5):1067–1075. Available from: http://www.tandfonline.com/doi/abs/10.1080/00045608.2012.659940

84. Rushton G, Peleg I, Banerjee A, Smith G, West M. Analyzing geographic patterns of disease incidence: rates of late-stage colorectal cancer in Iowa. J Med Syst [Internet] 2004;28(3):223–236. Available from: http://www.ncbi.nlm.nih.gov/entrez/query.fcgi?cmd=Retrieve&db=PubMed&dopt=Citation&list_uids=15446614.

85. Rushton G, Lolonis P. Exploratory spatial analysis of birth defect rates in an urban population. Stat Med. 1996;15(7–9):717–26.. Available from: http://www.ncbi.nlm.nih.gov/entrez/query.fcgi?cmd=Retrieve&db=PubMed&dopt=Citation&list_uids=9132899

86. Beyer KM, Rushton G. Mapping cancer for community engagement. Prev Chronic Dis. 2009;6(1):A03.

87. Cai Q, Rushton G, Bhaduri B. Validation tests of an improved kernel density estimation method for identifying disease clusters. J Geogr Syst. 2012;14(3):243–64.

88. Tiwari C, Rushton G. A spatial analysis system for integrating data, methods and models on environmental risks and health outcomes. Trans GIS. 2010;14(s1):177–95.

89. Mendez DD, Hogan VK, Culhane J. Institutional racism and pregnancy health: using home mortgage disclosure act data to develop an index for mortgage discrimination at the community level Public Heal Rep (Washington, DC) 2011;126: 102–114.

90. Beyer KMM, Zhou Y, Matthews K, Bemanian A, Laud PW, Nattinger AB. New spatially continuous indices of redlining and racial bias in mortgage lending: links to survival after breast cancer diagnosis and implications for health disparities research (manuscript submitted).

91. Bemanian A, Beyer KMM. Measures matter: the local exposure/isolation (LEx/Is) metrics and relationships between local level segregation and breast cancer survival. Cancer epidemiol biomarkers prev.

92. Massey DS, Denton NA. The dimensions of residential segregation. Soc Forces. 1988;67(2):281–315.

93. ZHOU Y, Bemanian A, Beyer KMMM. Housing discrimination, residential racial segregation, and colorectal cancer survival in southeastern Wisconsin. Cancer Epidemiol Biomark Prev [Internet] 2017; cebp.0929.2016. Available from: http://cebp.aacrjournals.org/lookup/doi/10.1158/1055–9965.EPI-16-0929.

94. Thomas SB, Quinn SC, Butler J, Fryer CS, Garza MA. Toward a fourth generation of disparities research to achieve health equity. Annu Rev Public Health 2011;32:399–416. Available from: http://www.ncbi.nlm.nih.gov/entrez/query.fcgi?cmd=Retrieve&db=PubMed&dopt=Citation&list_uids=21219164.

95. Williams DR, Mohammed SA. Racism and health II: a needed research agenda for effective interventions. Am Behav Sci. 2013;57(8):1–27.. Available from: http://www.ncbi.nlm.nih.gov/pubmed/24347667

96. Williams DR. Race, socioeconomic status, and health the added effects of racism and discrimination. Ann NY Acad Sci. 1999;896(1):173–88.

Chapter 16
Rural-Urban Disparities in Breast Cancer: Six Suppositions and Future Directions

Sara McLafferty

Abstract Disparities in breast cancer outcomes between rural and urban populations are of great interest as environmental, social, and technological processes unevenly affect rural and urban landscapes. This chapter examines research on rural-urban disparities in breast cancer. The first section briefly reviews recent literature on variations in breast cancer incidence, stage, survival, quality of life, treatment and costs in rural and urban areas. The next section critically evaluates this work by presenting six suppositions about rural and urban places and populations. Each supposition discusses a key issue concerning how rural and urban categories and disparities are defined, measured, and analyzed. I argue that rural and urban are complex, heterogeneous categories that are difficult to define and that change over time complicates our understanding of breast cancer disparities. The complexity, heterogeneity, and dynamism of urban and rural places and populations give rise to unequal and varying BC outcomes. In addition, people's differing experiences of urban and rural places strongly influence important risks and exposures, while also affecting access to diagnosis and treatment facilities, leading to people- and place-based heterogeneity in breast cancer outcomes. Implications for future research on rural-urban disparities are discussed.

Keywords Rural · Urban · Breast cancer · Disparities

16.1 Introduction

Rural-urban disparities in breast cancer have attracted increasing attention among cancer researchers and policy-makers. Research shows that people living in rural areas differ from those living in urban areas along a wide range of breast cancer metrics including incidence, diagnosis, treatment, risk behaviors, and outcomes.

S. McLafferty (✉)
Department of Geography and GIScience, University of Illinois at Urbana-Champaign,
Champaign, IL, USA
e-mail: smclaff@illinois.edu

© Springer Nature Switzerland AG 2019   379
D. Berrigan, N. A. Berger (eds.), *Geospatial Approaches to Energy Balance and Breast Cancer*, Energy Balance and Cancer 15, https://doi.org/10.1007/978-3-030-18408-7_16

Recent commentaries describe rural residence as a cancer "risk factor" ([42], p. 1657) that is "often overlooked" ([21], 119) in research on health disparities. Similarly, the distinctive breast cancer risks of urban populations and the wide inequalities in cancer outcomes within and between cities have been extensively studied and compared to those in rural places [56]. Although this growing body of evidence offers valuable insights, it devotes limited attention to important conceptual and methodological issues, including how we define and characterize urban and rural place environments and how we identify and model their associations with breast cancer risks and outcomes.

Rural and urban are widely used, but imprecise, terms that describe the geographical settings–place environments—in which people live, work, and interact. These settings are important for breast cancer risk and outcomes because they affect the kinds of people who live in a place; the services, hazards, and opportunities available to them; and their behaviors and interactions. The concepts of composition, context, and collective are critically important for understanding breast cancer disparities between urban and rural place environments [38]. *Composition* refers to characteristics of the people who make up a place's population. It includes social, demographic, and biological characteristics such as age, gender, income level, occupation, and education, that affect people's risk of developing cancer, their risk behaviors, and their ability to obtain effective diagnosis and treatment services. In contrast, *context* describes attributes of the local environment such as climate, transportation, and retail and health care services. Contextual factors affect breast cancer risk through diverse pathways, for example, by influencing people's exposures to environmental contaminants, their access to resources such as tobacco, green spaces, and alcohol that may be healthful or harmful for cancer risk, and the availability of health services like mammography screening that are essential for achieving optimal outcomes. In addition, breast cancer risks are influenced by *collective* factors – the interactions among people and population groups within a place. Social norms, social and political capital, and inter-group relations that unfold in places impact diverse health-related behaviors, knowledge, coping mechanisms, and experiences of vulnerability and marginalization via processes like racial discrimination.

Researchers increasingly view context and composition as interdependent and mutually constituted. The demographic, educational, and economic characteristics of a place reflect in part the place's resources, services, institutional, and environmental attributes [16]. At the same time, people's behaviors, social interactions, and institutions shape the places in which they are embedded. The dynamic interplay between composition, context, and collective is central to understanding the social and geographical drivers of BC in urban and rural settings.

This chapter begins with a brief summary of recent research on rural-urban disparities in BC. Several recent review articles have been published on closely related topics [36, 42, 47, 70], so to narrow the scope and to avoid duplication, this chapter only covers research on the United States, and it primarily focuses on recent literature. The review is organized around breast cancer outcomes including incidence, stage at diagnosis, mortality, etc. In the second section, I propose six suppositions that underpin and influence rural-urban BC research. The implications and challenges posed by each issue are discussed. The final section builds on the first two by highlighting future directions.

16.2 Research on Rural-Urban Breast Cancer Disparities

16.2.1 Incidence

Most recent evidence for the U.S. shows higher breast cancer incidence rates in urban than in rural areas. Analyzing data from the 18 SEER cancer registries, [8] observed higher incidence in metropolitan counties versus rural, non-metropolitan counties. Similarly, data from cancer registries covering 97% of the U.S. population reported in [27] show an increasing trend in breast cancer incidence with increasing urbanity (Fig. 16.1). The age-adjusted incidence rate in the most highly urbanized counties, those located within metropolitan areas whose population size exceeds one million, is approximately 17% higher than that in rural, nonmetropolitan counties. Urban disadvantage has also been reported in state-level studies, such as a recent investigation in Utah [24].

Less is known about the factors implicated in these rural-urban disparities in BC incidence. Although most studies adjust for important compositional factors such as age and race/ethnicity, the effects of contextual factors have not been widely studied. A recent analysis of county-level SEER data determined that county-level socioeconomic status and density of primary care physicians accounted for the observed rural-urban disparity in BC incidence [46]. Beyond socioeconomic factors, environmental contextual characteristics, such as exposure to endocrine

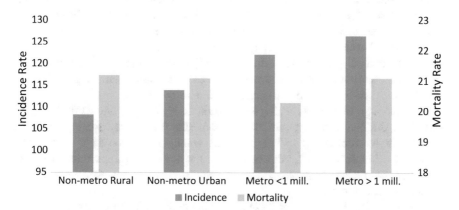

Fig. 16.1 Rural-urban gradients in age-adjusted breast cancer incidence and morality rates. Data are from [27]. Incidence data are for 2004–2013 and mortality data are for 2006–2015

disruptors and radiation are rarely considered in analyzing rural-urban gaps in incidence. Such "extrinsic" factors are thought to play a significant role in BC carcinogenesis [65], and their relationship to rural-urban variation warrants future research attention [70].

16.2.2 Stage

Stage at diagnosis strongly affects BC morbidity and mortality making it a crucial dimension of BC disparities. Rural-urban gradients in stage have been widely studied. It is hypothesized that rural women have higher rates of late (distant) stage diagnosis than urban residents because of the limited availability and accessibility of BC screening services in rural areas. However, evidence is mixed. A 2014 review and meta analysis of literature on BC stage and urban-rural location concluded that rural women were more likely than urban women to be diagnosed with breast cancer at a late stage [47]. However, the review covered diverse countries, with diverse urban and rural definitions, making it difficult to draw general conclusions.

Recent research for the U.S. offers mixed and conflicting evidence of rural-urban disparities in BC stage. A number of studies find evidence of rural disadvantage in late-stage risk including recent analyses in Nebraska [12] and Texas [51]. Others, however, observe no disparity in late diagnosis. Using national NAACCR data for 2009–2013, [69] identified higher rates of localized BC among urban residents than among rural residents, but no significant difference in rates of distant stage disease. Similarly, [28] analysis of registry data for 10 states, and state-level studies of California [9], New Hampshire [11] and South Dakota [67] found no significant difference in rates of late-stage diagnosis between urban and rural areas. In contrast, in Illinois [40] and Florida [37], higher late-stage risk was observed in urban areas.

Both contextual and compositional factors have been implicated in geographic disparities in BC stage. Henry et al. [28] found that age, race/ethnicity, health insurance coverage, and census tract poverty were strongly associated with stage, whereas travel time to mammography was not. National statistics also show strong racial and ethnic disparities in late diagnosis [45]. Other studies confirm that women living in socioeconomically disadvantaged areas have higher late stage risk [61]. Residential isolation and racial segregation also contribute to elevated risk of late/distant-stage diagnosis [17, 34, 44], as do state-level policy and regulatory contexts [43]. Although many researchers hypothesize that limited spatial access to mammography contributes to late-diagnosis among rural women with BC, the empirical evidence is weak, with several studies finding no association between spatial access and late-stage risk [28, 29, 62]. Screening rates, however, are inversely related to late diagnosis [3].

It is difficult to make sense of these conflicting findings due to differences in time period, study area, and rural-urban definition. Time is linked to period and cohort effects associated with changes in BC diagnosis. The past four decades saw rapid expansion of mammography screening, changes in age-related recommendations for screening, and changes in mammographic sensitivity, all of which have influenced stage at diagnosis. Incidence of localized BC is increasing due to better detection [64]. These period effects significantly affect incidence of both localized and distant-stage BC [19], and effects may differ between rural and urban areas due to differences in mammography availability and diagnostic capabilities and practices, as discussed late in this chapter.

16.2.3   Mortality and Survival

BC mortality and survival reflect complex diagnostic and treatment factors, along with cancer subtype and stage that are likely to differ between rural and urban settings. At the national scale, higher rates of BC mortality have been reported in rural than in urban areas [57]. During the past decade, BC mortality declined more rapidly in urban areas leaving rural areas with a slightly higher age-adjusted mortality rate than that found in urban metropolitan areas [27]. These broad comparisons, however, hide considerable spatial heterogeneity in BC mortality within both urban and rural areas. For example, the map of age-standardized BC death rates by State Economic Area in Fig. 16.2 shows high death rates in some rural areas within the central and southeastern U.S., but low death rates in rural areas in states such as Wyoming, North Dakota, and Maine.

Survival – the time-varying process between diagnosis and death, has also attracted attention in research on rural-urban disparities. Survival is complicated to analyze because it requires longitudinal data about disease progression within

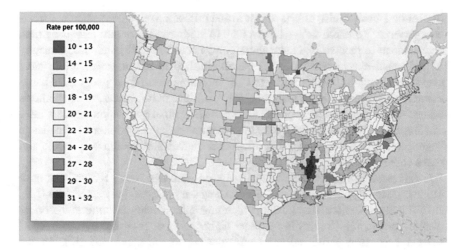

Fig. 16.2 Age-adjusted breast cancer death rate among females (2011–2015) by State Economic Area. (Source: National Vital Statistics System, 2018. More information is available at: https://gis.cancer.gov/canceratlas/data)

individuals over time. Research in Australia reveals a growing rural-urban gap in survival, despite survival gains overall [68]. In the U.S., the limited evidence on rural-urban differences in survival indicates little or no disparity [24, 49]. However, within cities, we find wide socioeconomic and racial inequalities in survival [55], and neighborhoods with very poor BC survival outcomes have been identified [7].

16.2.4   Quality of Life and Well-Being

Only a handful of studies have analyzed differences in quality of life and other psychosocial outcomes between rural and urban BC survivors. A US study based on a small sample of survey respondents (N = 46) found that rural BC survivors reported lower quality of life than urban respondents [52]. However, the study only considered a short time window (1 month) after treatment. A survey of cancer survivors in Alaska and Oregon showed varied patterns: In Oregon, rural cancer survivors reported more negative impacts, including worry and employment concerns than did those living in urban areas; however, the disparity was reversed in the Alaska sample [41]. Community characteristics played an important role in these disparities, including travel/access to services, care coordination, local resources, and social ties and interactions, an indication that contextual and collective factors are important for quality of life and well-being.

16.2.5   Screening, Treatment and Costs

Rural-urban location also affects access to and utilization of BC screening and treatment services. Research shows that women living in rural areas are less likely than other women to receive regular mammography screening [18] and BRCA testing [33], although the gap in the latter has diminished in recent years. While most researchers hypothesize that lower rates of screening result from geographic barriersand limited availability of mammography facilities in rural areas, this hypothesis has not received empirical support. Research shows that geographic barriers have little impact on rural-urban inequalities in mammography utilization and late-stage diagnosis [29, 63], suggesting that other characteristics of rural/urban people and places come into play.

   Geographic disparities in treatment between rural and urban BC patients have also been widely studied. Rates of mastectomy vary substantially across the U.S., and differences persist after adjusting for demographic, socioeconomic, and service-related factors [58]. Studies have found higher rates of mastectomy in rural BC patients, even after individual and contextual factors are controlled [32]. Boscoe et al. [10] observed that among women with early-stage disease, the likelihood of mastectomy increases with increasing distance from a radiation treatment center.An earlier study found that rural women were less likely to receive radiation therapy following breast conserving surgery for ductal carcinoma in-situ [54]. Insured women living in nonmetropolitan areas are less likely to receive BRCA testing than are women living in metropolitan areas and less likely to receive magnetic resonance imaging of the breast if a genetic mutation is detected [33].

Differences in the costs of treatment for BC patients have also attracted research attention. Medicare claims data for BC patients in the final 6 months of life showed that average treatment costs were 9% less for rural patients after adjusting for age, chronic conditions, and other factors affecting disease severity and service utilization [15]. Rural patients were less likely than their urban counterparts to use physician and home health care services, although rates of hospitalization were similar.

In sum, the large literature on rural-urban disparities in BC presents varying and sometime conflicting findings. Although some studies indicate poorer BC outcomes among rural versus urban residents, others point to urban disadvantage, especially in neighborhoods isolated by poverty, racial segregation, and limited access to quality healthcare. Findings also differ with the scale and geographic scope of the study, the time period considered, and the health outcome of interest. These varying findings raise broader questions about how rural and urban are defined, studied, and analyzed – issues discussed in the sections that follow.

The following sections propose six suppositions about urban and rural which describe salient aspects of rural and urban places and their implications for BC research. Each section discusses key issues, their relationships to BC research, current approaches to addressing them, and, if relevant, opportunities for future research.

16.3 Rural, Urban and Breast Cancer Research: Six Suppositions

16.3.1 Rural and Urban are Complex Categories

What are rural and urban? These concepts are easy to define at the extremes: The dense central cores of New York City and San Francisco are clearly "urban," and the sparsely-settled plains of central Wyoming are clearly "rural." But a wide and diverse range of settings exist in between. What makes places urban or rural, and how do we differentiate them?

Scholarship on rural/urban definitions suggests several key points. First, urban and rural are socially constructed categories that represent shared understandings of the settings in which people live and in which socio-economic and environmental processes unfold [22]. Conceptions of urban and rural vary from place to place and over time: there are well-known differences in urban/rural definitions among countries. The U.S. Census definition of urban areas has changed over time with shifts in settlement patterns and density and as the needs for and uses of these definitions have evolved [23, 25]. Similar kinds of differences in understandings of urban and rural exist at regional scales such as between states in the U.S. Second, urban and rural are relational concepts, defined in relation to each other and in relation to the context in which they are adopted [26]. We often define rural as: "not urban," an approach that skirts the messy task of identifying specific attributes of rural places. Finally, the rural-urban binary simplifies complex and diverse landscapes. Real-world land-scapes gradually shift from rural to urban with no clear dividing line. Thinking critically about the meanings and complexity of urban and rural categories is important for BC research because it forces us to consider the salient characteristics of rural and urban contexts and their links to BC outcomes.

16.3.2   Rural and Urban are Difficult to Define

The relational qualities of rural/urban give rise to varying definitions. In the U.S., several major rural-urban classification schemes exist, each using different criteria, numbers of categories, and so on. Varying definitions affect the results of cancer studies by impacting how geographical areas, and their corresponding cancer data, are categorized. Pruitt et al. [51] analyzed the impact of rural-urban classification schemes on geographic inequalities in late-stage BC in Texas. They found moderate to high agreement in results irrespective of the classification method used, an indication that in Texas, the classification methods are highly consistent. However, it is unclear whether these findings apply to other states and regions that have different rural-urban geographies.

Several recent papers review the major rural-urban classification schemes used in the U.S. [25, 42, 51, 62], so I do not provide a detailed analysis here; Table 16.1 outlines the main features of the classifications that are most widely used in U.S.-based BC research, noting differences in criteria, numbers of categories, and geographical scale.

The criteria used in classifying rural and urban areas are highly relevant for BC research. Most schemes rely on one or more of three primary criteria in designating rural and urban areas: population density, adjacency, and interaction [31]. *Density* captures the central distinction between rural and urban places, differences in the proximity and availability of people and human activities and interactions, but it fails to capture spatial dimensions that reflect where places are located relative to other places. These spatial dimensions are typically defined in relation to densely-settled, urban places, so identifying urban areas is a prerequisite to identifying rural. *Adjacency* describes a place's geographical proximity to or location within a metropolitan area, and *interaction* describes the place's flows/connections with urban settlement(s). Typically, these criteria are combined providing an overall index. But they can be viewed as separate components, each capturing a distinct dimension of rural-urban differentiation.

Although adjacency and interaction are often correlated, they are not the same – places can interact while not being adjacent, and they can be adjacent but not interact.

Table 16.1 Characteristics of Major Rural-Urban Classifications in the U.S

	#Categories	Scale	Population density/size	Adjacency	Interaction	
Index of Relative Rurality	Continuous	Country	Y	Y	N	https://purr.purdue.edu/publications/2960/1
National Center for Health Statistics 2013	6	Country	Y	Y	N	https://www.cdc.gov/nchs/data_access/urban_rural.html
Rural Urban Continuum Codes 2013	9	Country	Y	Y	N	https://www.ers.usda.gov/data-products/rural-urban-continuum-codes.aspx
Rural Urban Commuting Areas 2010	10 (with subcat)	Tract, Zipcode	Y	N	Y	https://www.ers.usda.gov/data-products/rural-urban-commuting-area-codes/
Urban Influence Codes 2013	12	Country	Y	Y	Y	https://www.ers.usda.gov/data-products/urban-influence-codes/
U.S. Census 2010	2	Country	Y	Y	N	https://www2.census.gov/geo/pdfs/reference/ua/Defining_Rural.pdf

An example of interaction without adjacency that is relevant for health research is the growing number of rural places that are attracting urban residents, both part-time and full-time, via the process of rural gentrification [20]. Located in regions traditionally considered as rural, these places often have educated and affluent populations with strong urban ties whose knowledge of and access to cancer services is on par with that of affluent urban residents. Another, albeit very different, example of interaction without adjacency is seen in rural communities that are home to prisons. Incarcerated populations housed in local prisons often come from urban areas, and flows of prisoners, family members, and personnel create strong urban interactions.

There are also examples of adjacency without interaction – urban neighborhoods and communities whose residents are isolated from the broader metropolitan region by poverty, lack of mobility, and other socio-spatial barriers. For example, poor urban residents who have limited access to transportation or face crime and violen ce in their local neighborhoods are often geographically isolated from BC screening and treatment services despite proximity [1, 50, 60].

Recently, multivariate measures of rurality have been developed to capture the multifaceted characteristics of rural and urban settings. Mao et al. [39] developed an innovative index that models rurality as a weighted linear combination of six variables representing demography, socioeconomic status, and settlement characteristics. Index values are estimated for 600 m grid cells revealing fine-grained geographic variation in rurality. Although this work represents an important step forward, it could be enhanced by incorporating spatial factors such as adjacency and interaction that underpin widely-used definitions of rural and urban. Another important contribution is the Index of Relative Rurality — a continuous measure of rurality based on a weighted average of four criteria – size, density, remoteness, and built-up area [62]. Applying this index to better understand rural-urban cancer disparities represents a promising future research direction.

16.3.3   Rural and Urban Places are Heterogeneous

Regardless of definition, urban and rural categories encompass highly diverse place contexts. Diversity within and among urban areas is well-documented. Wide demographic and socioeconomic inequalities exist among urban places affecting multiple dimensions of BC risk and outcomes. Environmental and social hazards, including air pollution, crime, and many others, are unevenly distributed, as are environmental amenities such as parks and recreational facilities. These have been shown to affect diverse BC-related exposures and risk behaviors such as obesity and physical activity leading to uneven geographies of BC risk. In addition, although compared to rural places, urban areas have greater availability of BC diagnostic and treatment services, these services vary greatly in availability and quality within cities, and access to services may be limited by economic, transportation, and social barriers that restrict people's ability to access them [60].

Although less well-documented than urban disparities, wide differences also exist among rural places in contextual and compositional factors that affect BC risk. Although many rural areas in the U.S. are experiencing population decline leaving a high concentration of older residents, some, particularly in the west and south, are growing rapidly and attracting young in-migrants [14]. Racial and ethnic population diversity is increasing rapidly in some rural communities with in-migration of Hispanic and Asian immigrants who work in local agricultural and manufacturing sectors. There are also wide socioeconomic inequalities among rural communities. Contrast the gentrifying rural towns located in places like western Montana and Vermont and on the fringes of large metropolitan areas with the impoverished rural communities found in parts of Appalachia and on Native American reservations [3]. In the latter areas, poverty, geographic isolation, and poor access to quality health-care place residents at high risk of poor BC outcomes. Environmental hazards and amenities also differ among rural communities. Some communities have distinctive hazards such as groundwater contamination from agricultural chemicals or mining operations that may be linked to BC or other cancer risks. In conclusion, these multiple and varying sources of geographic heterogeneity within urban and rural areas are critically important for BC research because they affect risks and pathways to BC outcomes.

16.3.4   People Experience Rural and Urban Places Differently

People's varying experiences of and responses to urban and rural places are also salient for BC research. People experience the same place differently depending on their age, gender, race/ethnicity, socioeconomic status, insurance coverage, daily mobility, and other interrelated dimensions of difference. Some population groups – low income, elderly, and people with disabilities – are often socially and spatially isolated in their residential communities due to restricted mobility. Socioeconomic status critically affects how people experience rural and urban places. Poverty has been linked to a wide range of BC-related experiences including access to healthy food and recreation and exposures to violence and environmental hazards that exist within the micro-geographies of rural or urban places. In contrast, high incomes facilitate mobility and enable travel to BC services and other health-promoting resources beyond a person's residential community [2]. Race and ethnicity also complicate experiences of place: In rural communities, for example, immigrants face special challenges due to occupational risks and linguistic and cultural barriers as compared to the majority white population.

Researchers are beginning to investigate how individual characteristic map onto rural-urban BC disparities. Illinois data from 1999–2003 (Fig. 16.3) show a markedly different rural-urban gradient in late-stage BC risk for black women with BC than for women of other race/ethnicities. Black women living in small towns and rural areas had an especially high risk of late diagnosis, whereas for other women, the percent diagnosed late was highest in Chicago, the most urban setting. A nationwide study of black-white disparities in BC mortality, found varying levels of racial

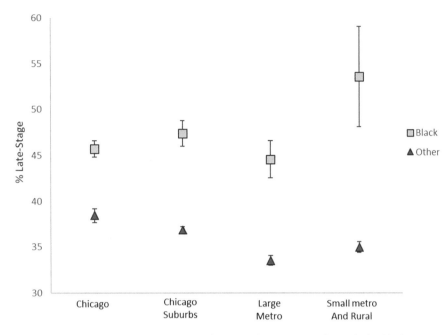

Fig. 16.3 Rural-urban gradients in percent late-stage breast cancer diagnosis for black women compared to women from other race/ethnic backgrounds, Illinois, 1999–2003

disparity, an indication that race intersects with place in affecting mortality risk [53]. Similar findings have been observed at the state level for other ethnic and racial groups [44]. These results point to varying experiences of rural and urban settings that reflect interlocking effects of economic, geographic and sociocultural factors in particular places. Efforts are also underway to analyze place-specific variables that differ for race/ethnic groups such as variables describing the concentration of one's own ethnic/racial group within the neighborhood of residence [44]. Extending this work to analysis of rural-urban disparities is an important area for future research investigation.

16.3.5 Analyzing Rural-Urban Disparities Raises Important Methodological Challenges

Rural and urban locations present distinctive methodological challenges for BC research. In rural areas, the small numbers problem – the fact that cancer rates based on small numbers of cases are unreliable, with high sampling variability – is a critical issue. Sparse populations in rural areas make breast cancer a relatively rare outcome, even when BC risk is high, so estimated incidence rates are unstable and unreliable. This problem is especially important when analyzing data for small areas such as counties and zip codes. For example, Hardin County, a rural county in southern Illinois, averages 3 breast cancer cases per year which is insufficient for estimating rates and trends. The small numbers problem can also emerge when analyzing subpopulations – populations defined by ethnicity, race, or geographic location — that may have distinctive cancer risks [59]. The uneven residential geographies of these groups further dilute sample sizes in rural and urban areas making it difficult to observe and analyze group-specific cancer needs and barriers.

To address the small numbers problem, researchers often aggregate data spatially by grouping data for adjacent counties or for groups of counties, but spatial aggregation smooths out contextual variation. Another approach is temporal aggregation which involves combining data for multi-year time intervals; however, this approach ignores cohort and period effects that reflect technological and diagnostic changes and socioeconomic trends. Innovative spatial and spatiotemporal Bayesian statistical methods have been developed to address the small numbers problem [66], but these methods still can be constrained by sparse data in rural areas.

Geographical scale of analysis is also important for research on rural-urban disparities. Most studies rely on cancer data for fixed geographic units such as counties, zip codes or census tracts, but results vary depending on the number, sizes and locations of units used. This issue – the modifiable areal unit problem (MAUP) – has been well documented in a variety of research contexts including cancer. A related issue is that the geographic units used often do not correspond to contexts that are causally meaningful for the question of interest, a problem known as the uncertain geographic context problem (UGCoP) [35]. For example, in rural areas, people's BC-related environmental exposures and access to health services do not correspond with county boundaries: some people travel across county boundaries for work, shopping, and social interactions; others may be restricted to small zones near the home due to age, immobility, or infirmity. While it is impossible to predict each individual's daily activity space in detail, creating person- and place-specific measures that represent well the geographic contexts people experience in everyday life and that affect health outcomes should be a high priority.

In urban BC research, efforts are already underway to address the MAUP and UGCoP by developing spatially continuous measures of contextual characteristics and by incorporating spatial relationships in statistical modeling. Researchers have used innovative spatial measures of residential segregation [5, 6] and spatial access to health services [63] to describe place contexts. In addition, a growing number of studies use context-dependent methods like spatial regression analysis, spatial multilevel modeling, and geographically-weighted regression to represent spatially autocorrelated errors and spatial interactions that extend across area boundaries. Although they do not capture interpersonal differences in geographic contexts, these methods make a significant advance by modeling spatial associations between nearby places. Tailoring these spatial measures and methods to rural contexts, where population demographics intersect with sparse settlement patterns and uneven transportation networks to create distinctive local geographies, is an important topic for future research investigation.

Another key methodological challenge is to integrate people and place more closely in analyzing rural-urban disparities. At the population level, researchers have addressed this by estimating rates or models separately by population group and by rural-urban setting. However a more rigorous approach is to model interactions between people and places directly; for example, by analyzing cross-level interactions in multilevel modeling. At the individual level, BC research should take advantage of data from GPS-enabled devices to characterize people's daily movements through space and time and their resulting contextual exposures. These data have been applied in analyzing BC risk factors such as obesity and physical activity, but opportunities exist to use them more broadly in studying issues that are affected by daily mobility such as utilization of diagnostic/treatment services and social support among cancer survivors.

16.3.6 Rural and Urban Places are Dynamic

Rural and urban places change over time affecting a wide range of BC risks, risk behaviors, exposures and outcomes. As noted earlier, rural places have varying trajectories: In the U.S., some are gaining population and economic activity, as they transition from rural to urban. At the same time, other rural places are losing people, becoming increasingly isolated. A recent comparison of rural-urban county designations over time found that 15% shifted between rural and urban designation from 2003–2013 based on the RUCC classification scheme [13].

Mobility, movement of people through space and time, is another key dimension of rural-urban dynamics. Flows of people intersect with changing rural and urban place environments to affect BC risks, behaviors and outcomes. The importance of daily mobility has already been noted, but longer-term residential mobility also has implications for research on rural-urban disparities. Migration is especially relevant in studying breast cancer incidence and etiology given the potentially long time lag between environmental exposures and BC outcomes. Over the last century, the U.S. has seen sustained rural to urban migration implying that some urban BC cases have their roots in rural place environments. In addition, ongoing population movements from urban core areas to suburban and exurban communities mean that the nature of "urban" exposures continues to evolve. These migration effects are only beginning to attract attention from BC researchers. Innovative space-time methods have been developed to investigate clustering of cancer cases in space and time based on detailed residential histories [30]. These methods can tell us not only about early co-occurrence of people who develop BC later in life, but also about critical time periods in a person's life when environmental exposures have the largest impact. An application of the methods to assess space-time clustering of BC in Denmark identified an area of persistently high risk during the study period [48]. In subsequent multivariate analysis, the cluster greatly diminished when socioeconomic and reproductive characteristics of the local population were controlled.

Another significant dimension of rural-urban dynamics concerns changes in health care availability and practices. Rural and urban places differ fundamentally in the geographic availability and accessibility of BC diagnosis and treatment services, but these change over time reflecting broader economic and political processes. Most health care innovations originate in urban areas where medical research infrastructure, businesses, and talent concentrate. Urban health care providers are often early adopters of effective innovations and technologies, and over time, the innovations spread to rural health care providers via a process known as hierarchical spatial diffusion. Research by Arrington et al. [4] documents diffusion from urban to rural areas in the adoption of sentinel lymph node biopsy for BC staging, as rural residents lagged urban residents in receiving SNLB when needed. The changes in screening recommendations and treatment practices discussed earlier also may undergo spatial diffusion from urban to rural areas.

Varying time lags in adoption of effective BC diagnostic and treatment services are especially relevant for studies of rural-urban disparities in BC stage, survival, and mortality because the services impact early diagnosis and longer-term outcomes. As effective technologies and practices diffuse from urban to rural areas, the rural-urban gap should diminish. However, continuing development and adoption of new innovations in urban areas complicates analysis of trends by perpetuating urban advantage. Nationally, there is little rural-urban disparity in late-stage BC, and both geographical contexts have experienced similar trends since the early 2000s [27], but research on other outcomes – mortality and morbidity – is needed to assess the effects of changing diagnostic and treatment services and treatment protocols in diverse urban/rural contexts.

16.4   Summary and Conclusions

The six suppositions complicate our understanding of rural-urban disparities in BC, raising key questions about what rural and urban mean; how they are measured and analyzed; and the complex pathways linking them to BC outcomes. The diverse and conflicting findings of current scholarship should not come as a surprise: the complexity, heterogeneity, and dynamism of urban and rural places and populations give rise to unequal and varying BC outcomes. Although many studies point to evidence of rural disadvantage, research also highlights strong disadvantage in many urban neighborhoods where vulnerable populations and adverse place characteristics combine to heighten BC risk. In addition, growing concentrations of low-income groups, immigrants, and other vulnerable populations in suburban and exurban areas result in new BC geographies that blur the distinctions between rural and urban contexts.

Although rural and urban are useful descriptive categories, concerns about heterogeneity and definition raise important questions about their use in understanding breast cancer risks and outcomes. Focusing on causally relevant characteristics of rural and urban places will provide more specific evidence about how and why BC concentrates in specific places and populations. These characteristics might include dimensions like population density and interaction, but it is also important to dig even deeper to assess distal and proximal determinants of BC that underlie these dimensions such as spatial access to healthcare and residential segregation/isolation. Innovative spatial and space-time data and methods will be critical in these efforts by capturing key contextual characteristics describing interactions within and among geographic zones at different scales and in different contexts. These methods include multilevel and spatiotemporal approaches along with geographically-varying and context-aware methods that directly model geographic variability in underlying associations.

Analyzing the interacting associations between people and places is another priority for BC research on rural-urban variation. The fact that different people experience the same place differently underlies some of the observed heterogeneity of findings on rural-urban variation. Population-level studies should take advantage of approaches like analyzing cross-level interactions and spatial, context-aware modeling while utilizing and developing BC datasets that include linked individual and contextual variables. Although these data raise important privacy concerns, access to them can be restricted to secure data centers as is done for many governmental datasets. Individual-level studies are also needed to capture person-place interactions, especially in rural, suburban, and exurban contexts where ongoing research is sparse. GPS-based tracking and direct exposure assessments will be crucial in these efforts for describing short term changes in behaviors and exposures, while longer-term changes will entail use of linked data on residential histories and historical contextual changes. Technological developments in monitoring devices and high performance computing have made these investigations feasible, even for large sample sizes.

Finally, researchers need to think more deeply about the processes underpinning rural-urban variations in BC outcomes and changes over time. GPS-based tools tell us where people travel and the environments they experience, but do not reveal why these interactions occur. Understanding the behavioral, socioeconomic, and institutional processes that affect people's cancer-related exposures and decisions, along with the services, places, and opportunities they have access to, is a key topic for future work. For research on rural-urban disparities, the latter includes processes like diffusion of health services, urban sprawl, and business location decisions.

From early exposures and risk behaviors to diagnosis and treatment to long term outcomes such as survival and well-being, breast cancer outcomes differ greatly from person to person and from place to place. Compositional, collective, and contextual factors that vary across rural and urban settings are central to these outcomes. The complexity, heterogeneity, and dynamism of these settings calls for nuanced approaches that focus on vulnerable people in vulnerable places.

References

1. Ahmad F, Mahmood S, Pietkiewicz I, et al. Concept mapping with South Asian immigrant women: barriers to mammography and solutions. J Immigr Minor Healt. 2012;14(2):242–50.
2. Alford-Teaster J, Lange JM, Hubbard RA, et al. Is the closest facility the one actually used? An assessment of travel time estimation based on mammography facilities. Int J Health Geogr. 2016;15:8. https://doi.org/10.1186/s12942-016-0039-7.
3. Anderson RT, Yang T-C, Matthews SA, et al. Breast cancer screening, area deprivation, and later-stage breast cancer in appalachia: does geography matter? Health Serv Res. 2014;49:546–67. https://doi.org/10.1111/1475-6773.12108.
4. Arrington AK, Kruper L, Vito C, et al. Rural and urban disparities in the evolution of sentinel lymph node utilization in breast cancer. Am J Surg. 2013;206:674–81.
5. Benmanian A, Beyer KMM. Measures matter: the local exposure/isolation (Lex/Is) metrics and relationships between local-level segregation and breast cancer survival. Cancer Epidemiol Biomark Prev. 2017;26(4):516–24.
6. Beyer KMM, Zhou Y, Matthews K, et al. Breast and colorectal cancer survival disparities in Southeastern Wisconsin. Wis Med J. 2016a;115(1):17–21.
7. Beyer KMM, Zhou Y, Matthews K, et al. New spatially continuous indices of redlining and racial bias in mortgage lending: links to survival after breast cancer diagnosis and implications for health disparities research. Health Place. 2016b;40:34–43.
8. Blake KD, Moss JL, Gaysynsky A, et al. Making the case for investment in rural cancer control: an analysis of rural cancer incidence, mortality, and funding trends. Cancer Epidemiol Biomark Prev. 2017;26:992–7. https://doi.org/10.1158/1055-9965.EPI-17-0092.
9. Blair SL, Sadler GR, Bristol R, Summers C, Tahir Z, Saltzstein SL (2006), Early cancer detection among rural and urban Californians. BMC Public Health, 6:194. https://doi.org/10.1186/1471-2458-6-194
10. Boscoe FP, Johnson CJ, Henry KA, Goldberg DW, Shahabi K, Elkin EB, Ballas LK, Cockburn M. Geographic proximity to treatment for early stage breast cancer and likelihood of mastectomy. Breast. 2011;20:324–8. PMID: 21440439
11. Celaya MO, Berke EM, Onega TL, Gui J, Riddle BL, Sherala SS, Rees JR. Breast cancer stage at diagnosis and geographic access to mammography screening (New Hampshire, 1998–2004). Rural Remote Health. 2010;10(2):1361. PMID: 20438282
12. Chandak A, Nayar P, Lin G. Rural-urban disparities in access to breast cancer screening: a spatial clustering analysis. J Rural Health. 2018;35:229–35. https://doi.org/10.1111/jrh.12308.
13. Cohen SA, Kelley L, Bell AE. Spatiotemporal discordance in five common measures of rurality for US counties and applications for health disparities research in older adults. Front Public Health. 2015;3:267. https://doi.org/10.3389/fpubh.2015.00267.
14. Cromartie J. Rural areas show overall population decline and shifting regional patterns of population change. Amber waves, 2017 Available at: /www.ers.usda.gov/amber-waves/2017/september/rural-areas-show-overall-population-decline-and-shifting-regional-patterns-of-population-change/
15. Crouch E, Eberth JM, Probst JC, et al. Rural-urban differences in costs of end-of-life care for the last 6 months of life among patients with breast, lung, or colorectal cancer. J Rural Health. 2018;35:199–207. https://doi.org/10.1111/jrh.12301.
16. Cummins S, Curtis S, Diez-Roux AV, et al. Understanding and representing 'place' in health research: a relational approach. Soc Sci Med. 2007;65:1825–38.
17. Dai D. Black residential segregation, disparities in spatial access to health care facilities, and late-stage breast cancer diagnosis in metropolitan Detroit. Health Place. 2010;16:1038–52.
18. Doescher MP, Jackson JE. Trends in cervical and breast cancer screening practices among women in rural and urban areas of the United States. J Public Health Manag Pract. 2009;15:200–9.

19. Gangnon RE, Sprague BL, Stout NK, et al. The contribution of mammography screening to breast cancer incidence trends in the united states: an updated age-period-cohort model. Cance Epidemiol Biomark Prev. 2015;24:905–12. https://doi.org/10.1158/1055-9965.EPI-14-1286.
20. Ghose R. Big sky or big sprawl? Rural gentrification and the changing cultural landscape of Missoula, Montana. Urban Geogr. 2004;25(6):528–49.
21. Gilbert PA, Larouche HH, Wallace RB, Parker EA, Curry SJ. Extending work on rural health disparities: a commentary on Matthews and colleagues' report. J Rural Health. 2018;34:119–21.
22. Halfacree KH. Locality and social representation: space, discourse and alternative definitions of the rural. J Rural Stud. 1993;9:23–37.
23. Hall SA, Kaufman JS, Ricketts TL. Defining urban and rural areas in U.S. epidemiologic studies. J Urban Health. 2006;85:162–75.
24. Hashibe M, Kirchoff AC, Kepka D, et al. Disparities in cancer survival and incidence by metropolitan versus rural residence in Utah. Cancer Med. 2018;7(4):1490–7.
25. Hart LG, Larson EH, Lishner DM. Rural definitions for health policy and research. Am J Public Health. 2005;95(7):1149–55.
26. Heley J, Jones L. Relational rural: some thoughts on relating things and theory in rural studies. J Rural Stud. 2012;28(3):208–17.
27. Henley SJ, Anderson RN, Thomas CC, et al. Invasive cancer incidence, 2004–2013, and deaths, 2006–2015, in nonmetropolitan and metropolitan counties – United States. MMWR. 2017;66(14)
28. Henry KA, Boscoe FP, Johnson CJ, et al. Breast cancer stage at diagnosis: is travel time important? J Community Health. 2011;36:933–42, PMID: 21461957.
29. Henry KA, Sherman R, Farber S, et al. The joint effects of census tract poverty and geographic access on late-stage breast cancer diagnosis in 10 US States. Health Place. 2013;21:110–21, PMID: 23454732.
30. Jacquez GM, Kaufmann A, Meliker J, et al. Global, local and focused clustering for case-control data with residential histories. Environ Health. 2005;4:4.
31. Isserman A. In the national interest: defining rural and urban correctly in research and public policy. Int Reg Sci Rev. 2005;28(4):465–99.
32. Jacobs LK, Kelley KA, Rosson GD, et al. Disparities in urban and rural mastectomy populations: the effects of patient- and county-level factors on likelihood of receipt of mastectomy. Ann Surg Oncol. 2008;15:2644–52.
33. Kolor K, Chen Z, Grosse SD, et al. BRCA genetic testing and receipt of preventive interventions among women aged 18–64 years with employer-sponsored health insurance in nonmetropolitan and metropolitan areas – United States 2009–2014. MMWR. 2017;66(15):1–11.
34. Kuo TM, Mobley LR, Anselin L. Geographic disparities in late-stage breast cancer diagnosis in California. Health Place. 2011;17(1):327–34.
35. Kwan M. The uncertain geographic context problem. Ann Am Assoc Geogr. 2012;102:958–68. https://doi.org/10.1080/00045608.2012.687349.
36. Leung J, McKenzie S, Martin J, McLaughlin D. Effect of rurality on screening for breast cancer: a systematic review and meta-analysis comparing mammography. Rural Remote Health. 2014;14:2730.
37. MacKinnon JA, Duncan RC, Huang Y, et al. Detecting an association between socioeconomic status and late stage breast cancer using spatial analysis and area-based measures. Cancer Epidemiol Biomark Prev. 2007;16:756–62. https://doi.org/10.1158/1055-9965.EPI-06-0392.
38. Macintyre S, Ellawa A, Cummins S. Place effects on health: how can we conceptualize, operationalize and measure them? Soc Sci Med. 2002;55:125–39. https://doi.org/10.1016/S0277-9536(01)00214-3.
39. Mao L, Yang J, Deng G. Mapping rural-urban disparities in late-stage cancer with high-resolution rurality index and GWR. Spat Spatio Temporal Epidemiol. 2018;28:15–23.
40. McLafferty S, Wang F, Luo L, Butler J. Rural-urban inequalities in late-stage breast cancer: spatial and social dimensions of risk and access. Environ Plann B Plann Des. 2011;38:726–40.

41. McNulty JA, Nail L. Cancer survivorship in rural and urban adults: a descriptive and mixed methods study. J Rural Health. 2015;31:282–91.
42. Meilleur A, Subramanian SV, Plascak JJ, Fisher JL, Paskett ED, Lamont EB. Rural residence and cancer outcomes in the U.S.: issues and challenges. Cancer Epidemiol Biomark Prev. 2013;22(10):1657–67. https://doi.org/10.1158/1055-9965.EPI-13-0404.
43. Mobley LR, Kuo TM, Watson L, et al. Geographic disparities in late-stage cancer diagnosis: multilevel factors and spatial interactions. Health Place. 2012;18:978–90.
44. Mobley LR, Kuo T-M, Scott L, Rutherford Y, Bose S. Modeling geospatial patterns of late-stage diagnosis of breast cancer in the US. Int J Environ Res Public Health. 2017;14(5):484. https://doi.org/10.3390/ijerph14050484.
45. Mobley LR, Kuo T-M. Demographic disparities in late-stage diagnosis of breast and colorectal cancers across the USA. J Racial Ethn Health Disparities. 2017;4:201–12.
46. Moss JL, Liu B, Feuer EJ. Urban/rural differences in breast and cervical cancer incidence: the mediating roles of socioeconomic status and provider density. Womens Health Issues. 2017;27(6):683–91.
47. Nguyen-Pham S, Leung J, McLaughlin D. Disparities in breast cancer stage at diagnosis in urban and rural adult women: a systematic review and meta-analysis. Ann Epidemiol. 2014;24:228–35.
48. Nordberg RB, Meliker JR, Ersball AK, Jacquez GM, Poulsen AH, Raaschou-Nielsen O. Space-time clusters of breast cancer using residential histories: a Danish case-control study. BMC Cancer. 2013;14:255. https://doi.org/10.1186/1471-2407-14-255.
49. Parise CA, Caggiano V. Regional variation in disparities in breast cancer specific mortality due to race/ethnicity, socioeconomic status, and urbanization. J Racial Ethn Health Disparities. 2017;4:706–17.
50. Peipins LA, Graham S, Young R, Lewis B, Foster S, Flanagan B, Dent A. Time and distance barriers to mammography facilities in the Atlanta metropolitan area. J Community Health. 2011;36(4):675–83.
51. Pruitt SL, Eberth JM, Morris ES, Grinsfelder DB, Cuate EL. Rural-urban differences in late-stage breast cancer: do associations differ by rural-urban classification system? Tex Public Health J. 2015;67(2):19–27.
52. Reid-Arndt SA, Cox CR. Does rurality affect quality of life following treatment for breast cancer? J Rural Health. 2010;26(4):402–5.
53. Rust G, Zhang S, Khusdeep M, Reese L, McRoy L, Baltrus P, Caplan L, Levine R. Paths to health equity: local area variation in progress toward eliminating breast cancer mortality disparities, 1990–2009. Cancer. 2015;121(16):2765–74.
54. Schootman M, Aft R. Rural-urban differences in radiation therapy for ductal carcinoma in-situ of the breast. Breast Cancer Res Treat. 2001;68(2):117–25.
55. Schootman M, Jeffe DB, Lian M, et al. The role of poverty rate and racial distribution in the geographic clustering of breast cancer survival among older women: a geographic and multi-level analysis. Am J Epidemiol. 2009;169:554–64.
56. Sighoko D, Hunt BR, Irizarry B, Watson K, Ansell D, Murphey AM. Disparity in breast cancer mortality by age and geography in 10 racially diverse US cities. Cancer Epidemiol. 2018;53:178–83.
57. Singh GK, Williams SD, Siahpush M, Mulhollen A. Socioeconomic, rural-urban, and racial inequalities in US cancer mortality: part 1—all cancers and lung cancer and part II—colorectal, prostate, breast, and cervical cancers. J Cancer Epidemiol. 2011:1–27. https://doi.org/10.1155/2011/107497.
58. Smith GL, Xu Y, Shih YT, et al. Breast-conserving surgery in older patients with invasive breast cancer: current patterns of treatment across the United States. J Am Coll Surg. 2009;209:425–33.
59. Srinivasan S, Moser RP, Willis G, Riley W, Alexander M, Berrigan D, Kobrin S. Small is essential: importance of subpopulation research in cancer control. Am J Public Health. 2015;3:S371–3.

60. Tarlov E, Zenk SN, Campbell RT, Warnecke RB, Block R. Characteristics of mammography facility locations and stage of breast cancer at diagnosis in Chicago. J Urban Health. 2009;86(2):196–213.
61. Tatalovich Z, Zhu L, Rolin A, et al. Geographic disparities in late stage breast cancer incidence: results from eight states in the United States. Int J Health Geogr. 2015;14:31. https://doi.org/10.1186/s12942-015-0025-5.
62. Waldorf B, Kim A. Defining and measuring rurality in the U.S.: from typologies to continuous indices. Commissioned paper for the workshop on commissioned paper. Washington, DC: National Academies of Sciences Workshop on Rationalizing Rural Classifications; 2015.. http://sites.nationalacademies.org/cs/groups/dbassesite/documents/webpage/dbasse_168031.pdf
63. Wang F, McLafferty S, Escamilla V, Luo L. Late-stage breast cancer diagnosis and health care access in Illinois. Prof Geogr. 2008;60(1):54–69.
64. Welch HG, Passow HJ. Quantifying the benefits and harms of screening mammography. JAMA Intern Med. 2014;174(3):448–54. https://doi.org/10.1001/jamainternmed.2013.13635.
65. Wu S, Powers S, Zhu W, et al. Substantial contribution of extrinsic risk factors to cancer development. Nature. 2016;529:43–7. https://doi.org/10.1038/nature16166.
66. Yasaitis LC, Arcaya MC, Subramanian SV. Comparison of estimation methods for creating small area rates of acute myocardial infarction among medicare beneficiaries in California. Health Place. 2015;35:95–104.
67. Yin Y, Wimberley MC. Geographic variations of colorectal and breast cancer late-stage diagnosis and the effects of neighborhood-level factors. J Rural Health. 2017;33:146–57.
68. Yu XQ, Luo Q, Kahn C, et al. Temporal trends show improved breast cancer survival in Australia but widening urban-rural differences. Breast. 2015;24:524–7.
69. Zahnd WE, Fogleman AJ, Jenkins WD. Rural-urban disparities in stage of diagnosis among cancers with preventive opportunities. Am J Prev Med. 2018;54:688–98.
70. Zahnd W, McLafferty S. Contextual effects and cancer outcomes in the United States: a systematic review of characteristics in multilevel analyses. Ann Epidemiol. 2017;27:739–48.. e3.

Chapter 17
Microenvironmental Influences on Team Performance in Cancer Care

Michael A. Rosen, Sadaf Kazi, and Salar Khaleghzadegan

Abstract Effective delivery of cancer care requires coordination across many professional and organizational boundaries. Breakdowns in coordination within this complex system underlie many quality of care issues. The interactions of care team members and multi-team systems matters to patient, staff, and organizational outcomes. Maturing the evidence-base for interventions and management strategies for teamwork and coordination within cancer care requires a robust toolset of measurement approaches suited to research and operational challenges. In this chapter, we provide an overview of the science of teams and traditional methods employed measure aspects of teamwork and coordination. We then review emerging unobtrusive and sensor-based methods and use cases for their application in cancer care delivery system research and operations.

Keywords Teamwork · Team dynamics · Team performance measurement · Unobtrusive measurement · Sensor-based measurement · Patient safety · Quality · Implementation science · Improvement science

17.1 Introduction

The continuum of cancer care encompasses numerous discrete types of care, and transitions between each [1]. This complex system requires coordination between a wide range of professionals with distinct roles, sets of domain expertise, and capabilities. The work of caring for cancer patients is inherently interdependent, with nurses, providers, patients and their loved ones, therapists, technicians, allied health professionals and administrators all playing a role in effective outcomes. The challenges coordinating this care have been documented extensively [2, 3]. Additionally, there is growing evidence that the manner in which organizations

M. A. Rosen (✉) · S. Kazi · S. Khaleghzadegan
Armstrong Institute for Patient Safety and Quality, Johns Hopkins University
School of Medicine, Baltimore, MD, USA
e-mail: mrosen44@jhmi.edu

© Springer Nature Switzerland AG 2019   399
D. Berrigan, N. A. Berger (eds.), *Geospatial Approaches to Energy Balance and Breast Cancer*, Energy Balance and Cancer 15, https://doi.org/10.1007/978-3-030-18408-7_17

manage these interdependencies, impacts patient, workforce, and organizational outcomes [4]. Interdependent work is managed in teams, and consequently, how organizations manage their teams matters.

In this chapter, we explore the concept of an organizational microenvironment and the influence of factors within this environment on the interactions of team members and the impact this may have on staff, patient, and organizational outcomes. The overarching goal of this chapter is to discuss existing and emerging methods for understanding team interactions across the continuum of cancer care and how these methods may be applied to challenges of researching and managing care in complex delivery systems. First, we define the team microenvironment in cancer care and connect this concept to the broader science of teams. Second, we provide a brief review of traditional and well-established methods for measuring aspects of the team microenvironment. Third, we outline key capabilities for the next generation of sensor-based and unobtrusive measures of team interaction. Fourth, we discuss specific applications of these methods in cancer care research and practice.

17.2   The Science of Teams Across the Cancer Care Continuum

In this section, we briefly review the science of teams to provide a conceptual framework for organizing key issues of coordination and teamwork.

17.2.1   Teams, Teamwork and Team Performance

Loose terminology has hampered progress in the multidisciplinary teams literature [5]. Therefore, we define key concepts used throughout the chapter. A *team* is defined as a set of two or more people interacting dynamically to manage interdependent work in the pursuit of shared and valued goals [6]. *Teamwork* refers to the interaction of team members in action (i.e., processes while engaged in task performance), transition (i.e., preparing for or reflecting on team task performance), or interpersonal processes (i.e., management of relationships within the team [7], and contrasted with *taskwork*, the work of team members in pursuit of individual task completion. *Team performance* refers to the outcomes of interaction and includes task performance (e.g., safety, quality, and efficiency), learning, and affective outcomes (e.g., trust and vitality). Research on work teams has generated an extensive set of theories to explain various aspects of interaction and performance [8]. Much of this literature can be broadly organized using an Inputs (i.e., relatively stable factors about the team, it's task and context [9, 10], Mediators (i.e., team interaction process and emergent states [11] and Outcomes framework.

17.2.2   The Microenvironment of the Care Delivery Team

Teams matter to cancer care delivery, from issues of team leadership and end of life decision making [12], to shared leadership in the transition from oncology to primary care teams [13], to the role of shared mental models in a wide range of multi-disciplinary care team situations [14, 15]. In this chapter, we define the *team microenvironment* as the collection of factors that exert influence on the social interactions of people participating in care delivery. This encompasses team inputs as well as the behavior of team members and those surrounding the team (e.g., local or system leadership). A more detailed understanding of how the microenvironment influences team interactions, and ultimately care outcomes, will provide the basis for interventions to better manage complex care delivery systems.

17.3   Traditional Methods for Understanding the Team Micro-Environment

Generating an evidence-based approach to managing teams within the cancer care continuum requires a tool kit of measures. Traditional methods such as survey [16] and observation [17] have been developed and well-validated for many care settings. We provide a brief review to these tools and key findings below.

17.3.1   Survey-Based Methods

Survey methods continue to be the workhorse measurement method for the social and organizational sciences. These methods involve asking team members to provide ratings about themselves as individuals, the team, or the larger organization or setting. Survey methods are well suited for capturing attitudinal constructs (e.g., mutual trust, collective orientation, psychological safety) due to their inherently subjective nature as well as constructs considered to be stable attributes of teams or their members (e.g., team inputs such as personality) due to the typically low time resolution of survey-based methods (i.e., it is rarely practical to have research participants complete lengthy survey measures). However, self-report methods can be applied to the vast majority of team related constructs including perceptions of teamwork [18], and team cognition [19]. This flexibility is one of their core strengths as a method along with well-established methods for developing and validating survey-based measures. The limitations of self-report methods in general and specifically for assessing team interaction are well documented also. Self-perceptions of performance tend to be inflated (i.e., the 'Lake Wobegon effect'), even more so for novices in a domain than for experts [20]. This means that respondents with lower levels of competence with teamwork behaviors will be more likely to have inflated self-ratings. This creates challenges when attempting to detect change over time. A final practical challenge involves achieving an adequate survey response rate so results can be interpreted appropriately.

17.3.2 Observation-Based Methods

Observational approaches have long been the paragon for measuring teamwork processes: when measuring teamwork skills, "there is no escaping observation" [21]. Observational approaches involve external raters providing judgments on what the team or team member's *do* during the course of a performance episode. Observation is valued for its objectivity (i.e., not relying on participant perceptions) and capability of linking team behaviors with situational events. Yet observation is not solely limited to the study of team processes. Measures could include a number of descriptive elements such as team size, member roles, task duration, task type, and other items reflective of team inputs. Affective and cognitive attributes can be inferred through the interpretation of team behaviors as well. For example, the Observational Teamwork Assessment for Surgery (OTAS) tool measures teamwork constructs related to communication (behavior), coordination (behavior), cooperation/back up behavior (affect/behavior), leadership (behavior), and monitoring/situational awareness (cognition) [22]. Using OTAS, raters make judgments of a team's level of cooperation through behaviors such as a surgeon's responsiveness to nursing and anesthesiology requests. Similarly, verbalizations of requests for information regarding patient status and regular instrument counts would be indicative of monitoring/situational awareness [22].

While observation overcomes some of the biases intrinsic to survey research, it is not without its own limitations. Significant investment is also needed to ensure raters are accurately assessing performance. Rater training typically necessitates a full day of instruction and practice using the system, with some systems requiring as much as 20 hours to establish high levels of rater reliability [17]. On top of rater training itself, dedicated rater time is needed to observe teams in training and naturalistic settings. This may prove particularly challenging when observations are scheduled around unpredictable and/or low occurrence events.

17.4 A Framework for Unobtrusive Methods of Team Interaction Measurement

The traditional methods discussed above provide a strong foundation for empirical research; however, emerging unobtrusive or sensor-based methods can complement these [23]. In this section, we discuss four categories of methods that can be applied to understand the team microenvironment for cancer care: linguistic features of communication, paralinguistic features of communication, team physiological dynamics, and activity traces [24]. These methods are summarized in Table 17.1.

Table 17.1 Unobtrusive methods of measuring team microenvironment

Measurement focus	Description	Example measures	Benefits and challenges
Activity tracing	Use of wearables and environmental sensors to capture physical activity and geospatial location, and collaboration tools (e.g., emails) to capture byproducts of interaction	In a pediatric ward, workers responsible for environmental cleaning had more instances of proximity to other individuals than nurses, physician, and patients [68]	Does not require responses from participants
			Unknown error structure (reliability and bias) to many of the data collection methods
Team Physiological Dynamics (TPD)	Continuous assessment of individual team members' autonomic and central nervous systems dynamics when they are performing as a team [56]	In a process control task team cardiovascular activity accounted for 10% of the variance in team performance [66]	High temporal resolution of data
			Substantial demands during data analysis
Linguistic communication	Assessing communication content, including frequency of word category use, emotional valence, semantic similarity, etc.	Latent sematic analysis metrics such as communication density and lags can be used to describe communication patterns of high performance teams [35]	Low data collection burden on researchers and participants
			Automation of speech recognition can speed up analysis
Paralinguistic communication	Measuring vocal features (e.g., pitch, tempo), communication flow, gestures, postures, facial expression, gaze behavior, etc.	Poor performing aircraft pilot crews had higher mean recurrence speech rate [47]	Can provide context to interpret data acquired from other sources (e.g. physiology, verbal communication)
			Substantial demands during data analysis

17.4.1 Linguistic Features of Communication

Team communication is a critical process [25]. Linguistic aspects of communication include the words used to communicate information. This is most commonly measured using self-report and content analysis of communication. Content analysis traditionally involves the manual coding of transcripts in order to categorize some unit of communication [26]. We focus here, on emerging methods of linguistic analysis that do not rely on burdensome manual coding of interactions: dictionary-based lexical analysis, supervised learning, and generative (or unsupervised learning) methods [27].

Lexical or dictionary-based methods use pre-defined lists of words and phrases associated with known constructs. The rate at which these key words or phrases appear in the team's communication are used to assign the team (or segments of its communication over time, or subsets by team member) to categories or measure the extent to which a construct is present in the team's communication. Linguistic Inquiry and Word Count (LIWC; [28]) is a well validated example of this approach.

However, there is a growing variety of tools available, particularly for sentiment analysis which quantifies the emotional valence and intensity communication content [29]. Dictionary-based methods like LIWC provide measures of domain independent language use such as verb tense or pronoun use. This has the advantage of being broadly applicable across teams and tasks; however, it does not capture any domain specific or technical content in language use. In a laboratory studies, linguistic style matching (e.g., the degree to which team members mimic one another's use of function words or speech rate) positively predicts small group cohesion, cooperation, and performance [30]. Lexical analysis has shown predictive validity for teams in more complex real-world tasks as well. Sexton and Helmreich [31] found patterns of general language use (e.g., use of first person plural) amongst commercial aircrews correlated with error rates. Similarly, Fisher and colleagues [32] found that both general patterns of language use and task domain specific communication are related to team performance outcomes for spaceflight teams.

Supervised learning methods use a variety of machine learning techniques to automate the process of coding text [33]. These algorithms require a training set of documents that have been coded previously by humans and a validation process using a set of held out documents (i.e., not included in the training set). Supervised learning methods are appropriate when using a well-defined coding scheme and it is feasible to code a subset, but not the complete set, of documents. Therefore, supervised learning methods can be viewed as a means to reduce the burden of manual interaction coding.

Generative (or unsupervised learning) methods are latent variable modeling techniques applied in machine learning and natural language processing (NLP) tasks. These approaches work from previously unclassified documents. As a person generates a document or speech, he or she has in mind certain ideas (i.e., the subject about which they are writing or speaking). The idea(s) that person has in mind influence the likelihood of words chosen to describe that idea [34]. Generative modeling identifies a set of topics (i.e., the latent variables that produced a set of documents or speech acts) that describe a set of documents. Latent Semantic Analysis (LSA) is one such generative modeling technique that infers expected relations between contextual usages of words in a discourse. LSA algorithms were able to predict team performance outcomes with a reasonable degree of accuracy (i.e., correlation of $r = .63$ between performance scores predicted by LSA algorithms and actual team performance scores [35, 36], and show that high performing teams have more semantic similarity [37].

These three methods each have the potential to contribute to a team interaction measurement system in different ways. Dictionary-based methods are highly generalizable and relatively easy to use, but do not capture context specific characteristics of speech. Supervised learning methods require pre-existing categories, large training sets of coded documents, and a complex validation process; however, they can greatly expand the throughput of a human coding team. Generative models (Topic Modeling, LSA) require no initial coding, but are atheoretical and model diagnostics are currently under developed [38]. There are active research communities developing each of these types of methods, and undoubtedly they are growing in power and ease of use.

17.4.2 Para-Linguistic Features of Communication

Paralinguistic aspects of communication are infrequently researched *within work team settings*. However, there is an extensive literature team researchers can draw from to better measure, understand and improve team communication [39]. This work details approaches for capturing vocal features, communication flow, gesture and posture, and facial expressions and gaze behavior.

Vocal features potentially important to the measurement of team communication include pitch, tempo, and energy [40]. These communication features have been validated as indicators of personality, perceptions of speaker competence, and persuasiveness [41]. Prosody (i.e., attributes of speech delivery such as intonation, and stress) and voice quality discriminate between most and least dominant group members [42]. Charfuelan and Schroder [43] used Principal Components Analysis (PCA) and Support Vector Machine (SVM) to identify vocal features associated with other team factors such as speaker role. SVM and Naive Classifiers were used alongside human annotation and coding to estimate cohesion using nonverbal communication behavior [44]. Specifically, maximum overlap of speaking rate was significantly higher in cohesive teams, where team members were actively participating. Nonverbal cues like prosody, speaking activity, and variation in energy (loudness heard by ear), in addition to visual nonverbal features like head activity predict emergent leadership [45]. The use of machine learning techniques demonstrated that emergent leaders could be correctly identified between 72 to 85% of the time.

Communication flow involves the temporal dynamics of communication acts and is perhaps the most widely researched paralinguistic aspect of communication within work team settings. This can involve overall assessments of turn taking behavior (e.g., speech dominance of individual members vs. egalitarian sharing of turns; [46]), the degree of stability in turn taking behavior [47], or the occurrence of specific patterns of interaction [48]. Unobtrusive measures of communication flow can be derived from audio recordings, automated speech detection systems (which identify segments of communication from microphones but do not record the content of communication to protect privacy in work settings) and activity traces (e.g., email, paging, phone, chats, and access logs in shared information systems). For example, Cooke and colleagues employed an experimental paradigm using a push button to talk paradigm to track conversational flow [49]. Here, information from the communication device (who was selecting to talk to whom, and when) provided important information about team interaction. One study that was mentioned earlier also used different aspects of communication flow including pauses between individual turns, pauses between floor exchanges, turn lengths, overlapping speech, in addition to others, using supervised machine learning techniques [44]. Some significant findings for identifying highly cohesive teams include total pause time (represents how actively attentive members of the team are to one another), total overlap (which was expected to be negatively correlated with cohesion but turns out that overlap is feature of highly cohesive teams because it indicates good rapport when team members can finish one another's sentences), and other audio cues.

Gesture and posture includes the communication of intent, emphasis, and emotional states of team members [40]. Gesture and posture data can be generated through analysis of video data or instrumenting individuals with sensors to capture movement, position, and muscle activation. There have been few studies linking gesture and posture within teams to outcomes or other constructs. However, synchrony in postural sway negatively predicts team cohesion [50], authoritarian leaders are likely to move their arms more than considerate leaders, while considerate leaders are more likely to imitate posture changes and head nods of their team members [51], and mimicry is generally an indicator of group cohesion. These paralinguistic features of communication are another opportunity to expand team communication measurement toolbox.

Facial expression and gaze behavior can communicate attentional focus and emotional states within the team. Facial expressions can be coded from video data or measures of facial muscle activity. Gaze behavior can be captured through eye tracking systems or inferred from head position in video data. Interestingly, synchrony of facial expressions within a team measured via video analysis or facial muscle activity is positively predictive of task performance outcomes [52] and team cohesion [53]. Additionally, teams with low levels of synchrony in facial muscle activity were more likely to adapt their strategies across different performance episodes [53]. In airline crews, synchrony in gaze behavior, as an indicator of shared attentional focus, was predictive of performance outcomes [54]. In a study of student air traffic control teams, investigation of individual and team situation awareness (SA) suggested that eye tracking could be used to measure individual and team SA by using the co-occurrence of information seeking and acquisition to predict some aspects of simulation [55].

17.4.3   Team Physiological Dynamics

Team physiological dynamics (TPD) refers to the continuous assessment of physiologies of individual team members during team performance episodes [56]. TPD researchers study both central and peripheral nervous systems. Cardiac (e.g., [57]) and electrodermal measures (e.g., [58]) are most common, but there is also increasing use of measuring electroencephalographic activity (e.g., [59, 60]). Kazi et al. [56] identified three types of TPD based on statistical methods of analyzing and aggregating data from individual team members to make inferences about team dynamics. The first, physiological arousal, pools together or aggregates the overall physiological activation of individual team members in creating the overall team physiological measure. The second, describing compositional dynamics of convergence over time [61], or physiological synchrony, considers the degree of similarity in TPD over time. Research using compositional physiological dynamics commonly uses methods such as cross-correlations, coherence between the frequency of signals, etc., to aggregate TPD. Finally, compilational physiological dynamics [61] describes patterns of divergent processes. That is, individual team members' physiological dynamics may assume stable, predictable patterns over time, or may fail to be organized into meaningful patterns; this is referred to by the term physiological organization. Compilational dynamics are aggregated through methods such as cross recurrence quantification analysis [62]. In the absence of a clear theory of when compilation vs. composition are appropriate, it is practical to consider both dimensions because each may be appropriate in different circumstances.

TPD has been studied in connection to team inputs, processes and emergent states, and outputs. For example, Gorman and colleagues [37] found that neural physiological organization in experienced submarine operator teams is more diverse during the team performance episodes, which may be indicative of greater cognitive flexibility within the team. In addition, shifts in communication patterns within experienced submarine operator teams precedes changes in team neural physiological organization [37], suggesting that shifts in TPD are at least partly driven by reactions to patterns of communication within the team.

The nature of the findings of existing research on process and output variables are complex and depend on aggregation method (e.g. [57, 63]). For example, cross correlation-derived cardiac physiological synchrony before [64] and during the task [65, 66] predicted better task performance. However, Strang and colleagues [50] found that physiological synchrony (using cross correlation) and physiological organization (using CRQA) were not associated with task performance, instead finding lower cardiac physiological organization aggregated through cross-fuzzy entropy, to be associated with better performance.

The use of unobtrusive sensors to measure physiological changes when working in a team offers a promising avenue for understanding the effects of teamwork on individual health and well-being. There is a small, but growing body of literature documenting changes in physiological dynamics when working in teams.

17.4.4 Activity Traces

Activity trace methods include a broad range of technologies that capture physical location and movement or extract information from existing technologies that can characterize patterns of work and coordination. Technology frequently moderates team interactions (e.g., communicating asynchronously through electronic health record documentation, use of email or paging systems). These interactions leave data that can be mined to describe and evaluate those interactions. Additionally, healthcare workers are increasingly instrumented with devices for the explicit purpose of tracking their activities (e.g., real-time locating systems in acute care settings).

Badges equipped with radiofrequency identification (RFID) and infrared sensors are increasingly used for location and activity tracking for research and operational aims. These sensors are used to measure a variety of constructs from workload [67], to interaction patterns that can enable the transmission of nosocomial infections [68]. Rosen et al. [67] studied intensive care unit nursing workload by combining data from unobtrusive, sensor-based measures with observations and self-report data including focus groups and perceptions of physical and mental exertion. The researchers used three types of sensors: RFID and infrared sensors that measured location and proximity; accelerometers that measured body movement and activity; and two-directional microphones that measured features of speech and environmental sounds. In addition to these measures, the researchers also collected data on patient census during each shift, and patient acuity. Results showed that perceptions of mental and physical workload were influenced by different types of variables. Higher perceptions of mental exertion was predicted by (1) environmental noise in patient rooms; (2) spending more time in non-service areas that had high activity levels; and (3) an interaction between the number of patients on insulin drip and high levels of 'burstiness' of speech, which described periods of irregular patterns of speech activity, i.e., high-intensity speech occurred close together or there were periods of no-to-sparse speech activity, instead of more even distribution of speech activity. Higher perceptions of physical exertion were predicted by (1) environmental noise in service areas containing medications, nutrition, and other supplies for patients; (2) unpredictable physical movements that occurred closely together; (3) an interaction between longer time speaking outside of main work areas and more time spent at nursing stations; (4) a negative interaction between environmental noise in service areas higher activity in patient rooms; and (5) average speech level at nursing stations and average patient load.

Isella et al. [68] used RFID to measure the transmission of nosocomial infections on a pediatric unit in which many patients were diagnosed with respiratory infection. Physicians, nurses, ward assistants who were responsible for environmental cleaning, transporting patients, and distributing food, patients, and caregivers wore sensors that detected proximity of contact. The sensors measured three variables: (1) number of distinct people that the person "interacted" with, i.e., was in face-to-face proximity to for at least 20 s; (2) the number of total contacts during the day, including repeated contacts with the same individual(s) at different points of time throughout the day; and (3) the duration of total contact. Results showed that ward assistants had highest median values on all three variables (distinct contact = between 5–6; total contacts = 99.5; duration = approximately 1 h), followed by nurses. Patients and caregivers, on the other hand, had lowest median values. Nurses, physicians, and ward assistants had dense interaction networks, indicating a variety of cross-training interaction. In contrast, patients and caregivers largely interact with each other. The researchers also found that patients interacted most frequently and for the longest duration with nurses. This pattern of interaction indicates nurses as potentially vulnerable to contamination by the infection and at risk for transmitting contamination.

Proximity sensors have also been used in conjunction with other methods such as email communication to study interaction patterns. Olguín Olguín et al. [69] instrumented 22 office workers with badges capable of detecting activity and face-to-face interactions, and also measured email interaction over the course of 20 working days. They found that office team members who work in close proximity exchanged fewer emails. Higher frequencies of interaction, including face-to-face and email communication, was associated with lower job satisfaction.

17.5 Applications to Cancer Care

The new approaches described above are maturing rapidly, and can help address key challenges in cancer care delivery. In this section, we discuss three use cases, or areas of application to demonstrate the applicability of these methods to research and operational work. These use cases span the levels of analysis from dyadic interactions between physicians and patients, to traditional team structures, and larger organizational units.

17.5.1 Physician and Patient Interaction

The quality of the interaction between a physician and a patient impacts perceptions of care and psychological adjustment [70, 71]. Traditionally, measures of this interaction use methods of self-report or manual coding of communication [72]. This has limited the availability of data for the purposes of research (i.e., what specific aspects of the interaction are most important?) and improvement (e.g., giving healthcare workers feedback on their patterns of interaction and how to improve). However, the advances in natural language processing and paralinguistic speech analysis introduced above can be applied to this form at team interaction and effectively scale team interaction analysis for linguistic and paralinguistic aspects of communication. This can be an invaluable tool for developing measures around the challenging issues of shared decision making, respect and dignity, and disparities and for generating interventions to train and coach effective interactions [73].

17.5.2 Acute Care Team Interaction Patterns

Coordination of care failures represent risks at all phases of the continuum of care (e.g., delayed diagnoses or test follow-up). However, episodes of acute care often expose patients to immediate, active, and severe threats to safety (e.g., medication errors, hospital acquired infections, device related errors). Intensive Care Units (ICUs) represent a disproportionate share of this risk due to the acuity of the patient population and the complexity of care delivered in these settings. ICU unit strain (i.e., time varying demands for critical care services) can stretch and overwhelm the capacity of a unit to effectively care for patients [74]. ICU team functioning can be assessed through observation for the purposes of research and developmental feedback [75], but the sensor-based approaches introduced above can greatly improve the timeliness of workload assessments and yield real-time information about team interactions and system failures.

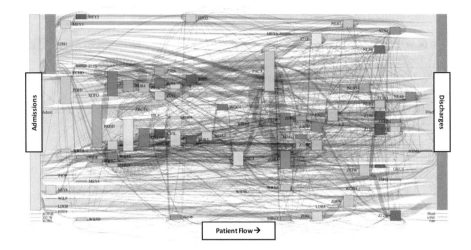

Patient Flow →

Fig. 17.1 Map of Multi-Team System interdependencies generated from activity trace data. This figure represents 3 months of patient care transitions (limited to patients' physical movements) through a large academic medical center. All transitions are within one physical location, a large hospital complex. Each node in the map is a physical location. The larger the node, the more patients moved through that location. Each line represents patient movement between two locations. The thicker the line, the more patients moved between those two locations. Units with higher upstream complexity reported worse patient care transitions

17.5.3 Multi-Team System Functioning

A multi-team system (MTS) comprises two are more teams interacting interdependently to achieve shared goals. These organizational structures are complex, and difficult to manage, but they do pose potential benefits such as adaptability [76]. Activity trace approaches can be a valuable approach to identifying coordination demands across the care continuum [77]. For example, Fig. 17.1 illustrates a map of MTS interdependence within a large academic medical center. This map was generated from activity trace data of patient movements within the hospital, and clearly illustrates the complexity of care delivery processes. Metrics derived from activity trace data such as these can be used to identify effective and ineffective patterns of coordination, drive organizational redesign efforts, and real-time management of patient flow (e.g., detecting patients on risky or atypical trajectories and intervening).

17.6 Conclusions

The team microenvironment in cancer care delivery systems comprises the collection of factors that exert influence on the social interactions of people in that system. The science of teams can be used to understand how the microenvironment impacts team interactions and care outcomes. In addition to traditional measures of interaction such as surveys and observations, newer methods using unobtrusive measurement techniques can also be used to capture team interactions based on geospatial location, activity tracing, team member physiologies, and team communication. There is great potential in using these newer assessment methods to build sophisticated data-driven management systems to capture facets of the microenvironment that are especially pertinent to cancer care delivery such as the quality of interactions between the physician and the patient, interaction pattern between members of the cancer care delivery team, and their coordination patterns. Additionally, the growth in remote surveillance technologies for healthcare and telemedicine increase the instances where healthcare teams are coordinating efforts from geographically separated locations or in asynchronous ways. Virtual teams such as these have been studied within the corporate world, but far less work has been conducted on these teams that span the micro- and macro-environments of cancer care delivery.

Acknowledgement This work was partially funded by a grant from the National Aeronautics and Space Administration (Grant # NNX17AB55G; PI: Rosen).

References

1. Taplin SH, Price RA, Edwards HM, et al. Introduction: understanding and influencing multi-level factors across the cancer care continuum. J Natl Cancer Inst Monogr. 2012;2012:2–10.
2. Walsh J, Harrison JD, Young JM, et al. What are the current barriers to effective cancer care coordination? A qualitative study. BMC Health Serv Res. 2010;10:132.
3. Walsh J, Young JM, Harrison JD, et al. What is important in cancer care coordination? A qualitative investigation. Eur J Cancer Care (Engl). 2011;20:220–7.
4. Rosen MA, DiazGranados D, Dietz AS, et al. Teamwork in healthcare: key discoveries enabling safer, high-quality care. Am Psychol. 2018;73:433–50.
5. Nestel D, Walker K, Simon R, et al. Nontechnical skills: an inaccurate and unhelpful descriptor? Simul Healthc. 2011;6:2–3.
6. Salas E, Cooke NJ, Rosen MA. On teams, teamwork, and team performance: Discoveries and developments. Hum Factors. 2008;50:540–7.
7. Marks MA, Mathieu JE, Zaccaro SJ. A temporally based framework and taxonomy of team processes. Acad Manag Rev. 2001;26:356–76.
8. Mathieu JE, Wolfson MA, Park S. The evolution of work team research since Hawthorne. Am Psychol. 2018;73:308–21.
9. Bell ST. Deep-level composition variables as predictors of team performance: a meta-analysis. J Appl Psychol. 2007;92:595–615.
10. Stewart GL. A meta-analytic review of relationships between team design features and team performance. J Manage. 2006;32:29–55.
11. LePine JA, Piccolo RF, Jackson CL, et al. A meta-analysis of teamwork processes: tests of a multidimensional model and relationships with team effectiveness criteria. Pers Psychol. 2008;61:273–307.
12. Waldfogel JM, Battle DJ, Rosen M, et al. Team leadership and cancer end-of-life decision making. J Oncol Pract. 2016;12:1135–40. https://doi.org/10.1200/JOP.2016.013862.
13. Tremblay D, Latreille J, Bilodeau K, et al. Improving the transition from oncology to primary care teams: a case for shared leadership. J Oncol Pract. 2016;12:1012–9. https://doi.org/10.1200/JOP.2016.013771.

14. Page JS, Lederman L, Kelly J, et al. Teams and teamwork in cancer care delivery: shared mental models to improve planning for discharge and coordination of follow-up care. J Oncol Pract. 2016;12:1053–8.
15. D'Ambruoso SF, Coscarelli A, Hurvitz S, et al. Use of a shared mental model by a team composed of oncology, palliative care, and supportive care clinicians to facilitate shared decision making in a patient with advanced cancer. J Oncol Pract. 2016;12:1039–45.
16. Valentine MA, Nembhard IM, Edmondson AC. Measuring teamwork in health care settings: a review of survey instruments. Med Care. 2015;53:e30.
17. Dietz AS, Pronovost PJ, Benson KN, et al. A systematic review of behavioural marker systems in healthcare: what do we know about their attributes, validity and application? BMJ Qual Saf. 2014;23:1031–9.
18. Wageman R, Hackman JR, Lehman E. Team diagnostic survey: development of an instrument. J Appl Behav Sci. 2005;41:373–98.
19. Wildman JL, Salas E, Scott CPR. Measuring cognition in teams: a cross-domain review. Hum Factors. 2014;56:911–41.
20. Kruger J, Dunning D. Unskilled and unaware of it: how difficulties in recognizing one's own incompetence lead to inflated self-assessments. J Pers Soc Psychol. 1999;77:1121–34.
21. Baker DP, Salas E. Principles for measuring teamwork: a summary and look toward the future. In: Brannick MT, Salas E, Prince C, editors. Team performance assessment and measurement: theory, methods, and applications: Psychology Press; 1997. p. 331–56.
22. Russ S, Hull L, Rout S, et al. Observational teamwork assessment for surgery: feasibility of clinical and nonclinical assessor calibration with short-term training. Ann Surg. 2012;255:804–9.
23. Rosen MA, Dietz AS, Yang T, et al. An integrative framework for sensor-based measurement of teamwork in healthcare. J Am Med Inform Assoc. 2014;22:11–8.
24. Rosen M, Dietz A, Kazi S. Beyond Coding Interaction. Cambridge Handb Gr Interact Anal Cambridge Handbooks Psychol. Cambridge: Cambridge Univ Press; 2018. p. 142–62.
25. Marlow SL, Lacerenza CN, Paoletti J, et al. Does team communication represent a one-size-fits-all approach?: a meta-analysis of team communication and performance. Organ Behav Hum Decis Process. 2018;144:145–70.
26. Brauner E, Boos M, Kolbe M. The Cambridge handbook of group interaction analysis. New York: Cambridge University Press; 2018.
27. Grimmer J, Stewart BM. Text as data: the promise and pitfalls of automatic content analysis methods for political texts. Polit Anal. 2013;21:267–97.
28. Tausczik YR, Pennebaker JW. The psychological meaning of words: LIWC and computerized text analysis methods. J Lang Soc Psychol. 2010;29:24–54.
29. Gilbert CJHE. Vader: a parsimonious rule-based model for sentiment analysis of social media text. In: Eighth International Conference on Weblogs and Social Media (ICWSM-14). Available at 20 04 2016. 2014. http://comp.social.gatechedu/papers/icwsm14vaderhuttopdf.
30. Gonzales AL, Hancock JT, Pennebaker JW. Language style matching as a predictor of social dynamics in small groups. Commun Res. 2010;37:3–19.
31. Sexton JB, Helmreich RL. Analyzing cockpit communications: the links between language, performance, error, and workload. Hum Perform Extrem Environ. 2000;5:63–8.
32. Fischer U, McDonnell L, Orasanu J. Linguistic correlates of team performance: toward a tool for monitoring team functioning during space missions. Aviat Space Environ Med. 2007;78:B95.
33. Evans JA, Aceves P. Machine translation: mining text for social theory. Annu Rev Sociol. 2016;42:21–50.
34. Landauer TK, Foltz PW, Laham D. An introduction to latent semantic analysis. Discourse Process. 1998;25:259–84.
35. Gorman JC, Foltz PW, Kiekel PA, et al. Evaluation of latent semantic analysis-based measures of team communications content. In: Proceedings of the human factors and ergonomics society annual meeting. Los Angeles: SAGE Publications Sage CA; 2003. p. 424–8.

36. Martin MJ, Foltz PW. Automated team discourse annotation and performance prediction using LSA. In: Proceedings of HLT-NAACL 2004: short papers. Association for computational linguistics, 2004. pp 97–100.
37. Gorman JC, Martin MJ, Dunbar TA, et al. Cross-level effects between neurophysiology and communication during team training. Hum Factors. 2016;58:181–99.
38. Chuang J, Gupta S, Manning C, Heer J. Topic model diagnostics: assessing domain relevance via topical alignment. In: International conference on machine learning; 2013. p. 612–20.
39. Gatica-Perez D. Automatic nonverbal analysis of social interaction in small groups: a review. Image Vis Comput. 2009;27:1775–87.
40. Vinciarelli A, Pantic M, Bourlard H. Social signal processing: survey of an emerging domain. Image Vis Comput. 2009;27:1743–59.
41. Schuller B, Steidl S, Batliner A, et al. A Survey on perceived speaker traits: personality, likability, pathology, and the first challenge. Comput Speech Lang. 2015;29:100–31.
42. Charfuelan M, Schröder M, Steiner I. Prosody and voice quality of vocal social signals: the case of dominance in scenario meetings. In: Eleventh annual conference of the international speech communication association. 2010.
43. Charfuelan M, Schröder M. Investigating the prosody and voice quality of social signals in scenario meetings. Lect Notes Comput Sci (including Subser Lect Notes Artif Intell Lect Notes Bioinformatics). 2011;6974. LNCS:46–56. https://doi.org/10.1007/978-3-642-24600-5_8.
44. Hung H, Gatica-Perez D. Estimating cohesion in small groups using audio-visual nonverbal behavior. IEEE Trans Multimed. 2010;12:563–75.
45. Sanchez-Cortes D, Aran O, Mast MS, Gatica-Perez D. A nonverbal behavior approach to identify emergent leaders in small groups. IEEE Trans Multimed. 2012;14:816–32.
46. Woolley AW, Chabris CF, Pentland A, et al. Evidence for a collective intelligence factor in the performance of human groups. Science. 2010;330:686–8.
47. Gontar P, Fischer U, Bengler K. Methods to evaluate pilots' cockpit communication: cross-recurrence analyses vs. speech act–based analyses. J Cogn Eng Decis Mak. 2017;11:337–52.
48. Tschan F. Ideal cycles of communication (or cognitions) in triads, dyads, and individuals. Small Group Res. 2002;33:615–43.
49. Gorman JC, Hessler EE, Amazeen PG, et al. Dynamical analysis in real time: detecting perturbations to team communication. Ergonomics. 2012;55:825–39.
50. Strang AJ, Funke GJ, Russell SM, et al. Physio-behavioral coupling in a cooperative team task: contributors and relations. J Exp Psychol Hum Percept Perform. 2014;40:145–58.
51. Feese S, Arnrich B, Troster G, et al. Quantifying behavioral mimicry by automatic detection of nonverbal cues from body motion. In: Privacy, Security, Risk and Trust (PASSAT), 2012 International confernece on social computing (SocialCom) IEEE, 2012. pp 520–525.
52. Chikersal P, Tomprou M, Kim YJ, et al. Deep structures of collaboration: physiological correlates of collective intelligence and group satisfaction: CSCW; 2017. p. 873–88.
53. Mønster D, Håkonsson DD, Eskildsen JK, Wallot S. Physiological evidence of interpersonal dynamics in a cooperative production task. Physiol Behav. 2016;156:24–34. https://doi.org/10.1016/j.physbeh.2016.01.004.
54. Gontar P, Mulligan JB. Cross recurrence analysis as a measure of pilots' visual behaviour. In: Proceedings of the 32nd conference of the european association for aviation psychology. Groningen; 2016.
55. Hauland G. Measuring individual and team situation awareness during planning tasks in training of en route air traffic control. Int J Aviat Psychol. 2008;18:290–304.
56. Kazi S, Khaleghzadegan S, Dinh J, et al. Team physiological dynamics: critical review hum factors under review.
57. Fusaroli R, Bjørndahl JS, Roepstorff A, Tylén K. A heart for interaction: shared physiological dynamics and behavioral coordination in a collective, creative construction task. J Exp Psychol Hum Percept Perform. 2016;42:1297–310.
58. Guastello SJ. Physiological synchronization in a vigilance dual task. Nonlinear Dynamics Psychol Life Sci. 2016;20:49–80.

59. Stevens R, Galloway T, Lamb C. Submarine navigation team resilience: linking EEG and behavioral models. In: Proceedings of the human factors and ergonomics society annual meeting. Los Angeles: SAGE Publications Sage CA; 2014. p. 245–9.
60. Toppi J, Borghini G, Petti M, et al. Investigating cooperative behavior in ecological settings: an EEG hyperscanning study. PLoS One. 2016;11:e0154236.
61. Kozlowski SWJ, Klein KJ. A multilevel approach to theory and research in organizations: contextual, temporal, and emergent processes. In: Klein KJ, Kozlowski SWJ, editors. Multilevel theory, research, and methods in organizations: foundations, extensions, and new directions. San Francisco: Jossey-Bass; 2000. p. 3–90.
62. Knight AP, Kennedy DM, McComb SA. Using recurrence analysis to examine group dynamics. Group Dyn Theory Res Pract. 2016;20:223–41.
63. Järvelä S, Kivikangas JM, Kätsyri J, Ravaja N. Physiological linkage of dyadic gaming experience. Simul Gaming. 2014;45:24–40.
64. Elkins AN, Muth ER, Hoover AW, et al. Physiological compliance and team performance. Appl Ergon. 2009;40:997–1003.
65. Henning RA, Boucsein W, Gil MC. Social–physiological compliance as a determinant of team performance. Int J Psychophysiol. 2001;40:221–32.
66. Walker AD, Muth ER, III FSS, Rosopa PJ. Predicting team performance in a dynamic environment: a team psychophysiological approach to measuring cognitive readiness. J Cogn Eng Decis Mak. 2013;7:69–82.
67. Rosen MA, Dietz AS, Lee N, et al. Sensor-based measurement of critical care nursing workload: Unobtrusive measures of nursing activity complement traditional task and patient level indicators of workload to predict perceived exertion. PLoS One. 2018;13:e0204819.
68. Isella L, Romano M, Barrat A, et al. Close encounters in a pediatric ward: measuring face-to-face proximity and mixing patterns with wearable sensors. PLoS One. 2011;6:e17144.
69. Olguín Olguín D, Waber BN, Kim T, et al. Sensible organizations: technology and methodology for automatically measuring organizational behavior. IEEE Trans Syst Man Cybern B. 2009;39:43–55.
70. Arora NK. Interacting with cancer patients: the significance of physicians' communication behavior. Soc Sci Med. 2003;57:791–806.
71. Zachariae R, Pedersen CG, Jensen AB, et al. Association of perceived physician communication style with patient satisfaction, distress, cancer-related self-efficacy, and perceived control over the disease. Br J Cancer. 2003;88:658–65.
72. Venetis MK, Robinson JD, Turkiewicz KL, Allen M. An evidence base for patient-centered cancer care: a meta-analysis of studies of observed communication between cancer specialists and their patients. Patient Educ Couns. 2009;77:379–83.
73. Epstein RM, Duberstein PR, Fenton JJ, et al. Effect of a patient-centered communication intervention on oncologist-patient communication, quality of life, and health care utilization in advanced cancer: the VOICE randomized clinical trial. JAMA Oncol. 2017;3:92–100.
74. Bagshaw SM, Opgenorth D, Potestio M, et al. Healthcare provider perceptions of causes and consequences of ICU capacity strain in a large publicly funded integrated health region: a qualitative study. Crit Care Med. 2017;45:e356.
75. Dietz AS, Salas E, Pronovost PJ, et al. Evaluation of a measurement system to assess ICU team performance. Crit Care Med. 2018;46:1898–905.
76. Zaccaro SJ, Marks MA, DeChurch LA. Multiteam systems: an introduction. Routledge; 2012. p. 18–47.
77. Weaver SJ, Jacobsen PB. Cancer care coordination: opportunities for healthcare delivery research. Transl Behav Med. 2018;8:503–8.

Chapter 18
Opportunities and Challenges in Geospatial Approaches to Breast Cancer Prevention and Control

Tracy Onega

Abstract The utility of geospatial approaches to breast cancer control are known to be influential across the cancer control continuum, although they range broadly from residential histories, to wearable sensors, to healthcare service area delineation, and beyond. Advances in computational technologies, location-based data expansion, and cancer control research provide fertile ground for adapting and applying geospatial approaches to reduce the burden of breast and other cancers. However, key challenges exist that are slowing down our progress towards this end: (a) the tension between the democratization of data and computational specialization coupled with theory; (b) the need to move from observation and monitoring to intervening; (c) the need to integrate objective measures from tools such as GPS, accelerometry, and remote sensing with subjective aspects and individual utilities and (d) data privacy and security balanced with accessibility. These challenges may be met, at least in part, through opportunities related to: data collection, storage, sharing, and analytics; workforce/training; and research methods. Cross-disciplinary teams are advancing computational and theoretical approaches to understanding the interplay across these dimensions, but we need multidisciplinary teams to apply them to fully achieve progress in mitigating the burden of cancer and reducing disparities in its impacts. Suggested actions are laid out to guide researchers, policy makers, funders, and cancer centers.

Keywords Geospatial · Cancer control · Geoinformatics · Capacity-building · GIS · Big data · Team science · Mobile technology · Location data · Spatial methods

T. Onega (✉)
Departments of Biomedical Data Science, of Epidemiology, The Dartmouth Institute for Health Policy & Clinical Practice at the Geisel School of Medicine at Dartmouth, Lebanon, NH, USA

Norris Cotton Cancer Center, Lebanon, NH, USA
e-mail: tracy.l.onega@dartmouth.edu

© Springer Nature Switzerland AG 2019
D. Berrigan, N. A. Berger (eds.), *Geospatial Approaches to Energy Balance and Breast Cancer*, Energy Balance and Cancer 15, https://doi.org/10.1007/978-3-030-18408-7_18

18.1   Introduction

This volume illustrates the multidimensional and multifactorial nature of geospatial influences and approaches to studying breast cancer. While the focus on risk behaviors, environmental and contextual effects, and care delivery provides critical understanding of the geospatial impact of breast cancer for physicians, scientists, and public health researchers, these themes apply to other cancers as well, particularly those attributed to known risk behaviors and those amenable to screening such as colorectal, cervical and lung cancer. Geospatial measures themselves are heterogeneous constructs, representing both physical/locational information, as well as subjective factors related to sense of place and other qualitative measures. Also, the role of geospatial factors varies across the cancer control continuum from etiology, prevention, early detection, diagnosis, treatment, survivorship, and end-of-life. We are in a dynamic period for advancing computational and theoretical approaches to understanding the interplay across these dimensions. The utility of geospatial approaches to breast- and other cancers is well established and robustly illustrated in the prior chapters. Given the ubiquitous nature of geospatial information and its integration with mobile technology, the field seems ready to evolve to meet diverse challenges in the application of spatial data to problems in cancer control.

18.2   Challenges

The chapters in this book highlight a number of common challenges to advancing cancer prevention and control via geospatial approaches. Most prominently these include: (a) tension between the democratization of data and computational specialization along with theory; (b) moving from observation and monitoring to intervening; (c) need to integrate objective measures from diverse sensors and GIS data layers including GPS, accelerometry, Census data and many other sources with subjective aspects, individual utilities, and perceptions of the environment; and (d) privacy.

18.2.1   Tension Between Democratization of Data and Computational and Theoretical Specialization

Locational information has become pervasive through widespread use of sensor-based devices, smartphones, satellite, and other data. At the same time, most people consume location information routinely, and indeed, expect accurate, timely, and accessible geospatial information, such as from Google Maps. Publicly available geospatial data, and the ability to manipulate it, has become the purview of the average citizen – the democratization of data. Not only are tremendous volumes of geospatial data readily accessible via the internet, but even mapping – once the domain of trained GIS users – is readily achieved outside of formal, stand-along GIS platforms. For example, Excel has mapping capabilities, as does R. Therefore, expensive and specialized GIS tools can now be bypassed, allowing more users to manipulate geospatial data.

This new reality was demonstrated recently in my research team when a postdoc, trained as a cancer mechanisms biologist who was acquiring health services research experience in claims-based analysis – with no training in geography, GIS, or geospatial methods – produced a national map of physician referral networks across the U.S. [1] based on ZIP-code level Medicare claims information directly from her analyses using R and R spatial packages. This mapping capability was user friendly, seamlessly integrated with the R platform, and required no a priori knowledge of cartographic principles, map projections, scale/resolution, or ArcGIS/Spatial Network Analyst extension. Information technology (IT) is rapidly evolving, and for those of us who do not spend all of our time focused on geospatial science, we must avoid the hubris of prior expertise and embrace the multitudes of IT users who often are using the latest tools – and indeed, are likely driving the development of/ market for such tools made for general users. I was reminded of this point recently when, as a senior investigator, I was an invited lecturer to a prominent NCI Cancer Center to present on geospatial methods applied to cancer control. At the end of my talk, a graduate student in the audience was interested in my travel time analysis methods, and noted her use of Excel for geocoding, wondering if the Excel Geocoding Tool would be an appropriate starting point. Despite my two-decades of ArcGIS use, including for travel time analysis – I was not able to give her an informed answer on the new, readily-available, user-friendly tool, added as an extension in a ubiquitously-used platform with no prior GIS capabilities! I was grateful to her for informing me of the new Excel spatial utility and quickly investigated. The democratization of geospatial tools and capabilities is increasing, and the landscape of those tools needs to be monitored routinely to stay abreast of new resources.

At the same time, as noted in Chap. 4, complexity and/or size of geospatial data often brings the need for specialized computational skills, knowledge, and infrastructure. Geospatial methodologies, such as sensor data, generate large volumes of data with sometimes challenging data structures for analytic purposes. Similarly, geospatial data integration from heterogeneous sources can be fraught with difficulties and unknown quality. Data scientists are increasingly needed as part of geospatial research teams to most appropriately and accurately handle geospatial data.

Further, end users of geospatial data and simple mapping tools must not lose theoretical grounding, and must have basic knowledge of geospatial principles to ensure that a given approach is capturing what was intended. Wilson (Chap. 1) emphasizes this point and highlights some recent work summarizing key competencies in geospatial approaches to health. For example, having a basic understanding of the difference between geographic coordinate systems and projected coordinate systems is vital when moving from tabular data (e.g. latitude and longitude derived from a spherical [three-dimensional] geographic coordinate system) to a projected coordinate system for visual representation of geospatial information – i.e. a map, which is two-dimensional. For mapping and visualization, one must have either the good luck of using an appropriate pre-packaged utility, or an understanding of map projections and the forms of possible distortion (area, form, distance, direction) to make correct measurements or visualizations. This principle is exemplified in the often-used choropleth or dot density maps; a projection preserving areal properties, such as Mercator, is crucial to accurately depict such measures. While writing this chapter, I realized that I was remiss in not knowing the projection used by typical web-mapping utilities – I was a blind end-user! Google Maps uses a Spherical Normal variant of the Mercator projection, ostensibly because it allows more realistic street level views, with less distortion, even though 'zoomed out' views will have some distortion. The important point is to be a geospatially-informed end user (or producer) of geospatial tools, or assemble research teams that include such individuals. Because even though data is increasingly accessible and used, there is a tension with the need for specialized computational skills and geospatial knowledge.

18.2.2 Moving from Observation and Monitoring to Intervening

The studies presented in this volume demonstrate that the field of geospatial approaches to cancer control has matured to a point that offers increasingly nuanced measures. While there is still work to be done in improving *what* and *how* we measure geospatial impacts, it is clear – as noted by authors in prior chapters – that geospatial methods are poised to be used as interventional tools. Chapter 4 noted both the promise and current limitation of Just In Time Adaptive Interventions, which use spatial and temporal cues to elicit changes in behavior, although the settings/applications for which they are effective are yet to be fully determined. Similarly, e-Health sensors can delivery tailored messages about physical measures, such as heart rate, activity level, etc. These interventions are largely targeted at the individual/person level. However, geospatial methods could be used to design community-based interventions. For example, using classic methods from geography, location optimization analysis can be used for placement of public exercise areas for maximal impact. Also, with spatiotemporal analysis, time and place of health fairs could be better strategized to coincide with the highest volume of shoppers. Geospatial interventional approaches are poised to expand in the near future. At the same time, we can expand and refine geospatial approaches to observation and monitoring.

18.2.3 Integration of Objective Measures with Subjective Aspects and Individual Utilities

Objective geospatial measures, such as travel time, walkability, and food environments have been shown to have significant impact on cancer-related outcomes: accessing care, obesity mitigation, and healthy eating, respectively. Many elements of the built environment can be measured. However, the challenge remains to create measures than incorporate subjective, or individual-based, components into the geospatial. For example, measures of walkability could be refined by capturing daily activity structures and personal utilities. That is people are likely to walk more if there are walkable places to which they need/want to go, rather than simply having traversable surfaces in proximity.

Similarly, a sizable literature demonstrates the significance of travel time on utilization of specific cancer services, although some studies show no effect. Underpinning the travel time literature, is the notion that some degree of travel time represents a burden or barrier to the patient. While this is undoubtedly true for some individuals, there is no component of travel time that captures the subjective aspect of this measure. Thus, 60 min of travel time may exceed a researcher-defined threshold for "poor access", yet the patient may feel that this is not unduly long. In fact, preliminary work from a sample of 1000 individuals in Vermont and New Hampshire, shows that across 10 destination domains (e.g. grocery shopping, primary care, care for a serious condition, recreation, etc.), <u>willingness</u> to travel, self-reported in minutes, were <u>double</u> the self-reported actual travel time. Therefore, individuals did not travel as long as they were willing to, calling into question the degree to which travel time is a burden/barrier, although we recognize other potential opportunity costs [2]. When examining this effect by urban-rural categories (RUCA 4), we found the same trend, although rural individuals reported long travel times for both being willing and actually traveling. Integrating subjective aspects and personal utilities into geospatial measures would likely better capture potentially causal mechanisms compared to objective measures alone. However, the challenge is to develop such integrated measures and validate them for generalized use.

18.2.4 Privacy and Security

A fourth challenge in geospatial approaches to cancer control is privacy and security of individual data. For cancer research, there is often a need to link individual data from a variety of sources, such as cancer registries, electronic health records, and research-generated data. Location information can be particularly sensitive, and even ZIP code of residence is considered an identifiable field for HIPAA. Ambient data collection, such as public cameras and drones, presents new issues related to privacy for individuals around location information. Also, public availability of Twitter feeds and other social media data, may also threaten individuals' privacy.

Researchers can fully consent patients to studies that require geospatial data collection, although there are drawbacks, including: cost, patient time, low study recruitment, and biased sample for consenting/non-consenting. While full consent is appropriate and necessary in some cases, many studies cannot feasibly acquire consent for data collection and use. The challenges related to geospatial data and privacy are yet to be completely addressed. Federal legislation around geolocation privacy is being pushed forward, which may affect future methodologic approaches to cancer control. Additionally, efforts to increase access to geospatial data relevant to cancer control include the NCHS Research Data Centers [3], expansion of the US Census Federal Statistical Research Data Centers [4], and NSF funding of efforts to develop turnkey approaches to data enclaves for spatial analysis [5, 6]. Individual data privacy and security is paramount in research, but hopefully can be balanced by a set of policies that both protect privacy and allow research use of spatially identified data to advance cancer prevention and control.

18.3   Future Directions

Four of the common challenges discussed for geospatial approaches to cancer control will need to be addressed as the field advances. Several key areas will provide the backdrop for the future of the field: (a) data collection, storage, integration, and sharing; (b) data analytics; (c) capacity-building, and (d) research advances.

18.3.1   Data Collection, Storage, Integration, and Sharing

Technologies that enable collection of large volumes of data, novel data sources, and allow for new geoprocessing techniques are rapidly growing. Real-time spatio-temporal data has exploded in the past decade, even creating new industries, such as location-based services (LBS) used by major internet-map providers. For researchers, wearable devices and other sensors are leading to new data collection challenges, capabilities, and methods. A corollary to this phenomenon is that participation in the generation of geospatial has broadened considerably, such that most individuals use a device, usually a smartphone, which can generate spatiotemporal information, sometimes referred to as volunteered geographic information [7]. Spatiotemporal data needs to be more agile, timely, and coordinated at various scales and across industry, such integrating residential history to examine latency or the use of social media for tracking healthcare utilization or perceptions of care.

Data storage should move toward the big data framework in order to accommodate heterogeneous data from various sources. Some infrastructure investment may be required, such as a Hadoop cluster for parallel processing of massive geospatial data. New models of data storage are moving beyond the old forms of data warehouses to allow for heterogeneous data sources and structures to co-mingle and/or be centrally integrated; key examples are data lakes and data hubs. Data lakes are centralized repositories for storage of both structured and unstructured data at any scale [8]. Data hubs are similar to data lakes, but differ in that there is a hub and spoke model, rather than communally held in one system, requiring movement and indexing for integration [9].

Often used in conjunction with Hadoop, or other parallel processing systems, data lakes and data hubs can allow for unprecedented synthesis of myriad data sources, such as health care encounter data, mobile device data, population surveillance data, streetcam images, and remote sensing data. Example of data lakes and hubs in geospatial cancer control research are not yet prominent in the literature, underscoring the need to partner with computational and data scientist experts to expand our toolbox in cancer care research. Although data operating systems need to be adequately defined to yield productive data integration, the loose data architecture environment of data lakes and hubs could promote consolidation and sharing of data across institutions, which could help address the "small data" problem, which creates a host of cross-cutting challenges, some of them spatial. Small data limits research in cancer control for some underrepresented population subgroups due to: few, dispersed, or inaccessible individuals/observations [10].

18.3.2 Data Analytics

While advances in spatial data analysis and visualization is transforming sectors of the business world, spatial analysis tools are somewhat underutilized in health-related research. For cancer, travel time analysis and kernel density estimation are commonly used, but increasingly there is recognition that predictive modeling is a largely untapped analytic method [11] that can increase the impact of geospatial data in cancer control research. There is currently a growing use of machine learning and artificial intelligence analyses applied to geospatial data, which is likely to expand even further. Machine learning algorithms can be applied to geospatial data for such purposes as: change detection in neighborhoods, environmental contaminants, or health care facilities; identifying transmission (of disease) hotspots; and monitoring the diffusion of new medical technology, such as digital breast tomosynthesis (DBT).

In our recent work, we used a geoinformatics approach that integrated natural language processing (NLP) and machine learning into a GIS environment to monitor diffusion of DBT in near-real time without regard to geographic extent to inform more equitable access over time and space. Specifically, we used a Google Search Application Program Interface (API) [12] to identify the presence of DBT at a particular facility through Web content mining -combining natural language processing (NLP), machine learning – to ascertain unique instances of DBT locations and associated facility addresses. We then used Google Maps's API to resolve its location into 2-D coordinates, allowing for reverse geocoding, yielding latitude and longitude. The algorithm to extract DBT location information was assessed for accuracy using a sample of known DBT locations (precision: 92%, recall: 96%, F1-score: 94%) [13]. We imported the algorithm location results into a geodatabase framework as a spatial dataset for use in an ArcGIS environment, integrating with underlying population demographics (screening-age women, racial/ethnic composition, and other sociodemographics) allowing for a host of spatiotemporal analyses as well as geovisualization techniques. The main purpose of this work was to develop a way to monitor diffusion of DBT for breast cancer screening, which had some evidence for benefit over traditional mammography, but for which generalizable evidence was still accumulating; thus informing both the issues of equitable access and efficient resource allocation. Typically this type of analysis could be done using claims information, however, for DBT, as many new technologies, at the time of our work, there was no billable code with which to track use of the technology; thus necessitating monitoring facility-level adoption in near-real time using Web-content mining. The novel aspect of this work was combining known techniques from informatics with GIS and applying it to a breast cancer screening technology equity issue requiring near-real-time location information [13, 14].

The major limiting factor in this, and other emerging work using machine learning to analyze geospatial data is the limited workforce of individuals with training in informatics methods and the underlying programming and computational knowledge/skills to both apply them appropriately to geospatial research, and to advance methods in the expandingarena of geoinformatics as applied to health-related fields. Geoinformatics is defined as "the science and technology dealing with the structure and character of spatial information, its capture, its classification and qualification, its storage, processing, portrayal and dissemination, including the infrastructure necessary to secure optimal use of this information" [15]. This deficit of expertise and deficiencies in the training pipeline should be addressed with intentional capacity-building across the spectrum of geospatial methods as applicable to cancer prevention and control.

18.3.3   Capacity-Building

From this volume and from my experiences at an NCI Cancer Center working on geospatial approaches to breast cancer control, several insights arise concerning capacity-building for future work. From experience in my research group, and those of colleagues doing geospatial work within cancer control, the limiting factors seem to be largely related to content expertise and technical expertise. Other challenges include data that are appropriate, high-quality, sufficiently granular, and adequately private/secure, with computing resources (hardware or software) less of a limitation. While some projects require high-performance computing clusters, such as Hadoop, the majority do not require computing capacity beyond the typical research needs. At our NCI-designated Comprehensive Cancer Center, we have access to this capacity through our medical school's CTSA, although it is largely used for machine learning/artificial intelligence analyses of radiology and pathology digital images and requires a systems administrator with specialized knowledge and skills.

Most projects do require some technical expertise in data wrangling, software usage, and analytics. Capacity-building for technical expertise could be developed bi-directionally in existing Master degree programs. That is – GIS-based programs could partner with programs in health fields, and public health or health sciences programs could partner with GIS curricula. Further, the rapidly-expanding array of biomedical data science programs could offer health-related geoinformatics courses, or dedicated tracks (e.g. University of Southern California, Johns Hopkins, University of Illinois, and others). Developing cross-listed, interdisciplinary courses in such programs can facilitate a well-prepared cadre of geospatial cancer control researchers in the workforce. Also, for current research team members, a host of workshops and online tutorials are available to gain skills and knowledge with specific software platforms, such as R spatial packages and web-GIS techniques. Our cancer center has built cancer-focused geospatial capacity through the staffing of a 1.0 FTE Geospatial Resource, consisting of a Master's-prepared geospatial analyst/GIS technician. This resource has been a value-added feature of Cancer Center membership, providing: capacity to include geospatial elements into grant-funded work, mapping for studies/papers/pilot work, analytics for catchment area definition and surveillance, community outreach and engagement, and partnership with our clinical departments for identifying areas of service needs, quality improvement initiatives, and public relations.

Ideally, all projects have the content expertise to apply geospatial principles to cancer control research questions, with well-informed conceptual models and constructs. Capacity-building to ensure content expertise should focus on fostering and incentivizing inter-disciplinary teams of geographers, epidemiologists, health services researchers, clinicians, and others. Such a notion is now advocated under the rubric of team science, but strategies to build teams with geospatial and cancer control expertise should be cultivated. Examples of this have seen through NCI efforts, such as specific funding mechanisms [16] and national workshops/meetings [17], and will hopefully continue and propagate. These efforts, and some NCI-funded teams, include PhD-level geographers as well as epidemiologists, health services researchers, behavioral scientists, and clinicians. Teams including PhD-level geographers for geospatial-based research are vital, and parallel the model of PhD-level biostatisticians as research team members. Capacity building in geospatial approaches to cancer control will be important to advancing cancer care and to research through generating evidence to increase our understanding of critical issues, such as breast cancer, as well as the ability to apply the evidence through impactful interventions.

18.3.4 Research Advances

Methods to understand geospatial impacts on cancer are continually advancing. Three areas seem particularly likely to have a positive influence on cancer prevention and control, if focused advances are made: (a) space-time methods; (b) integration of geospatial and network analysis; (c) expansion of mixed methods.

18.3.4.1   Space-Time Methods

Geographers have been developing theories and integrative approaches to spatio-temporal measures [18, 19], in which correlations across repeated time measures and correlations across space need to be accounted for analytically. Jacquez (Chap. 2) presents examples and potential new directions in this area. Accounting both spatial and temporal correlations adds complexity to modeling, as does the difference in dimensionality for time (uni-dimensional – forward) and space (2- or 3-dimensional). While in the past, spatio-temporal analysis was used for such studies as evaluating incidence of late-stage breast cancer over time, now spatio-temporal analyses are more challenging with 'big data', such as accelerometer data adding computational complexity (e.g. Chap. 4).

18.3.4.2   Integration of Geospatial and Network Analysis

As noted in Chap. 14, geospatial aspects of health care delivery are influenced by more than just locations and proximity. Organizational structures, financial policies, and care delivery models, all play a role in cancer patients' trajectory through cancer care. Yet understanding and being able to measure access, utilization, care coordination, and outcomes across comparable units, is a mainstay of outcomes research. Typically, these units are based on county, as in Health Service Areas, or on utilization-based service areas (e.g. Hospital Service Areas). But as discussed in Chap. 17, diverse aspects of care are amenable to micro environmental and ultimately spatial analysis. At the same time, geospatial data are increasingly being harnessed for social network analyses based on a spatial data (such as Twitter feed content), with an associated locational attribute. The ability to combine social network analysis and geospatial analysis can yield novel insights into health, such as depression in newly diagnosed cancer patients, behaviors, such as cancer screening, and health care utilization, such as genomic testing. Expanding the methods related to coupling geospatial and social network analysis has begun in my research group [20] and others, and will provide exciting new possibilities for cancer control research.

18.3.4.3   Expansion of Mixed Methods

Geospatial measures are often based on a group-level, or areal unit, with the attribute for the unit being assigned to every individual within that unit. Two major limitations arise from this approach: (1). Ecological fallacy – i.e. erroneous attribution of a group-level measure/inference to individuals within that group; (2). Capturing a heterogeneous composite construct, which may obscure more granular causal factors. A good example is taken from Chap. 16 in which the construct of "rural" is discussed. Usually, rurality is determined by the designation for the geographic area in which one resides (e.g. ZIP, county). For a given individual, that group level attribute of rurality may not apply if they happen to live in the far, rural reaches of a county classified as metropolitan. Further, the mechanism by which rurality might be acting, such as social isolation or inadequate knowledge sharing, may not be represented by a coarse category of rurality. Mixed methods approaches to better understand *what* should be measured, *how* it should be measured, and to ensure quality measurement are needed. These challenges in rural health and in the analysis of small populations are of growing interest in public health research and at NCI [10, 21].

18.4   Conclusion

Geospatial approaches to breast cancer offer critical avenues for understanding and addressing issues across the cancer control continuum. We have seen examples of geospatial approaches related to risk reduction, incidence, early detection, treatment, mortality, survivorship, and disparities across the continuum. While there is no one single way that geospatial approaches can reduce the burden of breast cancer, the fundamental fact that all people and populations exist in physical space, leads to important spatial influences that are inseparable from the risk and experience of breast cancer. Table 18.1 offers ten suggestions to expand and promote geospatial approaches to cancer control. These may, in part, facilitate the pursuit of cancer control researchers to discover and apply evidence that prevents breast and

Table 18.1 Ten ideas for advancing geospatial approaches to cancer prevention and control

1	Promote training and hiring of spatially oriented researchers at NCI designated cancer centers
2	Form a network of cancer oriented spatial researchers to develop training opportunities via an application for an NCI R25 grant
3	Support bi- or triannual meeting or workshops focusing on Geospatial Approaches to Cancer Prevention and Control, including some skill-based, hands-on workshops (such as those conducted by: Research Data Assistance Center [ResDAC], North American Association of Central Cancer Registries [NAACCR] for SEER∗Stat software, etc.)
4	Develop standard area-based metrics to describe cancer center catchment areas
5	Expand research on rural cancer control with an emphasis on better measures of the platial and spatial features of rural areas influencing cancer control
6	Develop spatially informed interventions using sensor, GPS and GIS data sources allowing adaptive and granular incorporation of spatial data
7	Use qualitative and quantitative methods to develop spatially-based measures that capture person-centered dimensions of human-space-time interactions (analogous to patient-reported measures for health care, we could have person-centered spatial measures)
8	Make reconstruction of residential histories a routine aspect of cancer relevant cohorts and use these histories for better exposure assessment
9	Issue an RFA, or explicit funding mechanism to build geoinformatics capabilities/resources, requiring interdisciplinary teams of geographers, health scientists, and computer scientists
10	Periodically, devote special issues of cancer-focused journals to geospatial approaches to cancer control to raise awareness and understanding of the role they play in the field

other cancers and mitigates the impact of cases that do occur. This volume provides examples of *how* and *why* geospatial approaches contribute to this goal, but scientists across disciplines must further develop and evolve new approaches in order to better achieve this goal and to be responsive to emerging issues in the field. And to the extent that the old adage, "geography is destiny" applies to cancer control, spatial approaches will continue to be indispensable to fully address disparities in breast cancer.

References

1. Moen EL, Bynum JP, Austin AM, Skinner JS, Chakraborti G, Malley AJ. Assessing variation in implantable cardioverter defibrillator therapy guideline adherence with physician and hospital patient-sharing networks. Med Care. 2018;56(4):350–7.
2. Onega T, Weiss JE, Alford-Teaster J, Goodrich M, Eliassen MS, Kim SJ. Comparison of willingness to travel and self-reported travel times for health services and activities by ZIP code based rural-urban residential location. Health Place. 2019;
3. Centers for Disease Control and Prevention. Research data center. https://www.cdc.gov/rdc/index.htm. Accessed 30 Dec 2018.
4. United States Census Bureau. Federal statistical research data centers. https://www.census.gov/fsrdc. Accessed 30 Dec 2018.
5. Richardson DB, Kwan MP, Alter G, McKendry JE. Replication of scientific research: addressing geoprivacy, confidentiality, and data sharing challenges in geospatial research. Ann GIS. 2015;21(2):101–10.
6. National Science Foundation. A robust and reliable resource for accessing, sharing, and analyzing confidential geospatial research data. Award Abstract #1832465. https://www.nsf.gov/awardsearch/showAward?AWD_ID=1832465&HistoricalAwards=false. Accessed 30 Dec 2018.
7. Goodchild MF. Citizens as sensors: the world of volunteered geography. GeoJournal. 2007;69(4):211–21.
8. Amazon Web Services (AWS). https://aws.amazon.com/big-data/datalakes-and-analytics/what-is-a-data-lake/. Accessed 29 Dec 2018.
9. Wikipedia. Data hub. https://en.wikipedia.org/wiki/Data_hub. Accessed 30 Dec 2018.
10. Srinivasan S, Moser RP, Willis G, Riley W, Alexander M, Berrigan D, Kobrin S. Small is essential: importance of subpopulation research in cancer control. Am J Public Health. 2014;105(S3):S371–3. https://doi.org/10.2105/AJPH.2014.302267.
11. National Geospatial Advisory Committee (NGAC). Emerging technologies and the geospatial landscape. A report of the national geospatial advisory committee. 2016. https://www.fgdc.gov/ngac/meetings/dec-2016/ngac-paper-emerging-technologies-and-the.pdf. Accessed 30 Dec 2018.
12. Google. APIs Explorer. https://developers.google.com/apis-explorer/#p/. Accessed 30 Dec 2018.
13. Onega T, Kamra D, Alford-Teaster J, Hassanpour S. Monitoring of technology adoption using web content mining of location information and geographic information systems: a case study of digital breast tomosynthesis. JCO Clin Cancer Inform. 2018;2:1–10. https://doi.org/10.1200/CCI.17.00150.
14. Onega T, Alford-Teaster J, Andrews S, Ganoe C, Perez M, King D, Shi X. Why health services research needs geoinformatics: rationale and case example. J Health Med Inform. 2015;05 https://doi.org/10.4172/2157-7420.1000176.
15. Raju PLN. Fundamentals of geographic information systems. In: Workshop: satellite remote sensing and GIS applications in agricultural meteorology. India; 2003.

16. National Cancer Institute. https://grants.nih.gov/grants/guide/pa-files/PA-15-010.html. Accessed 29 Dec 2018.
17. National Cancer Institute. https://researchtoreality.cancer.gov/discussions/geospatial-approaches-cancer-control-and-population-sciences. Accessed 29 Dec 2018.
18. Kwan MP, Richardson R, Wang D, Zhou C, editors. Space-Time Integration in geography and GIScience; Research frontiers in the US and China. Dordrecht: Springer; 2015. ISBN 978–94–017–9205–9
19. Kwan MP. Beyond space (as we knew it): toward temporally integrated geographies of segregation, health, and accessibility. Ann Assoc Am Geogr. 2013;103:1078–86.
20. Moen EL, Kapadia NS, O'Malley AJ, Onega T. Evaluating breast cancer care coordination at a rural National Cancer Institute Comprehensive Cancer Center using network analysis and geospatial methods. Cancer Epidemiol Biomark Prev. 2018;28:455–61. https://doi.org/10.1158/1055-9965.EPI-18-0771.
21. Kennedy AE, Vanderpool RC, Croyle RT, Srinivasan S. An overview of the National Cancer Institute's initiatives to accelerate rural cancer control research. Cancer Epidemiol Biomark Prev. 2018;27(11):1240–4.

Index

Printed in the United States
By Bookmasters